The
NATURAL
HEALTH
HANDBOOK
FOR WOMEN

About the Author

Dr Marilyn Glenville PhD is a nutritional therapist, psychologist, broadcaster and author of the internationally best-selling *Natural Alternatives to HRT*, *Natural Alternatives to Dieting* and *Natural Solutions to Infertility*. She obtained her doctorate from Cambridge University and is the Chair of the Governing Council for the British Association of Nutritional Therapists and the Chair of Foresight (the association for the promotion of pre-conceptual care). She is also a Fellow of the Royal Society of Medicine.

For more than 20 years Dr Glenville has practised nutritional therapy in the UK and the USA, specialising in the natural approach to female hormone problems. She frequently advises health professionals and lectures at academic conferences held at the Medical Society and the Royal College of Physicians. As a respected authority on women's healthcare, she gives regular talks on radio and has often appeared on television and in the press.

Dr Glenville has been officially appointed by The Foods Standards Agency to be an observer on the Expert Group of Vitamins and Minerals. She is also the Chair of the steering group for the Nutritional Therapy Council, instigated by the Government to set national occupational standards for Nutritional Therapy in the UK.

She practises in London with two gynaecologists in St John's Wood and also at the prestigious Hale Clinic.

The
NATURAL
HEALTH
HANDBOOK
FOR WOMEN

*The complete guide to women's health
problems and how to treat them naturally*

MARILYN GLENVILLE PhD

PIATKUS

Copyright © 2001 by Marilyn Glenville

First published in 2001 by
Judy Piatkus (Publishers) Limited
5 Windmill Street
London W1T 2JA
e-mail: info@piatkus.co.uk

The moral right of the author has been asserted

*A catalogue record for this book is available
from the British Library*

ISBN 0 7499 2191 9

This book has been printed on paper manufactured with respect for the environment using wood from managed sustainable resources

Typeset by Palimpsest Book Production Limited
Polmont, Stirlingshire
Printed and bound in Great Britain by
MPG Books Ltd, Bodmin, Cornwall

To all those women who over the years have helped me learn and grow by listening to their problems. I now give this knowledge back to help those who need it

Disclaimer

The contents of this book are for information only and are intended to assist readers in identifying symptoms and conditions they may be experiencing. The book is not intended to be a substitute for taking proper medical advice and should not be relied upon in this way. Always consult a qualified doctor or health practitioner, especially if you are pregnant, taking the Pill or on any medication. Your situation will need to be looked at individually and you should not attempt to self-treat. The author and publisher cannot accept responsibility for illness arising out of the failure to seek medical advice from a doctor.

Contents

Contents

Acknowledgements

A book of this size and depth is not written without help and support. I would particularly like to thank Karen Sullivan who helped to make this book clear by asking questions, pointing out omissions and generally helping to make the book so readable. My thanks go to Rachel Winning, my editor at Piatkus, and all the staff at Piatkus who are extremely helpful and professional.

My special thanks to all those who supported me while I took the time away from the clinic to write this book, including Linda McVan, my practice manager, and also Bea, Trish and Ally. Also to my long-suffering family, my husband Kriss and my children, Matthew, Leonard and Chantell, who are now used to episodes of feverish writing and research.

Words cannot express the thanks I would like to extend to Women's Health Care in North London, and in particular to Yehudi Gordon and Talha Shawaf. These two consultant gynaecologists have embraced the concept of Integrated Medicine (the coming together of conventional and natural medicine) so that women can have a choice in the treatment of their problems and under the expert eye of Bill Smith, the ultrasonongrapher, can be monitored for the efficacy of that treatment. It is a pleasure working in that environment and I know that the women value the fact that they are being taken care of holistically, that they know they are listened to and heard, and that their treatment is a two-way communication between the patient and practitioner.

Introduction

This book is about women's health and those problems that are specific only to women. I have written it calling on my 20 years of experience of specialising in women's problems. Over time, it has become clear that when women come to see me they tell me that they not only want to know what natural remedies are available to treat their problem and get themselves back to optimum health, but they also want details of the conventional medical options as well. Quite rightly, many women feel that they want as much information as possible in order to be able to make an informed decision about which treatment to choose.

How Can This Book Help You?

This book is very different to anything you will have read before. It is a very specific, self-help book. What you will find, for each problem, is a carefully structured programme designed to help you gain relief from your health problems and help you to maintain optimum health in the future. The information presented is the accumulation of knowledge I have gained in working with thousands of women over the years, using nutrition and herbs to help them get their health back and stay healthy. It is this knowledge that I am passing on to you.

Maybe you've just been told that you have a problem, such as fibroids or endometriosis, for example, and that you need a hysterectomy or drugs. You may not be comfortable with this suggested treatment and wonder if there are any other choices. What you really want to know is what other options are open to you. Is a hysterectomy the only choice for your particular problem, or are there other medical options available? What about a more natural and non-invasive approach? Could nutritional medicine help? Is it effective? Is it appropriate for your problem? Can it get rid of your symptoms and help you to feel better?

This book lets you know what choices are available to you both naturally and medically. It takes you through the natural options that can be used for your health problem and then explains the medical approaches involving drugs or surgery that could also be used. It also helps you to plan a treatment strategy, whereby you may want to use both natural and medical treatments alongside one another. Alternatively, you may choose to 'go natural' for six months or so, and then have a medical check-up to see how effective this treatment has been.

There are many books available, with treatment plans involving long lists of supplements and herbs from which the reader is supposed to choose. However, I have often felt confused when reading such lists. How do you make the choice as to which ones are right for you, how much do you take and for how long?

This book is different. At the end of every section, you are presented with a treatment plan with simple, clear and specific recommendations to follow. These recommendations are the ones I use with many of the women who come to see me, and find to be the most effective and to make the most difference.

Other natural treatments such as acupuncture, homeopathy, osteopathy, aromatherapy, reflexology and hypnotherapy can be extremely helpful for many women's problems, and they can be used together with the recommendations made in this book. In fact, on many occasions, using these therapies can make those recommendations even more effective.

Natural medicine and conventional medicine are not mutually exclusive. You do not have to make a choice to use one or the other. You can, in fact, get the best of both worlds and use both of them to your advantage. That is what this book is all about. This approach is called 'integrated medicine' and, in years to come, this will be more and more the way medicine is practised. At the moment there are only a few clinics, such as the one I work in in London, where this approach is used. In these clinics you can have medical tests and investigations to diagnose a problem. At the same time, a consultation with a nutritional therapist can take place, and both the medical and the nutritional practitioners work together to map out a treatment plan. With something like a severe prolapse of the womb (uterus), for example, it may mean that corrective surgery is needed, in combination with nutritional medicine to get you back to optimum health as quickly as possible and to prevent it happening again. Another example may be heavy or painful periods, where a series of medical tests may show that there is nothing seriously wrong. Trying the natural approach, in this case, for three months or so, followed by a reassessment at the end of that time, can prove to be very effective in relieving the symptoms and correcting the problem.

If you can't find a clinic that operates an integrated medical approach, find a good doctor you can trust. If you've been told you need a total hysterectomy for fibroids, for example, get a second opinion. Most of the conditions discussed in this book are not life or death situations, so allow yourself time to think about the decision. Don't be rushed into anything. Before you make any decision, confirm with another doctor that the diagnosis is correct, and find out what your options are. If you get differing opinions between two doctors, find a third doctor whom you feel is objective.

If you have had a first opinion from a private doctor, remember that they are financially better off if you have more radical treatment. For example, hysterectomy may be offered instead of a D&C – dilatation and curettage, which is an operation where the neck (cervix) of the womb is dilated and the lining of the womb is lightly scraped, hence it is often called a 'scrape'. On the NHS or any state-funded healthcare, of course, the reverse can happen. Funds are tight, so conservative procedures may be offered to save the expense of invasive surgery. It is sad, if not frightening, that the course of treatment you are offered can be determined by the finances involved, rather than the most appropriate treatment for your condition at that time.

In fact, over the years I have seen many women who have told me that they later discovered, from other doctors, that the surgery they had was unnecessary. Of course, this is not always the case and there are many situations where surgery is essential. You just need to find out what is best for you. And, to reassure you, I know and work with some very wonderful, caring doctors who will always put the needs of their patients first and foremost.

The most important aspect of female health involves taking control of your problem. Find out all you can about the condition, and ask questions. Women have talked to me about feeling out of control, of being on a conveyor belt of treatment where they are just carried along without knowing enough about why each step is being taken. One woman who came to see me told me she had found a lump in her breast and had private medical insurance so she went to see a specialist. She was told that the lump was benign, but 'just in case it should change' she should have it removed. The specialist was going away on holiday within a couple of days so he suggested that she had it removed immediately. Everything was done so quickly that she was in a state of shock. She felt she had been sucked into the surgery without having time to think. The operation, unfortunately, was not performed well, and she cannot now lift her arm past the height of her shoulder. On reflection, she felt that she needed more time and fuller information to think about her options, and maybe get a second opinion. However, at the time she felt overwhelmed by the seeming necessity to have the lump removed almost immediately: not because it was life threatening, but because her specialist was going on holiday.

The relationship between doctor and patient has changed over the years. Previously patients would not ask questions or enquire about the possible side-effects of drugs or even whether there were other choices of treatment. The Internet has made us all more knowledge-able, and we all want to know what we are taking and why. More and more of us are demanding to know the results of tests, and want them explained in language that we can understand. It is no longer acceptable to be fobbed off by 'You wouldn't understand it' or 'Trust me, I'm a doctor'.

Women come to see me from all over the world and many bring along copies of all their test results, ultrasounds, X-rays, blood tests and other important information given to them by their doctors. In the UK, it was once impossible to get copies of these results. Now, thanks to the Patients' Charter, you are entitled to copies of your tests from your doctor. It is your right to see and have copies of them; you just need to ask.

It's vital when seeing your healthcare practitioner that you ask the following questions:

- What exactly is the problem?

- Can you draw a diagram for me?

- What caused the problem in the first place? ('Just one of those things' is not an acceptable answer.)

- Can I prevent it from happening again?

- If tests are indicated, what information will those tests give?

- Will that information alter the treatment options? (If not, why have the tests?)

- What choices of treatment do I have (surgery, drugs, nutritional therapy or other natural treatments)?

- How effective is that treatment?

- What are the risks or side-effects associated with that treatment?

- What happens if I have no medical treatment for six months?

- What is the worst that can happen?

If you know the time-scale that you are working with, then you have the flexibility to use more natural approaches in that time. For instance, one woman, with fibroids that were giving her extremely heavy periods, was scheduled for a hysterectomy. However, the waiting time for the operation on the NHS was about nine months. During that nine months, we worked together to change her diet, adding in vitamins and minerals to correct any deficiencies, and using herbs to help balance the hormones. After several months, and on the advice of her gynaecologist, she was able to cancel the operation as her condition had improved so much and was now manageable.

When faced with a health problem about which you have to make some important decisions, always bear in mind: it is your body, you have the right to know what is going on and you have the right to be fully involved in the discussions and decisions about the appropriate course of action for you.

With the information contained in this book you will gain the knowledge to help yourself and to ask the right questions and understand the answers given. This in turn will give you the confidence to choose the treatment you feel is best for you and you are most comfortable with and which can be seen to give you the best results.

Wishing you a long and healthy life.

Marilyn Glenville PhD

How To Use This Book

What You Must Read

No matter what health problem you have, you *must* read Chapter 1. It explains the role of nutrition and lifestyle in women's health. It is so important because without that basic foundation, everything else falls apart.

Nutrition is not alternative medicine. You have to eat; it is something you do every day. Nutrition is the actual foundation of your health – you are what you eat. The food you put into your mouth gives your body the 'fuel' it needs to make and control your hormones, repair your cells, destroy mutant cells and foreign bodies, fight infection etc. In fact, your body is dependent on what you eat in order to survive. What you eat governs how well you survive and the actual quality of your health. It governs whether your body has the ability to heal itself and keep itself in balance.

Over the last few years scientists have realised through research what a profound effect nutrition can have on our health and how it can be used both in prevention, as with cancer, and in controlling problems, as with heart disease.

Specific Health Problems

The second part of this book is divided up into chapters relating to specific women's health problems according to the organs affected.

Each problem is then split into a number of areas including:

• What the problem is

• What symptoms could you expect if you had this problem

• How would you get it diagnosed

• What causes this problem

• What could you expect from your doctor, i.e. what conventional treatments are available

• What natural treatments are available

• Integrated treatment plan – how you can combine the best of both worlds, conventional and natural

• A summary of what you should do.

PART 1

THE FOUNDATION OF GOOD HEALTH

CHAPTER 1

Nutrition and Lifestyle

What you eat can have a profound effect on your health. There are many female health problems, but most are triggered by the same mechanisms, including stress, hormone imbalance, nutritional deficiencies and toxins. By taking steps towards optimum health, the vast majority of women's health problems can be alleviated or, in many cases, eliminated altogether. Your diet and your nutritional status are crucial to this process and, as a result, you will find that this chapter is referred to in every single chapter of the rest of this book.

This chapter looks at the ways in which you can get back your health. The main route to good health lies in diet, but there are many other lifestyle factors, such as your environment, that need to be addressed as part of any successful treatment plan. Before any health problem can be treated – and I mean treated, not just suppressed – you need to address the fundamental basis of most health problems. These are outlined in this chapter, which forms the foundation of every treatment plan in the book. The recommendations outlined here are essential for the success of your treatment. It's perfectly possible to see a difference in your symptoms if you use only the advice specific to your problem. But that's not enough. What this book aims to do is to restore you to optimum health and well-being, so that you can experience the kind of good health that so few of us have.

Treating the Cause, Not Just the Symptoms

Imagine your health as a tree, with various symptoms attached to different branches. For example, you may suffer from a lack of energy, mood swings, headaches, weight gain, bloating, period problems, skin disorders and more. In theory, each of these 'symptoms' could be treated separately, as they are in conventional medicine. For example, you could be given painkillers to treat your headaches, the Pill to regulate your cycle, antibiotics for skin problems, and perhaps even antidepressants to deal with the emotional factors. You can be pumped up with all sorts of drugs, but once they are stopped, the problem will return. The reason for this is that most of conventional medicine is aimed at treating symptoms alone. The root cause is not addressed and the underlying problem remains, no matter how good medication makes you feel in the short term. Quite apart from that, many drugs have unacceptable side-effects, and in an attempt to feel better in the short term you may well be causing long-term damage to your overall health.

Beneath your symptom tree are the roots that feed and nourish the plant. The nourishment the tree gets determines how well the leaves on the branches grow and how it blossoms. It's clear that in order to affect the symptoms that appear on your branches, you need to do some work on the roots. That's the basis of natural medicine, which aims to get to the root cause – literally – of any health condition. This chapter will show you how to affect the health of your roots, so that your branches, and every symptom found upon them, will respond. If you make changes at root level, many symptoms will drop away without ever having had specific treatment. Even better, once your tree is healthy, you only need a simple maintenance programme to keep it that way.

Most medical students will get only a few hours of nutrition lectures in over six years of training, so you probably won't find any nutritional recommendations as part of your doctor's treatment plan. But nutrition is crucial. Everything that you eat can be turned into the fuel that your body uses to produce hormones, enzymes, blood, bone: in fact, every single cell in your body, and all the processes that take place, are determined by what goes into your mouth.

It took many years for the link between cardiovascular disease and nutrition to be established. Now the evidence is overwhelming. More research is now linking nutrition to cancer, growth disorders, mood and much, much more. In the future, further research will show that your diet plays a part in every aspect of your health.

It took, for example, 20 years for the benefits of folic acid in pregnancy to become known. The evidence that it could prevent spina bifida was around 20 years ago, but only recently was it recommended that women take it as part of a preconceptual plan. As a practising nutritional therapist, I find it extremely frustrating that nutrition is so undervalued. While it's satisfying to see that research is slowly turning in the right direction, there is still a great deal of information that should be made available for everybody. Twenty years is too long to wait for experts to confirm what many of us in the profession already knew.

And the evidence is there for the majority of female problems, too. What you eat can actually cause many health problems, and the reverse is also true: in other words, if you change your diet, you can alleviate many health problems.

Sadly, you may not ever have heard about the research that can affect your health on such a dramatic level. First of all, studies tend to remain lost in the corridors of the academic world. Most of them are not even comprehensible to the average person. But secondly, and most importantly, there is no vested interest in getting that knowledge 'out there'. Pharmaceutical companies do not stand to make a big profit if the cause of conditions currently treated by expensive drugs is found to be linked to something we eat. Similarly, nutritional supplements are never going to make the kind of money that drugs do; you cannot patent a nutrient so there is no commercial incentive to investigate and promote it.

Every woman needs the information that is already available to the readers of medical and scientific journals. You need that information now, and that's why this book has been written.

Natural Health Using Nutrition

Using nutrition as a form of treatment works quite differently from conventional medicine. The first aim is to work on the symptoms by addressing the underlying cause of the problem. The next stage – and here's the big difference – is to work on prevention. This approach works well with all of the problems discussed in this book, but the easiest way to see this in practice is to take the example of endometriosis.

A woman may have been told she has endometriosis and needs surgery in order to remove it, because the endometriosis is causing so much pain during her periods. The surgery will remove as much of the endometriosis as possible, but if the woman does not change anything regarding her diet or lifestyle, the endometriosis can grow back within a few months, because the underlying cause of the problem has not been addressed.

Why Are There So Many 'Women's Health' Problems?

Women are complex pieces of equipment. But that very complexity means we have more 'bits' that can go wrong. Because women have the ability to bear children, which requires a monthly cycle, we are automatically put on a roller-coaster of hormone changes each and every month. In comparison, men have a relatively steady stream of hormones once they get past puberty, and it continues at more or less the same rate until they die. This steadiness means that there is less potential for things to go wrong.

A doctor who deals with female problems is known as a gynae-cologist. What do you call a doctor who deals with male problems? Chances are you don't know. The equivalent doctor is called an androl-ogist, but they are few and far between. If a man has a problem with fertility, for example, he's likely to be sent to a urologist. There are more doctors for women because women *do* have more health problems.

Why You Need Food Supplements

Throughout this chapter and this book, you'll notice that food supplements are recommended. You may wonder why you might need them, particularly if you have a good diet. As you will see below, unfortunately, even the best diet can no longer supply us with everything we need, and supplements are no longer considered to be a little 'extra'.

The well-balanced diet is a myth. You simply do not get all the nutrients you need from your food. This was confirmed from a National Food Survey conducted in 1995, which found that the average person in Britain is grossly deficient in six out of the eight vitamins and minerals surveyed. Less than one in ten people receive the RDA (Recommended Daily Allowance) of 15mg for zinc, which is the most important mineral for female hormone problems. You need to supplement your diet because it is almost impossible to get all of the nutrients you need from food alone. For instance, our intake of selenium (34mcg) per day is now only half the amount it was in the daily diet 25 years ago. This amount is half the minimum 75mcg a day recommended for men and 60mcg recommended for women.

In order for your food to contain the nutrients it needs, the soil in which it was grown needs to be rich in nutrients. For instance, carrots will extract the minerals from the soil and you absorb those nutrients when you eat them. But the soil has been overfarmed to the point that it no longer contains the nutrients we need. Furthermore, pesticides and other chemicals reduce the nutrient content of foods, and then we go on and process the foods, stripping even more key nutrients from them. Extra chemicals put an additional strain on our bodies, which means that we need *more* of the key nutrients, and what we are getting in our daily diets represents *less*.

We have, as a culture, begun to eat far too many processed, convenience and refined foods that have been stripped of essential nutrients during the manufacturing process. For example, 80 per cent of zinc is removed from wheat during the milling process to ensure that a loaf of bread (for instance) has longer shelf life.[1]

Furthermore if you, like many people, have been dieting for a number of years – either restricting your food intake, or trying different diets, diet drinks or pills – you are more than likely to be deficient in a number of important vitamins and minerals.

The other reason why it is important to use supplements is that you want to achieve positive health benefits in as short a space of time as possible. Certain nutrients, depending on your problem, will help to speed up this process because they can help you to detoxify or strengthen your immune system.

It is absolutely essential that you get the best quality supplements for maximum absorption and effectiveness. Chapter 2, on natural medicine, explains what you should be looking for in a supplement and how to test if you are absorbing it well.

What You Should Eat

While much overused, the old saying 'you are what you eat' is definitely true. Your diet is the foundation of your health, so it is important that your food contains the right nutrients to keep you balanced and healthy, and to prevent health conditions from cropping up in the future.

Many of our female hormone problems are caused by an excess of oestrogen, so you need to aim to have the kind of diet that helps to control high levels of oestrogen. You also need to ensure you are eating foods that have an overall balancing effect on hormones.

I will list the main points of this hormone-balancing diet, and then go through them in detail to explain why they are so important. Later sections of the book will list specific dietary recommendations that will need to be implemented in order successfully to treat your problem.

The Hormone-Balancing Diet

1. Eat plenty of fruit and vegetables
2. Eat complex carbohydrates – wholegrains like brown rice, oats and wholemeal bread
3. Buy organic foods where possible
4. Eat phytoestrogens, including beans such as lentils, chickpeas and soya products
5. Eat oily foods, including fish, nuts, seeds and oils
6. Reduce your intake of saturated fat from dairy products etc.
7. Drink enough fluids
8. Increase your intake of fibre
9. Avoid additives, preservatives and chemicals, such as artificial sweeteners
10. Reduce your intake of caffeine
11. Reduce alcohol
12. Avoid sugar, both on its own and hidden in foods

1. Eat plenty of fruit and vegetables

These are important in your diet for a number of reasons. They contain a good range of nutrients, including vitamins, minerals, antioxidants and fibre. The vitamins and minerals are important because by giving your body the right nutrients, you are giving it the 'tools' to heal itself. Fresh produce is your best option – organic, if possible (see page 19) – but otherwise frozen vegetables are better than tinned if you can't always get fresh.

ANTIOXIDANTS

One of the most important things that fruits and vegetables can do is to supply us with antioxidants, which protect us against the effects of atoms called free radicals. Oxygen, which is vital for our survival, can also be chemically reactive. It can become unstable, resulting in the 'oxidation' of other molecules, which in turn generates free radicals. Free radicals are a rather complicated concept, but in a nutshell, they are chemically unstable atoms that can cause all sorts of damage in your body. Pollution, smoking, fried or barbecued food and UV rays from the sun can also trigger these free radicals.

Free radicals have now been linked to health problems, including cancer, coronary heart disease and premature ageing. They speed up the ageing process by destroying healthy cells and they can also attack the DNA in the nucleus of a cell, causing cell change (mutation) and cancer. We have protection against free radicals in the form of anti-oxidants, which occur naturally in the food which we eat. Vitamins A, C and E (the ACE vitamins), plus the minerals selenium and zinc, are all antioxidants and are contained in the following foods:

Sources of antioxidants

Vitamin A	Orange and yellow fruits and vegetables, such as carrots and pumpkins, fish
Vitamin C	Fruits (particularly citrus), green leafy vegetables such as broccoli, cauliflower, berries (such as strawberries, raspberries and blackberries), potatoes and sweet potatoes
Vitamin E	Nuts, avocados, seeds, vegetable oils and oily fish
Selenium	Brazil nuts, tuna, cabbage
Zinc	Pumpkin and sunflower seeds, fish, almonds

2. Eat complex carbohydrates

Carbohydrates give you energy and the amount of energy they provide depends on the form in which you eat them. Carbohydrates are starches and sugars, and they can either be 'simple' or 'complex'. The more complex the carbohydrate, the longer lasting the energy you get from it, and the bigger the health benefits.

Complex carbohydrates	Simple carbohydrates
Grains (wheat, rye, oats, rice, barley, maize	Honey
Beans (lentils, kidney beans, soya etc.)	White and brown sugar; glucose in soft drinks
Vegetables	Fruit

Simple carbohydrates (apart from fruit) are all refined foods, and this group also includes foods made from white flour, from which all the goodness has been stripped away. The difference between the two types of carbohydrates on the body is enormous. The complex carbohydrates can prevent you from feeling tired, balance your blood sugar and so minimise cravings, lower cholesterol, maintain an appropriate appetite and – as you will see in Chapter 5 on pre-menstrual syndrome (PMS) – help to balance your hormones.

BREAKFASTS

Muesli – choose a good sugar-free muesli and soak overnight in apple juice or orange juice.

Porridge Oats – buy organic and cook with water. Top with linseeds, sunflower or sesame seeds or mix in a teaspoon of sugar-free jam or a dash of pure maple syrup. When using small seeds such as linseeds or sesame seeds, it is best to crack the seeds in a grinder or pestle and mortar before you eat them, otherwise they can pass through you undigested.

Cornflakes – buy sugar-free organic cornflakes usually sweetened with apple juice, and have them with organic soya milk or organic cows' or goats' milk, rice milk or oat milk.

Grilled kipper – with grilled tomatoes and mushrooms. Avoid the artificially coloured kippers.

Wholemeal toast – with sugar-free jam or marmalade. Avoid diabetic preserves which contain sorbitol, choose only those made with pure fruit.

Natural live organic yoghurt – with your choice of fruit. Try bananas or strawberries.

Dried fruit – soaked overnight. When you buy dried fruit choose brands which do not have sulphur dioxide added. It is used to preserve the colour of apricots, for example, but they taste just as delicious without it.

Choose any other breakfast cereals which are sugar-free, and have them with organic soya milk, or organic cows' or goats' milk.

3. Buy organic foods where possible

Because the soil in which the organic fruit and vegetables has been grown has not been so depleted, organic produce usually contains more valuable nutrients. One of the practices of organic farming involves crop rotation, which ensures that the soil is enriched rather than depleted.

If you eat dairy foods, choose organic brands to avoid the harmful effects of antibiotics and other chemicals that may have been added to the animal's food. Out of all the dairy foods, yoghurt is the most beneficial for your health, but only when it contains a culture like *Lactobacillus acidophilus*, which is a natural inhabitant of the gut. This culture (bacteria) is important because it is one of the defences of the immune system, and helps to keep unhealthy bacteria and invaders, such as fungal infections and viruses, at bay. 'Live' yoghurts normally have this culture, but the cartons can be marked in a variety of different ways. 'Bio' usually means 'live' and will contain a culture like *lactobacillus,* but when yoghurts are heat-treated they lose their original culture, so you will not benefit from eating them.

Choose to buy organic free-range eggs. Free-range is certainly kinder to animals, but the birds can still be fed on an inappropriate diet, which can include chemicals and antibiotics, among other additives. Organic hens have a strict dietary regime, which includes no worrying additives.

If your budget is limited and you are unsure of what to prioritise in terms of organic produce, go for organic grains, as in porridge, brown rice and wholemeal bread. Even if this is the only organic part of your diet, it can make a huge difference. Grains are very small, so they can absorb more pesticides than other foods.

Remember that organic produce, such as carrots and potatoes, does not need to be peeled. Most of the nutrients of vegetables and fruits are concentrated just under the skin. Just wash and scrub them carefully, and prepare as normal.

GENETICALLY MODIFIED FOODS

This is the ultimate can of worms, and a subject that I have addressed in some detail in my book *Natural Alternatives to HRT* (Kyle Cathie, 1997). Genetic modification involves tampering with the DNA of a plant or animal. Even patent advocates of the process have to admit that it bypasses the natural evolutionary process, and we do not know yet what the price of that may be. For that reason, I suggest that everyone avoids buying, eating or using genetically modified products. Stick to organic: organic foods and other products that are not genetically modified.

---

4. Eat phytoestrogens

Phytoestrogens ('phyto' means 'plant') are substances that occur naturally in foods and they have a very interesting effect on our hormones. Calling them phytoestrogens would imply that we are adding yet more oestrogen into our bodies, but these plant oestrogens work in a special way. They have been shown to have a balancing effect on hormones.[2] One study showed that eating soya increased oestrogen levels when they were low and reduced them when they were too high. This could explain why soya beans can reduce hot flushes for women going through the menopause (when it is believed that there is an oestrogen deficiency), and reduce the incidence of breast cancer (often due to an excess of oestrogen).

Because these foods have a controlling effect on oestrogen, it is important to include them in your diet – particularly when you are suffering from a condition that is sensitive to excess oestrogen, such as fibroids, endometriosis, or lumpy and tender breasts. Research has also shown that phytoestrogens can help to produce lighter periods, and to lengthen the cycle in women whose cycles are too short.[3]

Phytoestrogens also have other positive benefits. Soya beans have been found to contain at least five compounds believed to inhibit cancer. The major research has focused on breast cancer because Japanese women have only one-sixth the rate of breast cancer that we have. It appears that when Japanese women move to the West, their rate rises to that of Western women.[4]

As well as these benefits on the hormones, phytoestrogens also have a positive effect on your cardiovascular health. Studies have shown that soya can lower the level of cholesterol, especially the 'bad' cholesterol (LDL) (see page 414).

These phytoestrogens are found in almost all fruit, vegetables and cereals, but they are most beneficial in the form of something called 'isoflavones', which are found in legumes such as soya, lentils, chickpeas etc. Beans are easy to use and they are great added to salads, soups and casseroles. Most beans (although not lentils) need to be soaked, sometimes overnight, before cooking. Alternatively, you can buy organic beans in tins from most supermarkets. Hummus is a dip made from chickpeas, and it is available ready-made from most supermarkets, or it is easy to make your own.

HUMMUS

SERVES 6–8
450g (1lb) chickpeas or 2 large (400g/14oz) tins of cooked
    organic chickpeas, drained
4 large garlic cloves
2 hot red chillies
juice of about 3 lemons
about 150ml ($\frac{1}{4}$ pint) tahini paste
85g (3oz) pitted black olives, plus a few for garnish
2 teaspoons ground cumin
about 1 teaspoon freshly ground sea salt
extra-virgin olive oil, to dress
a little paprika, to garnish
chopped flat-leaf parsley, to garnish

If using dried chickpeas, soak them overnight in water. Next day, discard the water, cover with fresh cold water and bring to the boil. Lower the heat, add one of the garlic cloves and the chillies and simmer

---

for 1 hour, until just soft. Drain, reserving the water and discarding the garlic and chillies.

Reserving a few whole chickpeas, put the rest in a food processor with the lemon juice, tahini paste, olives, cumin, 150ml ($^1/_4$ pint) of the reserved water (or plain water if using tinned chickpeas) and salt. Chop the remaining garlic, add to the processor and blitz to a coarse purée. The consistency should not be too smooth, with discernible pieces of chickpeas giving texture. Add more water if too dry. Adjust the flavouring with more tahini, lemon juice and salt to taste.

Spread the hummus on individual plates, forking circular ridges on the surface. Pour a little olive oil over and arrange a few whole chickpeas and olives on top, dust with a little paprika and garnish with the flat-leaf parsley. Can be served with warm wholemeal pitta bread.

This recipe is taken from my book *Natural Alternatives to HRT Cookbook* (Kyle Cathie, 2000).

There is still a great deal of confusion about soya, but there is no doubt that it can be a useful addition to your diet (see below).

CONFUSED ABOUT SOYA?

Soya has had some fairly bad press in the last few years, particularly with the growing concern about genetic modification, for which soya is a prime candidate. But what about the rest of the scare stories? You may have heard that soya can cause an underactive thyroid condition, or that it can be at the root of mineral deficiencies. There is also concern about aluminium levels in soya, which have been linked to Alzheimer's disease. For every story claiming health benefits for soya, there is another suggesting that it can damage health.

If you are confused, you are not alone. Many women have written to me over the past year, understandably perplexed about the findings and unsure whether they should be eating soya at all. For that reason, I'll take this opportunity to set the record straight.

First of all, it's important to remember that every study is funded, and that every sponsor will have a vested interest in the results of the study for which they pay. Soya is now a big industry, particularly in America, where it is used in margarines and salad dressings, and to feed animals, among other things. Its non-food uses include newspaper printing inks.

Many of the big companies behind the research are those that accept and use the process of genetic modification. They fund the research into soya in the hope that studies will find it completely safe or, even better, a wonder food that we simply can't do without. But then, the good publicity for soya tends to alarm big companies on the other side of the board: the pharmaceutical giants who stand to lose a lot of money if alternatives to HRT and other menopausal drugs are found. And what about the dairy farmers, who lose out when the population shifts to soya instead of milk and other dairy produce? Everyone has something at stake. Who do you believe?

QUALITY OF RESEARCH

The research citing the negative effects of soya has not been substantiated. In September 2000, the British Nutrition Foundation issued a press statement saying: 'Recent media coverage has raised a number of concerns about possible effects of soya products on health including thyroid abnormalities, mineral deficiencies, Alzheimer's disease and effects in women consuming soy products during pregnancy on the unborn child. In reality, for most of these there have been few published studies and much of the work cited to support many of these claims has been conducted in experimental animals, rather than humans. So, at the present time, these concerns remain speculative and unproven.'[5]

In some of the studies mentioned in the media, the animals were fed high amounts of *raw* soya flour for *five* years. In one study the scientists were looking at the effect of protease inhibitors on the pancreas. Proteases (including trypsin) are enzymes that dismantle proteins. The pancreas secretes trypsin, which enables your body to break down protein in the small intestine. Raw soya contains trypsin inhibitors, which could theoretically stop this process from happening. Out of 26 monkeys tested, only one showed even moderate pancreatitis (inflammation of the pancreas). The questions here are: Why use raw soya flour in tests and on animals? Which traditional culture eats raw soya?

Traditionally fermented soya foods, such as miso and soya sauce, are relatively free of protease inhibitors. In tofu, these inhibitors end up in the soaking fluid (which is then discarded), and not in the curd itself. Soya milk, which is made from whole soya beans, also involves a soaking process and again, the fluid is discarded after this process.

NOT ALL SOYA IS THE SAME

There is an enormous difference between whole soya beans and soya protein isolates (isolated compounds of soya), and this is where the confusion lies. Most of the studies, and therefore the arguments, are focused on soya protein *isolate*: in other words, a part of the soya plant and not the whole food.

Soya protein isolates are made in an industrial setting. The fibre from the soya bean is removed with an alkaline solution and then the beans are put into an aluminium tank with an acid wash. This is where the aluminium concerns come into play. You may remember an old cook's tip for cleaning out aluminium pans. It was suggested that cooking rhubarb in stained pans would 'wipe them clean'. And it worked. The reason? The surface of the aluminium was neatly absorbed into the rhubarb, an acidic fruit. It's the same premise at work here with the soya beans. When left to soak in an aluminium tank, they absorb aluminium. A very straightforward concept, and certainly relevant to soya protein isolates, but *not* whole soya foods. Furthermore, soya protein isolates undergo a number of other chemical treatments, which add nitrates to the end product. Nitrates are another concern, as they are now known to be potent carcinogens (cancer-forming agents).

This 'food', which no longer resembles the original soya bean, can then be made into anything, including textured vegetable proteins (with added 'chicken' or 'beef' flavours, for example), flavour enhancers in soups and sauces (as hydrolysed vegetable protein), lecithin (which is used as an emulsifier in products such as mayonnaise), and even infant formulas, children's snacks and some soya milks. The difference is that these products are not made with whole soya beans, but with powdered soya isolate. Even worse than the fact that these products have infiltrated a good part of our food supply is the concern that it is very difficult to guarantee that soya isolate is not genetically modified.

There is a fundamental and important difference between traditional (Chinese and Japanese) and Western-style soya foods, and the only way that you will ever be able to tell the difference is to read the label on the foods you propose to buy. Some manufacturers buy soya isolate powder and make it into soya milk by adding other ingredients. Other companies, such as Provamel, specify on the label that their products are made from whole beans, and they are also able to confirm that these beans are not genetically modified. One easy way to tell a whole soya product is when it has an 'organic' label. At the moment, if a food is labelled organic it is not genetically modified. In future it may be hard to tell if GM seeds are then grown organically. At present seeds must be organic and grown organically.

Up to 60 per cent of processed foods contain soya, including bread, biscuits, pizza and baby food and, in the majority of cases, the soya takes the form of soya isolate, and is not derived from whole soya beans.

Traditional soya foods can be broken down into two primary types:

- **Fermented**, including soya sauce (also tamari), miso, natto and tempeh. Tempeh is fermented in two days, but miso and soya sauce can take many months. The fermentation process aids digestion.

- **Unfermented** soya, including soya milk and tofu.

THE THYROID CONNECTION

Some foods are termed 'goitrogens', which means that they have the ability to block the uptake of iodine from the blood. Iodine is essential for thyroid function, and a deficiency can be the cause of an underactive thyroid condition. Therefore, any food that is a goitrogen will make an underactive thyroid problem worse. Soya is one of those foods, but so are turnips, cabbage, peanuts, pine nuts, Brussels sprouts, broccoli, kale and millet. If you are diagnosed with a severe underactive thyroid problem you will normally be told to restrict your intake of these foods. When eaten raw, and in excess, problems can occur.

There is an abounding myth that when something is good for you, a lot must be even better. I see this belief illustrated a great deal in the field of nutrition, where people tend to believe that extra quantities of herbs or vitamin supplements will enhance the effect. This is nothing but a myth – and it can be dangerous. Very often the effects of a food or supplement are most beneficial at a specific, often small dose. This myth has, not surprisingly, spread to soya. Once the positive effects became clear, people moved in droves to get as much as they could. As a result, you can now buy soya in almost every imaginable form. In fact, there are now available snack bars that are nothing more than *raw*, ground soya beans. Remember the experiment with the monkeys? The same goes here. Soya is not meant to be eaten raw, and it is not meant to be eaten in excessive quantities. Certainly any goitrogen, of which soya is one, will affect thyroid function in a serious way if it is eaten in this manner.

PHYTATES

Some studies have showed that soya beans are high in phytic acid, which blocks the uptake of essential minerals, such as calcium, magnesium, iron and zinc. However, what these studies don't tell us is that phytates are, in fact, present in the bran or husks of *all* grains and legumes. Muesli is a good example of a phytate-rich food. It must be soaked before being eaten, or the phytates it contains will block the uptake of minerals. So we should pour milk, water or juice over our muesli and leave it for about 20 minutes before eating. But has there been an outcry against muesli? Is it on the danger list? Phytates are contained in soya beans, but for there to be a serious effect on nutrient uptake, you would have to consume abnormally large quantities.

WHAT SHOULD YOU EAT?

Do eat soya products – they are good for you! But eat them in their traditional form, choosing products such as miso, tofu or organic soya milks. These foods are healthy, and they can have a dramatic effect on your health, particularly during the menopause. Avoid 'gimmicky' soya bars and snacks unless you know they are made from the whole bean, and even then make sure that the beans are not raw or genetically modified.

Variety is the key to a healthy diet, and it's important to remember that soya is only one of many phytoestrogens (see page 20). Phytoestrogens are found in other legumes such as lentils, chickpeas, garlic, celery, seeds (including linseeds, sesame seeds and sunflower seeds), grains such as rice and oats, certain fruits, vegetables, alfalfa and mung beansprouts, and herbs such as sage, fennel and parsley. For further information on the different types of phytoestrogens (isoflavones, lignans and coumestans) and how to eat a healthy diet cooking with these foods see my *Natural Alternatives to HRT Cookbook* (Kyle Cathie, 2000).

WHAT ABOUT PHYTOESTROGEN SUPPLEMENTS?

This is where I think you need to be cautious. Traditional cultures have eaten phytoestrogens in the form of soya, lentils, chickpeas, grains and other foods for thousands of years, but the use of phytoestrogens (or isoflavones) in tablets or capsules is relatively new. Nobody knows yet what the long-term effects of taking supplements like these might be. Supplements never offer the same beneficial effects that complete foods can. Foods contain a variety of different elements, including fibre, water and nutrients that do not appear in dried supplements. We found out, for example, that removing the active ingredients of herbal products and making them into pharmaceutical drugs brought with them a whole host of side-effects that simply did not occur when the herbs were taken whole. The problem is that we do not know if the same holds true here.

My recommendation is to use soya or red clover supplements in the short term to help combat the symptoms of the menopause (including hot flushes and irritability). At the same time, however, you should also make changes in your diet and start to include phytoestrogens in your cooking.

SEX HORMONES

Sex hormone-binding globulin (SHBG) is a protein produced by the liver that binds sex hormones, such as oestrogen and testosterone, in order to control how much of them are circulating in the blood at any one time. If you have the correct amount of this SHBG there will be a balancing effect on the hormones, ensuring that just the right amount is circulating in your body. Phytoestrogens help to stimulate the production of SHBG.[6]

---

5. Eat oily foods, including fish, nuts, seeds and oils

Does this seem like an odd suggestion? Oil is traditionally associated with fat, and if you listen to the scare stories in the media, fat is something that should never pass our lips. In fact, most women follow, or have followed, a low-fat or no-fat diet for health benefits (weight loss is one). But this pervading myth can do more damage than you'd think.

First and foremost, let me set the record straight. We all need fats. Saturated fats are not good for us, and they can lead to a variety of health problems. However, some fats are not only important, but essential for health – even more so when you are trying to rectify a female health problem, particularly if it is hormone-related. These essential fats are, not surprisingly, known as 'essential fatty acids', or EFAs.

Do you get any of these symptoms?

- Dry skin
- Cracked skin on heels or fingertips
- Hair falling out
- Lifeless hair
- Poor wound healing
- Dandruff
- Depression
- Irritability
- Soft or brittle nails
- Allergies
- Dry eyes
- Lack of motivation
- Aching joints
- Fatigue
- Difficulty losing weight
- High blood pressure
- Arthritis
- Pre-menstrual syndrome (PMS)
- Painful breasts

The above are all signs of an essential fatty acid deficiency. EFAs are found in foods such as nuts, seeds and oily fish. These essential fats are a vital component of every human cell and the body needs them to balance hormones, insulate nerve cells, keep the skin and arteries supple, and to keep the body warm.

Unsaturated fats
Saturated fats are the fats that we need to avoid (see page 30). The focus should be more on unsaturated fats, and these can be broken down into two types: monounsaturated and polyunsaturated.

1. Monounsaturated fats (Omega 9 fats) are not classed as essential fatty acids, but they can have health benefits. They are called monounsaturated because, chemically speaking, they have only one double bond. Olive oil, for example, is high in monounsaturated fats, which has been found to lower LDL ('bad' cholesterol) and raise HDL ('good' cholesterol), which is one of the factors contributing to the low rate of heart disease in the Mediterranean.

2. Polyunsaturated fats can be split into two types:

- Omega 6 oils are found in nuts and seeds (they can go stale fairly quickly, so make sure your supply is fresh), and also in evening primrose, starflower and borage oil. These essential fatty acids help prevent blood clots and keep the blood thin. They can also reduce inflammation and pain in the joints, and so are vital in preventing arthritis.

- Omega 3 oils are found in fish oils and linseed (flaxseed) oil, and also to some extent in pumpkin seeds, walnuts and dark green vegetables. These oils can help lower blood pressure, reduce the risk of heart disease, soften the skin, increase immune function, increase metabolic rate, improve energy, help with rheumatoid arthritis and alleviate eczema. Oily fish includes mackerel, tuna, sardines, herrings and salmon. A small portion of salmon (115g/4oz) can contain up to 3,600mg of Omega 3 fatty acids, while the same sized piece of cod will contain only 300mg.

The Department of Health recommends that we should double our intake of Omega 3 oils by eating oily fish two to three times a week. More and more research suggests that it is vital to supplement these fatty acids, not relying solely on diet. The quantities needed are listed in the recommendations for each particular health condition throughout this book.

'GOOD' PROSTAGLANDINS

The body makes beneficial prostaglandins (hormone-like substances) from these essential fatty acids. These prostaglandins help to prevent inflammation, regulate the immune system and reduce abnormal blood clotting. They play a major role in helping with endometriosis and period problems so they are extremely important when thinking about women's health.

Unfortunately, your body produces 'bad' prostaglandins from saturated fats (see below), which cause inflammation, and can cause swelling and pain.

Choosing an EFA supplement

Don't be tempted to supplement your diet with cod liver oil capsules. In the sea, fish can accumulate toxins and mercury, which pass through their livers (the organ responsible for detoxification). Extracting the oil from the liver of the fish is likely to provide higher quantities of these toxins than the oil taken from the body of the fish.

If you are vegetarian or prefer not to take fish oil, the other way to get those Omega 3 fatty acids is by taking linseed oil capsules. Linseed oil, also called 'flaxseed oil', contains both Omega 3 and some Omega 6 essential fatty acids.

Warning

Some of the symptoms listed under EFA deficiencies can also be caused by a thyroid imbalance, so it is worth seeing your doctor for a check-up.

---

6. Reduce your intake of saturated fat

Saturated fats are not essential for your health – in fact, this is one type of fat you could do without. These fats come mainly from animals, and are contained in foods such as meat, eggs and dairy products. They are also present in tropical oils, such as palm and coconut. Saturated fats can be detrimental to your health, especially when consumed in large amounts.

For one thing, saturated fats can contribute to weight gain. The more saturated a fat becomes, the harder it is to digest, so it becomes deposited in the body. Butter, coconut oil and palm oil are the saturated fats most easily assimilated by the body, so they are less harmful. Fats from beef, lamb and pork are the hardest to digest because they are hard at body temperature. Being overweight is a risk factor for many health conditions (see Chapter 13), but one of the most distressing problems for women is that it can reduce fertility.

Saturated fats can also block other nutrients. They interfere with your body's absorption of the essential fatty acids that are essential for health.

A diet high in saturated fat is now known to stimulate oestrogen overproduction, so it follows that eliminating animal products (the richest source of saturated fats) can help to do the opposite.[7] If you can't cut out saturated fats completely, take an *acidophilus* supplement, which helps to ensure that 'old' hormones are reabsorbed.

Finally, the saturated fats in red meat and poultry produce hormones called prostaglandins. These aren't the healthy prostaglandins that can be created by essential fatty acids (see page 29). The particular prostaglandin produced from saturated fats is highly inflammatory and can cause swelling and pain. This hormone can trigger muscle contraction and constriction in the blood vessels, so it can increase period pains, endometriosis-related cramps and the spread of endometrial tissue.

MARGARINE VERSUS BUTTER

Hydrogenated vegetable oil is listed in the ingredients of most margarines and also many fast foods, crisps, biscuits and crackers. The process of hydrogenation (which makes a fat more solid and spreadable) changes the essential unsaturated fats contained in the food into trans fatty acids, which have been linked to all sorts of problems, including an increased rate of heart attack, and an inability to absorb essential fats.[8]

For this reason, I recommend using butter (most supermarkets now sell organic butter) in moderation or unhydrogenated margarine (look on the label) obtained from healthfood shops, rather than ordinary margarine. Although margarine is manufactured from polyunsaturated fats, these 'good' fats become 'trans fats' in the hydrogenation process. These have a plastic-like quality and your body struggles to try to eliminate them. Why put your body under extra pressure to deal with a substance that you do not really need to eat? You want to make things easy for your body so that it functions efficiently and by doing so has the resources to heal itself.

Choosing and using Oils

Oils can easily become damaged, so it's essential that you take care when choosing, storing and using them. If oils are overheated, left in sunlight or reused after cooking, they are open to attack by free radicals (see page 17), and these have been linked to cancer, coronary heart disease, rheumatoid arthritis and premature ageing.

- To prevent free radicals from forming, always choose cold-pressed, unrefined vegetable oils or extra-virgin olive oil. A number of supermarkets now have organic oils, which are better still, because no chemicals will have been used in their production. Unfortunately, standard supermarket oils are manufactured and extracted with chemicals and heat. This destroys the quality of the oil and the nutritional content. Store your oil away from sunlight and do not be tempted to reuse it after heating.

- Do not fry polyunsaturated fats as they can become unstable when heated. Use olive oil or butter for frying. Olive oil, which is a monounsaturate, is less likely to cause free radicals (see page 17), and butter will not cause free radicals because it is a saturated fat. Reduce the cooking temperature to minimise the chances of free radicals forming. Keep all fats to a minimum when frying — try to bake, steam, roast or grill instead.

7. Drink enough fluids

Your body is made up of approximately 70 per cent water and this is involved in every bodily process, including digestion, circulation and excretion. It helps transport nutrients and waste products in and out

---

LUNCHES

If you are working and have a limited choice of food for lunch you could have sandwiches a couple of days a week and take something slightly more substantial on the others.

Sandwiches – choose wholemeal bread. Wholemeal pitta can also make a change from sliced bread. Suggestions for fillings:

- tahini and freshly sliced apple
- mashed avocado with a sprinkling of sesame seeds
- tuna and salad
- egg and cress
- avocado and salad
- hummus and salad
- bean sprouts and tahini
- tofu mashed with a little miso and salad
- miso, tahini, lettuce and a squeeze of lemon.

Jacket potatoes – with sweetcorn/tuna/salad/hummus

Soups – make home made ones with any combination of vegetables and beans or buy some good tinned organic soups available in the supermarkets and healthfood shops.

Smoked mackerel and salad

Leftovers – some lunches such as soups, can be made from left-overs from the meal the night before, for example, stir-fried rice and vegetables.

of the cells. We can survive without food for about five weeks, but we can't live without water for longer than five days.

Most of us do not drink enough fluids and, ironically, women who suffer from water retention tend to restrict their liquid intake thinking that the less they drink, the less their bodies will retain. Actually, the opposite is true. If you restrict fluids your body will try to compensate and retain liquid, just in case it is in short supply. You should aim to drink around six glasses of water a day, which should take the place of less healthy drinks, such as canned soft drinks, coffee, sugary drinks, etc. An excellent start to the day is a cup of hot water with a slice of lemon. It's good for the liver, and it works by kick-starting and cleansing. Herbal teas can be counted as part of your liquid intake but other drinks, such as coffee or black tea, can't.

Tap water can be contaminated with impurities such as arsenic, copper and lead, all of which can occur naturally and leach into the

A BOTTLED WATER BUYER'S GUIDE

- **Spring water** – May have been taken from one or more underground sources and have undergone a range of treatments such as filtration and blending.

- **Natural mineral water** – Is bottled in its natural state (without treatment). It has to come from an officially registered source, conform to purity standards, and carry details of its source and mineral analysis on the label.

- **Naturally sparkling water** – Must come from an underground source with enough natural carbon dioxide to make it bubbly.

- **Sparkling (carbonated water)** – Has carbon dioxide added to it during bottling (as with ordinary fizzy drinks).

water from the pipes. Other substances, such as pesticides and fertilisers, can leach into the water from the ground. Get a filter (either a jug filter or one plumbed in under the sink) and use water from that for cooking vegetables and making hot drinks. A filter cannot eliminate every impurity but it is better than nothing.

If you are unsure about your water supply, or if you have lead pipes or a lead tank, then you can ask your environmental health department or water supplier to test the water for you. Your public library should have a copy of the Drinking Water Inspectorate's annual report, which gives details of the monitoring of the water supply and when water has exceeded 'maximum permitted levels'.

8. Increase your intake of fibre

Everybody tends to think of fibre and its effects on the bowels, but it does more than simply prevent constipation. Fibre plays a major role in balancing our female hormones. The fibre contained in grains and vegetables reduces oestrogen levels and seems to work by preventing oestrogens that are excreted in the bile from being reabsorbed back into the blood. In other words, 'old' oestrogens do not enter the bloodstream again (thus preventing an excess of oestrogen in the body). Studies show that women who eat a vegetarian diet (high in fibre) are able to excrete three times more 'old' oestrogens than women who eat meat as well. Meat–eaters also reabsorb more oestrogen, which can cause havoc with overall health. There are many problems associated with excess oestrogen, including breast cancer, fibroids and endometriosis.

There are two main types of fibre: soluble and insoluble. Insoluble fibre is found in whole grains and vegetables, while soluble fibre is found in fruits, oats and beans. Soluble fibre helps to control cholesterol because it binds with some of the cholesterol and fat in the food you eat. Fibre can also be useful when you want to lose weight because it helps digestion, increases your feeling of fullness and removes toxins from the body.

Fibre does have a very beneficial effect on the bowels because it binds water and increases the bulk of the stools, so that they are easier to eliminate from the body. Fibre also prevents food from putrefying inside your body, which can give you symptoms such as bloating and flatulence.

DINNERS

These can include:

- brown rice and stir-fried vegetables
- grilled fish with salad and green vegetables
- tuna bake with pasta, sweetcorn and tomato sauce
- bean casserole
- fish pie, with fish and mashed potato
- vegetable and lentil curry
- tofu and vegetable risotto.

Many ideal recipes including those for sugar-free desserts can be found in my book *Natural Alternatives to HRT Cookbook* (Kyle Cathie, 2000).

---

9. Avoid additives, preservatives and chemicals

The aim is to eat your food in its most natural state without added chemicals in the form of additives, preservatives and artificial sweeteners. The overall aim of this book is to encourage optimum health and, in doing so, address any hormonal imbalances. For this reason, it is important that you avoid any chemicals in food or drinks. So you will need to read the labels and avoid foods or drinks that have a long list of chemical-sounding ingredients.

You may be tempted to substitute sugar with artificial sweeteners in order to cut calories. Don't. If a food or drink is described as 'low sugar', 'slimline' or 'diet', it will usually contain an artificial sweetener. These sweeteners have been linked to mood swings and depression, and it has been found that people who regularly use artificial sweeteners tend to gain weight because they can slow down the digestive process and increase appetite.

Avoid any foods or drinks containing artificial sweeteners. They can be added to yoghurts, fizzy drinks, desserts, salad dressing, confectionery, jams and many other foods, so read those labels.

10. Reduce your intake of caffeine

Caffeine has a diuretic effect on the body, depleting valuable stores of vitamins and minerals that are essential for a healthy hormone balance. Caffeine in tea, coffee, chocolate, and caffeinated soft drinks acts as a stimulant and causes a fast rise in blood sugar, followed by a quick drop, which contributes to the roller-coaster ride of blood sugar swings (see page 39). Avoid them whenever possible; even better, cut them out of your diet completely. Substitute them with herbal teas and grain coffee, spring water and diluted pure fruit juices.

It is a good idea to eliminate caffeine gradually. Suddenly giving up coffee, for example, can cause a variety of unpleasant withdrawal symptoms, such as headaches, shaking and muscle cramps. Wean yourself off gradually by substituting some of your cups of coffee for herbal teas or grain coffee, and take the coffee out slowly.

METHYLXANTHINES

Methylxanthines are a family of substances found in coffee, black tea, green tea, chocolate, cocoa, cola and decaffeinated coffee as well as medications that contain caffeine, such as headache remedies. These methylxanthines have been linked to a benign breast condition called fibrocystic disease – this comes and goes with the cycle, and can give symptoms such as tender, lumpy and swollen breasts. Many women experience breast discomfort in the week before a period and for some women they can be very uncomfortable.

---

11. Reduce alcohol

Keep alcohol to a minimum, particularly while you are correcting a health problem. A couple of units a week is really the maximum allowable intake while you are healing. It is important that you have at least a couple of days a week free from alcohol to give your liver a 'break'. Where your problem is more 'oestrogen specific', such as endometriosis and fibroids, alcohol should be eliminated completely while you are working to alleviate the symptoms (see Chapter 6).

Alcohol takes its toll on your liver (see page 37) and can compromise its ability to detoxify your system, which is one of its main roles. It also contributes to blood sugar imbalance (see page 38) and it acts as an anti-nutrient, which means that it blocks the good effects of your food by depleting vitamins and minerals. Alcohol can also interfere with the metabolism of essential fatty acids, which are absolutely crucial for your health. It is also full of calories – a glass of wine gives 100 calories and a pint of beer around 200 calories.

You may be wondering how this all fits in with the idea that red wine is good for you. Certainly the French eat even more saturated fat than we do and yet their heart disease rate is lower than in the US and the UK. Grapes contain an antioxidant called 'resveratrol', which decreases the 'stickiness' of the blood platelets and keeps blood vessels from narrowing. Resveratrol is mainly contained in the skin of grapes, which is why red wine seems to be more effective than white (red wine includes grape skins and pips, whereas white wine is only made from the flesh). Scientists have even compared the effect of alcoholic and non-alcoholic red wines, and found that the non-alcoholic version is actually better for the heart.[9]

In the long term, once you have achieved optimum health, the best approach is to keep alcohol in moderation and save it mainly for the weekend or special occasions. Do not drink every night and when you do, don't have more than two glasses of wine or beer. And don't save up all your units for one binge!

TAKE CARE OF YOUR LIVER

With any female problem, especially those that are connected with hormone imbalances, such as fibroids, endometriosis or polycystic ovary syndrome, it is also important that your liver is functioning at optimum level. The liver is the waste disposal unit of the body, not only for toxins, waste products, drugs and alcohol, but also for hormones. If the liver is not functioning efficiently, old hormones can become accumulated. These old hormones are left over after each menstrual cycle, but unless they are deactivated by the liver, they can return to the bloodstream and cause all sorts of problems.

The liver deals with oestrogen so it can be eliminated safely from the body. Oestrogen is not just one hormone, but a group of hormones. Oestrogen includes three hormones: oestradiol, oestrone and oestriol. Oestrogen is secreted by the ovaries in the form of oestradiol and the liver metabolises oestradiol to oestrone and oestriol. The liver's ability to efficiently convert oestradiol (the most carcinogenic oestrogen) to oestriol is very important because oestriol is the safest and least active form of oestrogen.

The liver also performs other important functions that have a bearing on your health. Among its many tasks are the storage and filtration of blood, the secretion of bile and numerous metabolic functions, including the conversion of sugars into glycogen, which is the form in which carbohydrates are stored in your body. It plays a vital part in metabolising fat (breaking it down properly) and it helps to use up fat to produce energy. The liver also helps to optimise thyroid function.

OPTIMISING LIVER FUNCTION

As well as avoiding substances that can compromise your liver, such as alcohol, you can also take substances to help liver function. The B vitamins are especially important because they are essential for the liver to be able to convert oestradiol into the harmless oestriol.

Milk thistle (*Silybum marianum*) is an excellent herb for the liver. A number of studies have shown that it can increase the number of new liver cells to replace old, damaged ones.[10]

12. Avoid sugar

Sugar is a problem because it can make you gain weight, which then increases oestrogen production and creates a hormone imbalance. The more sugar you eat, the more insulin your body releases. The more insulin is released, the more of your food is converted into fat, and your body therefore fails to break down previously stored fat. Fat stored on your body is a manufacturing plant for oestrogen, so it is important not to carry too much excess weight.

Sugar is also 'empty calories'. It does not give you anything of nutritional value. So when you are trying to nourish your body and give it the right tools to correct a health problem you don't want to eat foods that have a negative effect on your health.

Fluctuations in blood sugar, especially low blood sugar, can cause a number of symptoms including irritability, aggressive outbursts, depression, fatigue, dizziness, crying spells, anxiety, confusion, inability to concentrate, headaches, palpitations, forgetfulness and lack of sex drive.

When you eat any food in its refined form you digest it very quickly. Refined foods are no longer in their 'whole' state and have been stripped of their natural goodness by various manufacturing processes. Two of the most widely used refined foods are sugar and white flour.

If digestion is too fast, glucose enters the bloodstream too rapidly. This also occurs when you eat any food or drink that gives a stimulant effect, such as tea, coffee or chocolate. The initial stimulating 'high' quickly passes and you plummet down to a 'low', in which you feel tired and drained. So, what do you need? Another stimulant, like a cup of coffee or bar of chocolate to give you a boost.

If there is a long gap between your meals your blood glucose will drop to quite a low level, leaving you feeling the need for a quick boost like a cup of coffee. When the glucose level falls too low, adrenaline is released by the adrenal glands to get your liver to produce more glucose to rectify the imbalance. You can then end up with too much glucose in the blood, which means that your pancreas has to secrete more insulin in order to reduce your glucose levels. Your body is then on a roller-coaster ride of fluctuating blood sugar levels.

If you continually ask your pancreas to produce extra insulin, it will literally become exhausted and unable to cope with the demands. You then have the opposite problem – high blood sugar (hyperglycaemia) – because your body is not producing enough insulin to deal with the glucose. The extreme form of this is diabetes. With this condition, insulin is supplied from outside the body in order to control glucose levels.

It is important that you keep your blood sugar in balance, not only to eliminate any health problems but also to keep you in good health and prevent problems for the future.

HOW TO BALANCE YOUR BLOOD SUGAR

To help maintain a steady blood sugar level during the day, aim to eat complex carbohydrates as part of your main meals, and make sure that you eat little and often during the day. Sometimes just an oat cake can be enough between meals to keep eating urges at bay.

If you find the symptoms associated with low blood sugar are worst first thing in the morning or if you wake during the night with heart pounding and you are unable to get back to sleep, then it is very likely that your blood sugar level has dropped overnight and adrenaline has kicked into play. Eating a small, starchy snack, like half a slice of rye bread, one hour before going to bed, will help to alleviate these symptoms.

Remember to make sure your complex carbohydrates are unrefined. In general, this means choosing brown instead of white. For example, eat wholewheat bread, brown rice and wholemeal flour as opposed to their white versions, which have been refined and stripped of essential vitamins, minerals, trace elements and valuable fibre.

- Do eat unrefined complex carbohydrates including wholewheat bread, potatoes, brown rice, millet, oats, rye etc.

- Do dilute pure fruit juice

- Always eat breakfast. Porridge or oatmeal is a good choice

- Do eat small, frequent meals no more than three hours apart

- Do reduce, preferably avoid, stimulants including tea, coffee, chocolate, smoking and canned drinks that contain caffeine

- Don't eat refined carbohydrates. Avoid 'white' in general. Remember that white flour is in many things, such as cakes, biscuits, pastries and white bread

- Don't eat sugar or the foods it is found in, including chocolate, sweets, biscuits, pastries and soft drinks

Lifestyle Factors

Xenoestrogens

Xenoestrogens ('foreign oestrogens') are oestrogen-like chemicals from pesticides or plastics that have been linked to health problems (see below). In the wild, some of these problems have been dramatic. For example, some fish are growing both male and female sex organs, and male alligators are becoming feminised, with hormonal levels altered to the extent that it is making reproduction difficult. There's no doubt that everyone is affected by xenoestrogens, and they may be at the root of more health problems than are currently known.

Xenoestrogens are stored in body fat, and can affect men and women differently. Overweight people tend to have higher concentrations because xenoestrogens are lipophilic – which means that they love fat!

The increasing levels of xenoestrogens in our environment have coincided with an earlier onset of puberty. In 1900 the average age for puberty to begin was 15. Now some girls as young as eight are growing breasts and pubic hair. It has been found that girls can enter puberty almost a year earlier if their pregnant mothers had higher levels of two synthetic chemicals, PCBs and DDT, while they were pregnant.[11]

Women with higher concentrations of certain pesticides in their bodies run a greater risk of developing breast cancer than women with lower levels.

A startling discovery was made by Professor Ann Soto in Boston, USA. She was studying breast cancer cells stored in large incubators. One day the cancer cells started to divide and multiply as if oestrogen had been present. When the laboratory changed the test-tubes on the incubators the cells stopped dividing. It turned out that nonylphenol, a synthetic oestrogen similar to those widely used in paints, toiletries such as skin creams, agricultural chemicals and detergents, had been used in the manufacture of the tubes and was being leached into the breast cell culture, causing the cells to be stimulated. Consider the implications if the moisturiser you have been using on your body – in particular your breasts – contained this chemical.

What can you do about this?

- There are 3,900 brands of insecticide, herbicide and fungicide approved for use in the UK, and some fruit and vegetables are sprayed as many as ten times before they reach the supermarket shelves. What's the answer? Buy as much organic as you can afford.

- Avoid, as far as possible, food and drinks in plastic containers or wrapped in plastic. Don't store any fatty foods (such as cheese or meat) in plastic wrap. Because xenoestrogens are lipophilic (fat-loving), they will tend to migrate into foods with a high fat content. Remove food from plastic packaging as soon as possible.

- Reduce your intake of saturated fats. There are two reasons for this. First of all, you will lay down fat stores that will present a welcome home for xenoestrogens, and second, the fat you take in is likely to contain xenoestrogens from the animal's environment.

- Do not heat food in plastic, especially in a microwave oven.

- Increase your intake of fibre (see page 34), which helps to prevent the absorption of oestrogenic chemicals into your bloodstream.

- Eat more cruciferous vegetables, such as broccoli, Brussels sprouts, cabbage and cauliflower. These are high in a substance called 'indole-3-carbinol', which helps to prevent toxic oestrogen from being absorbed in your body, while at the same time encouraging its elimination.

- Eat phytoestrogens (see page 20), such as soya, chickpeas and lentils, which can reduce the toxic forms of oestrogen in your body.

- Buy 'natural' cleaning products for your home, to reduce the number of potentially xenoestrogenic chemicals in your household.

- Use natural toiletries – in particular, anything that is rubbed into your skin (see page 48).

Exercise

The benefits of regular exercise cannot be exaggerated. Exercise helps to keep your bowels working efficiently, which means you are eliminating waste products that your body doesn't need. It also improves the function of the immune system, the lymphatic system and your body's ability to keep blood sugar in balance. It stimulates thyroid gland secretion and helps to improve thyroid function, which has a direct effect on your metabolism.

Exercise releases brain chemicals called 'endorphins', which help us to feel happier, more alert and calmer. They can have a dramatic positive effect on women suffering from depression, stress and anxiety.

Exercise increases the circulation and also seems to lower LDL ('bad' cholesterol) and increase HDL ('good' cholesterol). Regular exercise can help to reduce high blood pressure.

Exercise can also have a direct effect on controlling your hormones, particularly oestrogen. A fascinating study reported in the US *Journal of the National Cancer Institute* showed that women who exercised for around four hours a week had a 58 per cent lower risk of breast cancer, and those who routinely exercised for between one and three hours a week had a 30 per cent lower risk.[12] The thinking is that regular exercise modifies a woman's hormonal activity in a beneficial way. We know that extremes of exercise alter the menstrual cycle dramatically

– many women athletes, for instance, don't have periods at all. So it is believed that moderate routine exercise suppresses the production (or overproduction) of hormones, reducing a woman's exposure during her lifetime. Some breast cancers are oestrogen-sensitive so it makes sense that if the hormone levels are more balanced then the risk of developing breast cancer will be reduced. Exercise is important if you suffer from problems caused by a hormone imbalance, such as fibroids and endometriosis, because it can help regulate oestrogen levels.

Exercise is also crucial for your bones (see page 425), especially as you get older, because it helps to keep up a good level of bone density.

Weight

Fat aids the manufacture of oestrogen, so when you are suffering from a problem that is caused by an excess of oestrogen (for example, fibroids or endometriosis), it is likely you will need to lose weight. Losing weight has also been found to be helpful in correcting poly-cystic ovary syndrome (see page 232).

If you are experiencing amenorrhoea (no periods; see Chapter 5), it is important to check that you are not underweight as too little body fat can cause your periods to stop. Oestrogen levels will fall as your weight is reduced.

The important thing to remember about weight is that you need to find a balance – in other words, your natural weight. Being over-weight (see Chapter 13) and underweight will have implications for your health, so the aim is to keep within the bounds of what is considered to be normal for your height and bone structure.

Smoking

There is a wealth of information available about the risks of lung cancer and emphysema, and most women are aware of the detrimental effects of smoking when pregnant, but unfortunately, more and more young women are smoking in the belief that it controls their weight and makes them look sophisticated. One study showed that women smokers are more likely to suffer a more severe and lethal form of lung cancer than men.

Smoking, however, does more than just affect the lungs. It has a huge negative impact on the female hormone system. Smoking has been linked with infertility in women[13] and it can bring on an early menopause because it brings down oestrogen levels to those more often seen in a menopausal woman.[14] This is especially important for older women who may be racing against time in an attempt to conceive.

This change in the hormones is also detrimental to your bones. It has been found that women who smoke are at greater risk of developing osteoporosis. In fact, smoking can reduce bone mass by up to 25 per cent.

Smoking depletes the level of vitamin C in your bloodstream so you can be lacking good levels of this very important antioxidant, which affects your body's ability to regenerate and, of course, maintain the immune system.

Tobacco contains more than 4,000 compounds, including carbon monoxide, oxide of nitrogen, ammonia, aromatic hydrocarbons, hydrogen cyanide, vinyl chloride, nicotine, lead and cadmium. When I do a mineral test on women who smoke (see page 70), they have high levels of cadmium, a heavy toxic metal. Cadmium can stop the utilisation of zinc, a mineral that is especially important for the reproductive system. Once you stop smoking, antioxidants such as vitamin C can be used to help eliminate the cadmium from your body.

If you need help to give up, then acupuncture and hypnotherapy can be extremely effective. Avoid using nicotine patches and gums as you can become addicted to them.

Stress

Our modern lifestyle creates stress in the shape of traffic jams, late trains, missed appointments, financial worries, work and family. Adrenaline is the hormone that most of us associate with stress. This hormone is released in a 'fight or flight' situation, and it has a powerful effect on the body. The heart speeds up and the arteries tighten to raise blood pressure. Your liver immediately releases emergency stores of glucose into your bloodstream to give you instant energy to fight or run. Then, because it is not necessary for immediate survival, your digestion shuts down. The clotting ability of your blood is also increased, to help prepare your body in the event of injury. This all means that you have been made ready to run faster, fight back and generally react more quickly than normal.

All this happens very quickly and it should, theoretically, last for a short space of time – long enough to get you out of danger. You could be stuck in a traffic jam, late for an appointment, becoming increasingly stressed and eating your lunch at the same time. Your stress response kicks in, just as it would if there was a real emergency situation. The difference is, of course, that in a life-threatening situation, you would have taken some action – run or fought. In the traffic jam you just sit there and seethe. What should be short-lived can go on for long periods of time. Digestion will have been shut down while you are trying to eat, which means that you will be getting little nutritional value from your food but, most importantly, perhaps, your risk of heart attack and stroke increases dramatically as your blood becomes thicker.

Adrenaline is also released when your blood sugar drops (see page 39), which means that you could literally be 'running on adrenaline', and will feel more and more stressed and unable to cope.

Stress can directly affect your reproductive system. Women going through a bereavement or other kind of trauma, for instance, can stop having periods.[15] The hormone prolactin can also be released when you are under stress and this hormone will prevent ovulation. It seems to be nature's way of protecting women from getting pregnant at a time when they would find it hard to cope.

Your immune system can also be compromised if you are under stress and it will not work efficiently. You will be more susceptible to infections and, when they do strike, you'll find they are more difficult to shake off.

If stress is a problem for you, it is important that you get your blood sugar in balance in order to reduce the amount of adrenaline released. Also, it would be worth learning some form of relaxation, stress management techniques or meditation, for example yoga or massage.

If stress is affecting your sleep then herbs can be very helpful. Valerian is a wonderful herb for helping with insomnia and it is classed as a sedative in herbal medicine. Passionflower (or passiflora) is another good herb for helping you sleep and can be used together with valerian for maximum effect. A cup of hot chamomile tea before bed can also be effective.

Aromatherapy oils such as bergamot, lavender and Roman chamomile can be added to a relaxing warm bath just before bed, and some women find that sprinkling the essential oil of lavender on to the pillow is restful.

Sleep

There is no doubt that sleep is important, and for a variety of reasons. As a society, we have pushed the waking day to the limits, and sleep has become a luxury, rather than the necessity that it is. If you are well rested, you'll be much better equipped – both emotionally and physically – to cope with the demands of a busy life. Inadequate sleep lowers the immune response. A recent study showed that missing even a few hours a night on a regular basis can decrease the number of 'natural killer cells', which are responsible for fighting off invaders such as bacteria and viruses. This will come as no surprise to those of us who succumb to colds and other illnesses when we are run down – normally after periods of inadequate sleep.

Even occasional sleeping problems can make daily life feel more stressful or cause you to be less productive. In fact, inadequate sleep is associated with poor memory, an inability to make reasoned decisions and to concentrate, as well as irritability and, of course, fatigue. You may recognise many of these symptoms alongside other health complaints. The answer is to get to bed early, and ensure that you are sleeping well. The herbs (see page 45) suggested for reducing stress can help if you find things difficult. It's also a good idea to cut out caffeine (see page 35), and to try some stress management techniques.

Keeping Well

There are many simple tips that can help to keep you well, above and beyond lifestyle changes. While they may seem to be precautionary, they can help to prevent health problems before they start.

Tampons

The vagina is normally an oxygen-free environment, which prevents the growth of certain bacteria. However, tampons can disrupt this environment, largely because air is trapped in the fibres. Oxygen is introduced into the vagina, so the possibility of bacteria and toxin overgrowth is increased. Furthermore, blood is held back by the tampon, which provides a nutrient source for bacteria to breed.

Tampons, especially super-absorbent brands, may dry out the vagina, making transfer of toxins into the bloodstream easier. Tampons are made from cotton and rayon, and higher absorbency tampons will normally contain more rayon, a derivative from wood-pulp, for better absorbency. Fifty per cent of the world's cotton is now genetically modified (GM), so unless the cotton is certified organic, tampons could contain GM cotton. The tampons could also contain chemicals such as pesticides, which have been used on the cotton.

Substances called dioxins are a potentially harmful by-product of the chlorine-bleaching process at paper and pulp mills. Dioxins are potentially carcinogenic and toxic to the immune system as well as the environment. We are exposed to dioxins in the environment from industrial emissions and car exhausts, and levels of dioxins are currently being monitored by the US Government's Environmental Protection Agency (www.epa.gov/ncea/dioxin) for their carcinogenic properties. Tampon manufacturers are now trying to make sure that the process of bleaching results in dioxin-free fibres, but the issues of pesticides and GM farming still exist.

We are exposed to many chemicals in the environment and the aim is always to reduce that exposure. This is one area where we need to pay particular attention. Tampons come into contact with delicate tissues that have direct entry to the bloodstream. Anything you put inside you can be easily transmitted. No risks should be taken.

It is now possible to buy 100 per cent organic cotton tampons and sanitary towels, that are non-chlorine bleached, GM free and 100 per cent biodegradable. My recommendation would be to use 100 per cent organic cotton sanitary towels most of the time to allow the blood to flow freely and to avoid introducing oxygen for bacteria to thrive. When needed (on holiday, or while swimming, for example) use 100 per cent cotton tampons. If you need to use other tampons, try to get away with the lowest possible absorbency.

TOXIC SHOCK SYNDROME (TSS)

TSS is a potentially fatal illness that has been associated with the use of tampons – particularly those with a high absorbency. It develops when *Staphylococcus aureus*, a common bacteria, starts to produce a toxin (TSST1) that is absorbed into the bloodstream, so TSS is literally a form of blood poisoning. The toxin overwhelms the immune system and attacks organs.

Scientists do not know what causes the bacteria to produce toxins, but it has been suggested that the tampon provides a surface for the bacteria to multiply, which is then fed by the blood supply. Higher absorbency tampons contain more rayon, which could react with the bacteria. In 1995, the *Journal of Infectious Diseases in Obstetrics and Gynaecology* published a study looking at 20 different kinds of tampons. They found that only the 100 per cent cotton tampons did not produce the TSST1 toxin, which is associated with TSS.

The symptoms feel like flu and can include sudden high fever, vomiting, diarrhoea, rash, sore throat, dizziness or fainting. If you suspect you have TSS, remove the tampon, use a sanitary towel and keep the tampon for analysis.

For prevention:

- Minimise the use of tampons
- Change your tampon regularly, every four to six hours
- Do not use a tampon when you do not have a period
- Use a lighter absorbency where possible
- Use 100 per cent cotton tampons

Anti-perspirants and deodorants

Your body sweats for a reason. Sweating is an essential process designed to eliminate waste products through your skin. Contained in this fluid, which is secreted by the sweat glands, is salt (sodium chloride) and urea. Sweating is your body's way of getting rid of nitrogenous waste and at the same time controlling your body temperature. The evaporation of sweat from the surface of your skin has a cooling effect on the body.

If you use an anti-perspirant, you prevent this natural process from occurring, and are effectively hampering the elimination process.

Furthermore, anything that goes on to the skin can be absorbed into the body. For example, hormone replacement therapy (HRT) or nicotine patches work by dispensing chemicals through the skin. It's an effective way of reaching the bloodstream. Unfortunately, anti-perspirants and deodorants contain chemicals that will be absorbed through the skin. As you will see in Chapter 9 on breasts, scientists are investigating the link between the use of deodorants and anti-perspirants and breast cancer.

Deodorants and anti-perspirants can also contain aluminium, which has been linked to dementia, because it has been found in patches of cell damage in the brains of people with Alzheimer's.

The answer is to buy a chemical-free, aluminium-free deodorant from a good healthfood shop. The ingredients will be listed so you can read what is in it. The deodorant will not stop the natural elimination process of sweating, but will prevent any odour. You could look out for deodorant crystals too, also found in healthfood shops.

So, the message is to eat well so that the foundation of your health is good and to help prevent problems in the future.

CHAPTER 2

Using Natural Medicine

This book looks at treating women's problems from both the conventional and the natural point of view. It is designed to present you with the choices you have available to you, in order that you can make an informed decision.

There are many differences between the conventional and natural ways of treating illness. One factor that may influence the health choices you make is the fact that natural medicine requires effort. It's certainly easier to pop a pill that reduces or removes any symptoms you may have. You can carry on with your lifestyle as it is, and push any issues affecting your health out of sight.

The natural approach involves a great deal of change. You will be asked to take responsibility for your health, looking at what you eat, your lifestyle, exercise and stress levels. The changes you will make are fundamental, and they involve a long-term commitment on your part. But these changes are well worth the effort involved. They will not only have an impact on the condition you are aiming to treat, but they will also offer you the opportunity of a healthy future. This is the cornerstone of preventative medicine. If you make changes now, you will be much more likely to prevent health problems both in the short term and the long term.

We are living in a time when degenerative diseases have become epidemic. Illnesses such as cancer, coronary heart disease, stroke, diabetes, arthritis and auto-immune conditions are on the increase, and they are the cause of death and disability in a huge percentage of the population. In the West very few of us die of 'old age'. We are dying of diseases that take time to manifest themselves in our bodies. They are not a 'natural' part of ageing, but the result of the way that we take care of ourselves over the years. For example, arthritis is a common feature of old age in the West. In other cultures, it simply does not exist to the same degree. Does the fact that it is common make it acceptable? I think not.

Natural medicine is about taking steps towards a healthy way of life – one that will prevent many of the diseases associated with old age, and help to encourage health on all levels.

The Aims of Natural Medicine

The first aim of natural medicine is to supply your body with the tools to heal itself. By ensuring that you have good levels of the correct nutrients, that you eat well, and that you use herbs, homeopathy or any other therapies to encourage overall health, your body can heal itself. Bodies have enormously profound healing energies and, given the right tools, they can correct any imbalances and restore good health. This is where natural medicine is so different from conventional or allopathic medicine. For example, if you were suffering from an infection, your conventional doctor would prescribe antibiotics, which kill off the bacteria. In natural medicine, the aim would be to stimulate and strengthen your immune system, so that your body can kill off the infection on its own.

What's the difference? The conventional approach leaves you weaker, as antibiotics tend to disrupt your system, killing off healthy bacteria that is part of your defence mechanism. Furthermore, your body has not 'learned' to fight off infection on its own, and chances are the exact same problem will occur again. By using the natural approach you will encourage your body to do the work, leaving it stronger and more able to address similar illness in the future.

It was Louis Pasteur who discovered the antibiotic properties of penicillin. In the early stages of his research, he said, 'In order for you to have a disease you have to have germs.' This encouraged the conventional approach to 'germs' and illness. Scientists were determined to find the 'germs' responsible, and to get rid of them. But, somewhere along the line, these scientists lost sight of the fact that our bodies can do this for themselves. If our bodies are strong and healthy, with our immune systems functioning at optimum level, we are much less likely to become ill and, when we do succumb, we heal that much more quickly. The emphasis clearly needs to be on keeping the body strong, rather than finding shortcuts to health.

Exposure to bacteria will not necessarily cause an infection. There has to be a weakness present in order for this to happen. In other words, it is the body's ability to fight its own battle that governs whether or not we succumb to illness.

Years after making his original statement, Louis Pasteur backtracked, saying instead, 'In a state of health, animals are shut off from the invasion of germs . . . The microbe is nothing, the terrain is everything.' What did he mean? If the terrain (your body) is healthy, disease cannot take hold. Interestingly, Louis Pasteur's work is considered to be a turning point in the treatment of disease, but his final message has been largely ignored. Conventional medicine isn't preventative. Natural medicine is.

The second aim of natural medicine is not just to suppress the symptoms, as is often the case in conventional medicine, but to identify and treat the cause. Symptoms are not the cause of the disease. A good way to understand this premise is the story of the hardworking doctors who are busy mopping up a floor that is quickly flooding. Water spills from the sink, where both taps are on full and the plug is in place. The doctors frantically treat the never-ending 'symptom' (the wet floor), while failing to address the cause. The natural approach would be to remove the plug and turn off the taps. Then the business of mopping up the water can begin. This process can take time, but the results are more permanent.

The third aim of natural medicine is to treat you as a whole person. We are not just a group of body parts. Everything works together and when one system is thrown out of balance, the others can and will be affected. You can see the conventional approach to treatment in a hospital setting. There are many different departments, clinics and specialities; for example, ear, nose and throat, gastro-intestinal, gynaecological, psychiatric and cardiovascular.

This is one of the main reasons why conventional medicine is not always effective in the long term. We are not separate 'bits'; we are whole people whose 'bits' interact constantly. So, if you are suffering from headaches and digestive problems, you would probably see two different specialists. There may only be one cause for the problems, but because they are being treated separately, there's much less chance that that cause will be uncovered.

There are also the emotional aspects to consider. Not only do our physical parts interact, but there is also a clear relationship between mind and body. Later in the book (see Chapter 5) you'll see that emotional stress can have a profound effect on your menstrual cycle. Natural medicine looks at interaction on every level. That's why it's so much more effective.

The fourth aim is prevention. Once you have treated a specific problem, you must continue to eat well and look after yourself in order to prevent problems in the future. It is much easier to prevent a problem than it is to treat it. All of us want to live a long life, but what point is there in living with crippling diseases? Quality of life is important both now and in the future. Taking steps to prevent problems now can make a big difference to the way you live your life in the future.

The fifth aim is to give you optimum health. By eating well, taking exercise and generally looking after yourself, you will look and feel healthy – both physically and emotionally. Many of us go through life with a series of niggling health problems. We wake up feeling tired all the time, which leads to feelings of depression. We don't feel 'ill', but we know we aren't '100 per cent'. But that's how we live our lives, and because everyone around us seems to suffer from the same niggling problems, we accept them as normal.

They are not. It's perfectly possible to feel 100 per cent. It's perfectly possible to feel fantastic. Natural medicine aims to give you optimum health in mind and body: the kind of health that gives you energy and encourages a feeling of well-being.

Remember that the role of the practitioner is very different in natural medicine. Natural health practitioners are different from conventional doctors in that they are not only there to treat a problem. Natural practitioners also help you to understand what factors can be affecting your health and they'll let you know what choices there are to make you better. Their job is to motivate you into taking responsibility for your own health.

You will need conventional expertise in obtaining a diagnosis and you want to find practitioners – both conventional and natural – whom you can trust for objective advice in order to make an informed decision about what is the best treatment plan for you and how the two approaches can be integrated.

Most of the advice offered in this book is based around nutritional therapy and herbal medicine, largely because that is what I use (with great success) in my own practice. But that doesn't mean there are no other options. There are a wide variety of exciting and hugely successful therapies now available and, in the hands of a good practitioner, they can make an overwhelming difference to your health and sense of well-being. Below you'll find details of some of the most commonly used and well-regarded therapies. There's no harm in experimenting. Many women find that they have a particular 'affinity' with a therapy, and that it works for them better than anything else. Take some time to find what works for you, and then stick with it until you get the results you want and deserve.

But remember that putting your health in the hands of a practitioner does not absolve you of your own personal responsibility. Embarking on any therapy requires commitment on your part, and you must be willing to make changes. The recommendations that you will find later in this book are all based upon making positive changes to affect your current and future health. Therapies can be used alongside this advice to great effect, but you need to work at the foundations of your health before you can expect miracles to happen.

The recommendations given in this book are known generally to help with a particular problem. But we are all individual and unique, and in natural medicine each person – even those suffering the same symptoms – is often treated differently. Follow the recommendations in this book and if the problem has not improved you then need to see a qualified practitioner for more individual help.

Your Choices

Nutritional therapy

Food is a powerful medicine that has a huge impact on the biochemical processes of your body. There is now an enormous amount of scientific knowledge showing the effects of food and nutrients on treating illness and preventing diseases, such as cancer. Nutritional therapy is not just about eating well. It is also about correcting any vitamin or mineral deficiencies (see page 71), improving digestive function (because you are what you eat, but also what you are able to absorb), balancing hormones naturally, and eliminating toxins and waste products.

It is important to remember that supplements are just what their name suggests – supplemental, or 'extra'. They are not a substitute for healthy food and a well-balanced diet. You cannot eat junk food, take nutritional supplements and hope to stay healthy.

The vitamins and minerals we require for our bodies to function work in harmony and most of them are dependent on each other to act efficiently. When you take any supplements you should always have a multivitamin and mineral as the foundation of the programme. This will provide a good range of nutrients to prevent a fundamental imbalance that can be caused by taking supplements on their own.

You then add in any extra supplements that relate specifically to your symptoms, as recommended at the end of each chapter of this book.

When it comes to buying supplements, you get what you pay for. You need to get good quality supplements for maximum absorption. Capsules (preferably vegetable ones instead of gelatine) are better than tablets. Capsules tend to be filled only with the essential nutrients, while tablets can include a variety of fillers, binders and bulking agents. Mineral supplements like calcium should be in the form of citrates, ascorbates or polynicotinates, which are more easily absorbed by the body. Chlorides, sulphates, carbonates and oxides should be avoided as they are not so easily assimilated and mineral supplements in this form may pass through the body without being absorbed, so it is always important to read the labels.

The other way minerals are made more digestible is by chelation (pronounced 'keylation'), where the mineral is 'hooked' on to an amino acid, which allows three to ten times greater assimilation than the non-chelated ones. (Good supplement companies include BioCare, Solgar, the Natural Health Practice and Lamberts.) Because there are so many different supplements on the market, some good and some not so good, it can be very confusing when deciding what to use.

A company called the Natural Health Practice asked if I would formulate some specific supplements according to the recommendations in this book. I insisted that these products would have to be of the highest possible standards and it was agreed that they would use only the most important ingredients at their highest effective dose to help achieve best results. These supplements also had to be in their most bio-available form to aid absorption and to be completely hypo-allergenic, free from genetically modified organisms, preservatives and additives and suitable for vegetarians. It has taken many months to achieve, but finally they came up with a range of supplements I am happy with. These supplements are mentioned at the end of the relevant chapters.

ABSORPTION TEST

If you are already taking supplements and you want to know how well they are being absorbed, do the following test. Place your supplement in a glass of warm vinegar for 30 minutes, stirring every few minutes. The warm vinegar roughly represents the conditions found in your gut. If the supplement does not dissolve after half an hour, then, as the critics say, 'you are paying an awful lot for nutritious urine'. In other words, your nutrients are probably coming out the other end in much the same form that they entered it! My recommendation would be to buy another brand.

Take any vitamins and minerals with food. You want your body to think they are part of your diet, so that they are better absorbed.

Herbal medicine

Herbs are the oldest form of medicine and have been used for healing in every single culture in the world, since the very beginning of time. Wise women have always played a central role in traditional cultures and knowledge about herbs was passed on from one generation to the next.

Herbs are, in fact, the foundation of numerous pharmaceutical drugs. Aspirin is based on an extract from willow, originally used for pain relief by the Native Americans. Up to 70 per cent of drugs in use today have their origins in plants, but Western pharmaceutical practice bears no relation to how native peoples the world over have used them. Modern drug companies only use the 'active ingredient' of the plant or herb in a pure form as the basis for the drug. Ancient peoples always, and continue to, use the whole plant. The advantage of using the whole plant is that the side-effects are minimal or entirely absent. That is the big difference between modern and herbal medicine.

For example, centuries ago the foxglove plant (*Digitalis purpurea*) was used for heart problems. In modern times, scientists have isolated the main active ingredient of the foxglove (digoxin) and put it into tablet form. However, by doing so, they have created a product with a real risk of side-effects. By using the whole plant, the active ingredient interacts with all the other constituents of the plant, which naturally contains 'buffer' ingredients that counteract any potential side-effects. Herbalists believe this is the proper way to use the healing powers of herbs and plants.

The easiest and most effective way to take herbs is in tincture form using approximately 5ml (1 teaspoon) three times daily in a little water. Try to get tinctures made from organically grown herbs, which will not contain pesticides or any other toxic ingredients. In the liquid form, herbs are already dissolved, which means that they can be absorbed (and therefore work) more quickly.

Dried herbs (in tablets or capsules) have to be digested and, once again, they will work only to the extent that your body is able to process and absorb them. Herbs are not like drugs. If drugs are stopped, the symptoms can return and then you are back where you started. Herbs may be aimed at easing symptoms, but they work at a more fundamental level. At the same time that the symptoms are being dealt with, the cause is being addressed. The symptoms disappear as your body becomes more balanced.

Other natural therapies

Homeopathy
The word 'homeopathy' comes from the Greek words *omio* meaning 'same' and *pathos* meaning 'suffering'. In other words, similar suffering. It reflects the key principle behind the homeopathic method – that a substance can cure the symptoms in an ill person that it is capable of causing in a healthy person.

Every single woman visiting a homeopath will be given a different set of remedies, according to her personal 'constitution' and her unique set of symptoms. Homeopathy is a system of medicine that supports the body's own healing mechanism, using specially prepared remedies. It is 'energy' medicine, in that it works with the body's own energies to encourage healing and to ensure that all body systems are working at optimum level.

Homeopathy is an extremely safe form of medicine, and it's safe for women of all ages, and during pregnancy. The remedy you take contains only the most minute quantities of a substance, so don't panic if you discover you've been prescribed something like Belladonna! While some homeopathic remedies can be used at home for 'acute' (short-term illnesses, such as colds and flu) health problems, it's essential that you consult a qualified homeopath for anything that you've had for a long time, or has become recurrent. A homeopath will take a very detailed history that looks at every aspect of you, including your health, symptoms, sleeping patterns, bowel movements, likes and dislikes, emotional factors and much, much more. Remedies are then prescribed, according to your individual requirements.

There are many homeopathic remedies used for women's health problems. For example, Sepia is indicated in some cases of prolapse, hormone problems, irritability, menstrual upsets, hot flushes during menopause, pain during intercourse and even low blood pressure. Another commonly prescribed 'female' remedy is Lachesis, which can be appropriate for headaches made worse by periods, hot flushes, PMS and period pains. It's one of the best 'menopause' remedies, and it helps to encourage balance.

Acupuncture

Acupuncture can be used alongside the other recommendations in this book in order to increase the effectiveness of the treatment. It can also be used alongside conventional treatment. It is an ancient system of Chinese medicine that dates back some 2,000 years and is based on the concept of Qi (pronounced *chee*), which is the body's natural energy. An acupuncturist aims to balance the flow of Qi along pathways called meridians. By inserting fine needles into the meridians the body's own healing response can be stimulated. Acupuncture can be particularly useful for correcting hormonal imbalances and problems such as fibroids and endometriosis. It's great for pregnancy and menopause symptoms, and can even be used to 'turn' a breech baby in the womb.

Aromatherapy

This is the use of essential oils found in the stem, flowers, leaves, bark, seeds or peel of aromatic plants. Once extracted, these become more concentrated and potent. Each essential oil has its own specific properties and works on two levels: through the sense of smell and by being absorbed into the bloodstream via the skin and lungs, where it has a therapeutic effect on organs, glands and tissue. Essential oils should be blended in a carrier oil, such as almond oil or diluted in water, before coming into contact with your skin (exceptions are lavender oil and tea tree oil). Drops of essential oils can be used directly in the bath.

Essential oils can be very useful for easing period pains, for example by adding lavender and chamomile to the bath. Other essential oils such as clary sage are useful for the symptoms of PMS as they help to lift the mood and balance your hormones. Rose oil is traditionally used to increase sperm count in men, although you may have a battle on your hands to get your partner into a rose-scented bath! Fennel can be helpful for water retention and can either be added to the bath or used as a massage oil. Other useful oils include the following:

- Jasmine, which can help to reduce period and labour pains, and relieve depression (including post-natal depression and depression during menopause).

- Juniper, which works on the kidneys and the urinary system, making it an excellent treatment for cystitis. It also helps to 'detoxify', so it can help with problems such as arthritis.

- Grapefruit oil works mainly on the liver and gallbladder, so can be useful for constipation, headaches and liverish complaints.

- Geranium has a cooling, regulating effect and it can help with conditions affecting the nervous system (restlessness and anxiety can be treated with this oil). It's also helpful for hot flushes and night sweats.

> **Warning:**
> Some oils, such as clary sage, are not appropriate for pregnancy. Check with a qualified practitioner before using any essential oils in pregnancy.

Massage
Massage is one of the oldest, simplest forms of therapy and is a system of stroking, pressing and kneading different areas of the body to relieve pain, relax, stimulate and tone the body. Massage does much more than make you feel good (although it helps!); it also works on the soft tissues (the muscles, tendons and ligaments) to improve muscle tone. Although it largely affects those muscles just under the skin, it is believed that it also reaches the deeper layers of muscles and possibly even the organs themselves. Massage also stimulates blood circulation

and assists the lymphatic system (which runs parallel to the circulatory system), improving elimination of toxic waste throughout the body.

There are many more therapies widely used in the treatment of women's health conditions. It's beyond the scope of this book to consider them all, but others that can be useful are reflexology and osteopathy.

CHAPTER 3

A Woman's Body

This book focuses solely on women's health and hormones, so it is important to establish, at the very beginning, what actually goes on in our bodies throughout our lives. It's surprising how few of us actually know where our reproductive organs are located (other than below the waist!), and fewer still understand the role of hormones and how they affect our bodies as we age.

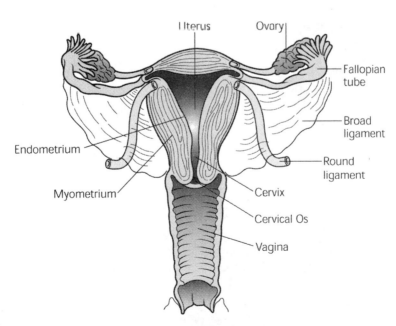

The female reproductive organs

The Female Organs

Throughout this book I will be referring to various parts of your body, and it helps to be clear about where exactly everything is, and how it sits in relation to everything else. The organs of the pelvis are like an intricately designed architectural structure. Every organ is kept in the right place by the organs and other structures around it. That's why when things go wrong (or begin to slip, as in the case of a prolapse; see Chapter 6), many organs are affected.

Your womb (uterus)

This is a hollow, pear-shaped organ and it is normally the size of your fist. It is composed of three layers: the endometrium, the myometrium and the parametrium:

- The endometrium is literally the lining of the womb, and this is what becomes thicker during the second half of your cycle, and during pregnancy.

- The myometrium is the muscular layer of the womb, and it is one of the strongest muscles of the body. These muscle fibres are responsible for the strong contractions that expel your baby from the womb during childbirth.

- The parametrium is the outermost layer of the womb, and it is composed of connective tissue.

The womb is suspended within the abdominal cavity, fixed only at its base by the ligaments from the cervix.

Your cervix

This is the part of the womb that protrudes into the vagina. It is sometimes called 'the neck of the womb'. The cervix changes quite dramatically during the menstrual cycle, according to the hormones that are being produced. Mucus-secreting glands (known as crypts) line the cervical canal and produce mucus continuously.

This fluid also undergoes important changes during the menstrual cycle. During the first half of the cycle (the follicular phase), the mucus is thick and sticky. It forms a plug over the cervix, which stops sperm entering. It also makes the vagina acid, which can kill off sperm within a few hours.

About three to four days before ovulation (the release of an egg or ovum from the ovary), as oestrogen levels increase, the mucus becomes clear, stretchy and there is more of it. Surrounded by this fertile mucus, sperm can live for up to seven days. Once ovulation has taken place and progesterone levels increase, the mucus again becomes thick and sticky (infertile mucus), protecting the cervix from sperm and also from any foreign bodies.

Your cervix also changes during the cycle. As your period ends, your cervix is located low in your vaginal canal and the opening is closed. If you were to reach in and touch it, it would feel like the top of a nose, or a rubber ball. As ovulation approaches and oestrogen levels increase, the cervix moves higher into the vaginal opening, making it more difficult to reach. It also begins to soften and open, resembling parted lips. This opening and rising helps the sperm to travel into the womb. After ovulation, the cervix lowers again, closes and becomes blocked with mucus to stop sperm entering.

Your vagina

This part of your body links your cervix and womb to the outside world. When you have a period, the blood from the womb lining leaves your body through the vagina. The vagina is muscular and it can stretch to many times its size during childbirth. It also stretches to accommodate an erect penis.

Your ovaries

Your two ovaries are the shape and size of large almonds. They sit on either side of the womb in your lower abdomen (around the top of the pubic bone). Your store of eggs is already in place when you are born. Most women are born with about 2 million egg follicles; by puberty there are about 750,000, and by the age of around 45, only 10,000 can be left. The rest have disintegrated over the years. Menopause (see page 400) occurs when your store of eggs runs dry.

The follicles on your ovaries begin to develop approximately three months before one is mature enough to release an egg at ovulation. In each menstrual cycle, about 20 follicles containing the developing eggs grow on the surface of the ovary. Generally only the biggest follicle continues to develop, which is why humans normally only have one baby at a time. The others degenerate and are reabsorbed. Sometimes two eggs are released from two separate follicles in one cycle and non-identical twins could be conceived.

Contrary to popular opinion, you do not ovulate from alternate sides every other cycle. The process can be quite random. You may, for example, ovulate from the same side for three months running, and then switch to the other. Which side ovulates is also dependent upon the health of each ovary.

Your Fallopian tubes

The Fallopian tubes were named after Gabriella Fallopio, who 'discovered' and named these passages that run between the womb and the ovary. These tubes serve as the passage through which the egg is carried from the ovary to the womb and through which sperm travel to reach the egg. Many people are unaware that the tubes are, in fact, open at one end. They are joined to the womb at the bottom, but literally hover over the ovary at the top. The Fallopian tubes literally have to catch the egg as it is released

To help that process, the end of the tubes closest to the ovaries have 'fimbriae', which are finger-like projections that waft around and sweep the egg as it is released from the ovary into the tube. Once in the tube, tiny hairs called 'cilia' propel the egg along towards the womb. The tube also rhythmically contracts, which helps to transport the egg.

The Female Hormone Cycle

Nature has designed our reproductive system to work in harmony with the hormones that are produced there, and in other parts of the body. These hormones are dependent upon each other and work together to ensure that everything works as a system. Despite the robust nature of many of our organs, the hormones are, in fact, very delicately balanced. The good news, however, is that imbalances can be easily restored, by undertaking simple changes in diet and other lifestyle factors, and by using vitamins, minerals and herbs.

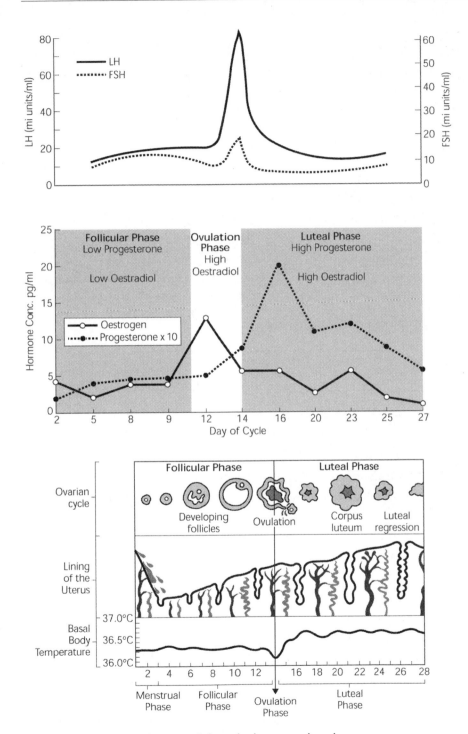

A normal female hormonal cycle

WHAT ARE HORMONES?

The word 'hormone' comes from the Greek word meaning 'urge on'. Hormones do just that – they are chemical messengers that are carried in the blood. Their job is to trigger activity in different organs and body parts. The reproductive hormones control your monthly cycle, and help to maintain a pregnancy.

OESTROGEN

Oestrogen is not just one hormone, but several grouped together under the umbrella term 'oestrogen'. For the sake of clarity, I will use the term oestrogen to include all of them. Oestrogen is the key hormone responsible ensuring that a woman matures from childhood through to adulthood. It causes the breasts to develop and produces the characteristic feminine shape.

Your body goes through the following stages each cycle:

1. The first day of your period is also the first day of your *next* menstrual cycle. On this day, FSH (follicle-stimulating hormone) is released from the pituitary gland.

2. FSH stimulates a group of follicles to grow on the surface of the ovary. These follicles will eventually produce eggs.

3. Over the next two weeks (known as the 'follicular phase' of the cycle), the eggs grow and mature. At the same time, oestrogen levels, which are produced by the ovaries, begin to increase.

4. As oestrogen levels increase, the pituitary gland decreases its production of FSH. A new hormone, known as LH (luteinizing hormone), is triggered. Fertile alkaline mucus is produced in the cervix to keep sperm alive, and to encourage their transport through the cervix and up towards the Fallopian tubes, where fertilisation will take place.

5. As LH surges, a mature egg (normally only one, but sometimes more) is released from a follicle and enters the Fallopian tube. This is known as ovulation.

6. The empty follicle becomes the 'corpus luteum' and produces a hormone known as progesterone. The second half of the cycle (called the luteal phase) has begun.

7. If fertilisation occurs, the fertilised egg will travel down the Fallopian tube and implant in the lining of the womb (known as the endometrium).

8. If fertilisation does not occur, the lining of the womb breaks down and is expelled. This is your normal monthly period. At the same time, there is a rapid and dramatic fall in the levels of oestrogen and progesterone. With this drop in hormone levels, the cycle starts all over again.

CAN YOU HAVE A PERIOD AND NOT OVULATE?

Yes, many women will not ovulate during a cycle and will not realise it unless they are usually aware of ovulation. This is even more common as a woman approaches the menopause or where there is a hormone imbalance and the egg is not being released. When ovulation does not happen the hormone progesterone is not produced in that cycle. It does not follow that if you are having periods you are automatically ovulating.

Nothing in Isolation

It's clear from the descriptions above that Nature has taken everything into consideration. Everything in our bodies fits and works together so precisely that it is easy to see how an imbalance of any sort – hormonal, nutritional, infectious etc. – could have a profound effect. If one part of your system is affected, everything else will be thrown slightly out of balance. It's also easy to see that an imbalance here will affect your whole body, because everything is dependent upon something else in order to function efficiently. Nothing works or operates in isolation. Here are some examples:

• Your pituitary gland controls the release of TSH (thyroid-stimulating hormone), which in turn helps to control the normal functioning of the thyroid gland. The pituitary gland also controls the release of a hormone, which in turn partially controls the activity of the adrenal glands. The pituitary also controls the release of FSH and LH, which in turn affect the production of hormones released by the ovaries.

- Your thyroid gland controls your metabolism and growth, and acts like a thermostat, controlling your body temperature and the speed at which it burns food. If your thyroid gland is underactive, this can, in turn, affect the balance of oestrogen to progesterone by decreasing the production of progesterone.

- Your adrenal glands produce hormones that help you cope with stress, regulate the balance of salt and water in the body, regulate fat, protein and carbohydrate metabolism, and also produce small amounts of the sex hormones, testosterone, progesterone and oestrogen. If your blood sugar drops too low (hypoglycaemia), then adrenaline is released in order to increase the blood glucose and correct the imbalance. But you then feel more stressed.

- Your pancreas secretes the hormone insulin that regulates the amount of sugar (glucose) in your blood. But if you have too much insulin then you can end up with too much testosterone because the insulin stimulates the ovaries to produce excess testosterone. If you have too much testosterone, your female hormones are then out of balance.

Everything in your body is interrelated. That's why it is so important to look at your health holistically. This is the approach taken by natural medicine. By getting yourself into optimum health, you will make an impact on every system in your body.

CHAPTER 4

Testing Your Health

Throughout this book, I provide details of tests that are useful for particular health conditions. For example, in the case of osteoporosis, the bone turnover urine test can be invaluable for measuring how well your bone is renewing itself. In the section on candida (see page 265), I discuss the tests available for yeast overgrowth. In each chapter, I have listed the most appropriate tests for each condition, and at the back of the book on page 507 you'll find details of how to obtain these tests by post. There are, however, other tests that can be undertaken to assess the general health of your body, and these are included here as well.

As you read through the women's problems discussed in this book, you will be aware that your health depends on a whole range of factors, such as diet, lifestyle, stress, age, exercise, job satisfaction, addictions (smoking, alcohol, coffee and even tea), leisure time, constitution and inherited strengths and weaknesses, relationships, sense of purpose and direction in life, your environment and many, many other things. Some of these areas we can control; others we cannot. What many of these tests can do, however, is pinpoint the areas where we are not in control, which gives us an idea of how to redress the balance. One of the first ways to do this is to assess your nutritional status.

Nutrition Tests

Modern life is incredibly busy, and most of us have little time to consider our diets carefully. Even when we do eat well, our food is still likely to be deficient in the vitamins and minerals we need to keep our bodies healthy and well balanced.

But there's more. Health also depends on how well we are able to absorb and digest the nutrients we eat. Problems such as lack of energy, insomnia, headaches, depression, mood swings, anxiety, low libido and many more, can be traced directly to deficiencies of specific vitamins and minerals.

Vitamins and minerals work in balance with one another. For this reason, it is vital that you take the right ones in the right amounts, in the right combinations and at the right times. You will notice that each supplement programme recommended in this book contains a multivitamin and mineral. This is because you need a good foundation, containing all of the key nutrients. All nutrients work in harmony, and if you take one on its own, such as zinc, for example, then you can affect the whole overall balance in your body.

Have you ever gone into a healthfood shop, looked at the array of supplements on the shelves and wondered what you should be taking? There are, in fact, scientific laboratory tests to evaluate your nutritional status.

Mineral analysis

There are many ways of testing nutritional status – for example, by using a sample of blood or sweat. But one of the most cost-effective and convenient ways is through a hair sample. Hair has been shown to reflect a good long-term record of our mineral and nutritional experience.[1] In fact, it's possible that hair samples will eventually be used to screen for potential diabetes or breast cancer. Work is being undertaken in Australia by Professor Veronica James at the University of New South Wales to analyse hair with a technique called X-ray diffraction.[2] As X-rays are fired through the hair they form a pattern on photographic film. From this pattern the researchers are able to pick up different information. For instance, sugar binds on to the hair filaments of a diabetic patient. It will therefore look different from a strand of hair from a person without diabetes.

Hair samples can also be used to test for drug use, such as cocaine, amphetamines and cannabis. This is helpful in forensic medicine and pathology, to determine whether someone was under the influence of drugs in an accident.

Because your hair cells are some of the fastest-growing cells in the body, they can 'lock' in information about your exposure to certain nutrients as they grow. In this way, your hair forms a permanent record of exposure to beneficial and toxic elements. Analysing hair is an excellent way to test for heavy toxic metals and is used in many medical studies to assess exposure to metals like mercury.[3]

Other ways of testing (using blood or urine, for example) can be less reliable, because the results are influenced by what you may have eaten. Also, your body tries to keep everything in balance. To do this, it tops up the levels of nutrients in your blood by taking them from elsewhere. For instance, if your blood calcium levels fall your body will pinch calcium from your bones to keep the level constant. A blood test may then suggest that your calcium levels are fine. But a hair analysis showing high levels of calcium would help identify the leaching of calcium from your bones. This information is particularly useful around the menopause, when maintaining bone density is crucial. If this leaching effect is seen in a hair test, recommendations can be given to slow this down.

However, like any testing medium, hair analysis has its limitations. For instance, when testing for nutrients it is important that your hair is not contaminated by tints, highlights or perms. And certain minerals (iron, for instance) are best tested by a blood sample. But levels of trace elements can be higher in hair, which makes them easier to analyse. Also, because hair doesn't need specialised sampling equipment or storage, this form of testing is accessible for women who are not conveniently near a qualified practitioner.

Hair can be used successfully to analyse calcium, magnesium, zinc, selenium, copper, manganese, chromium and also the toxic metals mercury, aluminium and cadmium levels.

Once the minerals have been analysed, usually together with a detailed questionnaire, a personalised programme of supplements can be offered. It is recommended that this programme is followed for a minimum of three to four months and then the hair is re-tested. Once your mineral and toxic levels are back to normal, it's recommended that you follow a maintenance programme and continue to eat well.

What can the mineral analysis show?

This analysis can show straightforward deficiencies of minerals such as low levels of zinc or selenium. Some of the minerals (such as copper) can be high, perhaps due to previous use of the Pill, IUD (coil), HRT or fertility drugs. High levels of copper are a concern as they are often associated with low zinc levels. Zinc is an important mineral in terms of the reproductive system. Keen swimmers should, however, beware! Swimming can confuse the analysis, showing unusually high levels of copper because pools can be treated with copper algicides that alter the levels.

The results of the mineral tests are given to you in the form of a graph so you can see how far your levels differ from the norm.

Apart from detecting imbalances in the minerals, your toxic metal levels may be too high. Two things will be required in this case. First of all, you will need to try to work out the source of contamination – and avoid it if possible. Secondly, you'll need to take specific nutrients, such as antioxidants, to eliminate these toxins from your body.

Nutritional questionnaire

This questionnaire is usually done in conjunction with the mineral analysis, and you are asked about your daily eating habits, your lifestyle, symptoms, health problems and risk factors. Each vitamin and mineral has certain deficiency symptoms so a lack of vitamin C, for example, can give you frequent infections, easy bruising, bleeding gums, slow wound healing. When you complete this comprehensive questionnaire you will be sent a detailed report showing the 12 vitamins (A, D, E, C, B1, B2, B3, B5, B6, B12, folic acid and biotin), 7 minerals (calcium, magnesium, zinc, iron, manganese, chromium and selenium) and essential fatty acids you need to take. This report will tell you what quantities you need in order to bring your body back into balance and optimum health.

Allergy/Food Intolerance Tests

There are two types of allergic reactions. Type A (classic allergy) is diagnosed when your reaction takes place immediately after contact with an allergen (such as peanuts). Type B (delayed allergy or intolerance) is diagnosed when the reaction takes place between one hour or four days after contact with the allergen. Common Type B allergens include dairy produce, eggs, wheat and sugar. Symptoms such as weight gain, bloating, water retention, fatigue, aching joints and headaches can all be due to a Type B allergy.

It is now possible to have a blood test (done privately) that analyses

217 different foods and food additives by measuring the release of certain chemicals that are responsible for the symptoms of food intolerance. You would then know the foods to which you are reacting, and these can be avoided for a short period of time. Unlike a Type A allergy, these foods would not have to be avoided indefinitely. While you are avoiding the foods, the aim would be to strengthen and correct any digestive problems, so that afterwards you can eat in moderation the foods to which you are intolerant.

When food is not being digested properly (see leaky gut test, below) food particles can leak out into the bloodstream. Instead of seeing these particles as food, your body views them as toxins and sets up an immune system reaction to them. This is often caused by sheer overload – in other words, eating too much of the same foods too often. Wheat is often a culprit, because you can have toast for breakfast, a sandwich for lunch, pasta for your evening meal and biscuits in between.

The test is analysed from a sample of blood and a kit can be sent to enable your practice nurse or doctor to take a small quantity of blood. This is sent to the laboratory and after it has been analysed you are sent an extensive personalised report outlining:

- foods that are highly reactive for you, those that are borderline and those that are OK

- recommendations of how to implement food changes and how to reintroduce the reactive/borderline foods safely at a later date.

Leaky gut test

Tracking down the foods to which you may be sensitive is only solving half the problem. Why has the problem developed in the first place? What happens when you reintroduce the offending foods? The answer lies in the state of your intestines, the gut and its capacity to process food properly. And allergies and food intolerances are often a sign that all is not well with your digestive system.

This is very important because if your intestines are not functioning properly you may not be absorbing nutrients efficiently, which means you can become deficient in vital vitamins and minerals. This test, conducted on urine, can check the state of your digestive system.

All food must be broken down by the digestive system, passed into the bloodstream and dealt with successfully by the body's lymphatic system. If this doesn't happen properly, the body 'sees' normal food as an antigen, a toxin, and sets up an immune system reaction to deal with it. At the same time, this undigested food is sitting around fermenting and putrefying. Large spaces can develop between the cells in the gut wall and food molecules can then pass into the bloodstream. This is called leaky gut or 'intestinal permeability' and can result in the overgrowth of candida (see page 265).

Initially it is important to stop eating the offending foods, which will help to alleviate the symptoms and make you feel better. Then the whole environment of the gut needs to be healed as well, in order to get the intestinal bacteria back in balance again so that you can stay healthy and prevent the symptoms recurring.

This condition has only recently become widely recognised and this very effective, non-invasive urine test is relatively new. It can be done in your own home with a kit that is posted to you. Two urine samples are required. The first one is a pre-test sample and the second is taken six hours after drinking a special liquid containing two marker molecules. When the samples are analysed, the amount of the marker molecules detected by the laboratory will give a strong indication as to how permeable (in other words, how leaky) your gut is. Once you have this information you can then decide what the best course of action will be in order to heal your intestines.

Female Hormone Test Using Saliva

This is a very simple test that is done at home and then sent to the lab for analysis. A total of 11 saliva samples are collected over one cycle at specific times. The levels of the hormones oestrogen and progesterone are mapped for that month to provide a pattern which can reveal:

- early ovulation

- anovulation (no ovulation)

- problems with the phasing of the cycles such as a short luteal phase (second half of the cycle)

- problems with maintaining progesterone levels.

This test can be done even if you have an irregular menstrual cycle and is very useful if there is a suscpicion that you have a hormonal imbalance between oestrogen and progesterone.

Osteoporosis Risk Evaluation (Bone Turnover)

This is a special non-invasive urine test that was developed in the US. Osteoporosis literally means 'porous bones' or bones that are filled with tiny holes. In bones affected with osteoporosis, new bone formation does not keep up with bone loss (this is called bone turnover), which causes the bones to become more brittle. This urine test assesses your bone turnover by measuring biochemical markers in the urine that are excreted as bone breaks down. If your bone turnover is higher than it should be, you can get advice to slow down the rate of loss (see Chapter 12).

Stress Index

This test looks at your stress levels by measuring the secretion of hormones from the adrenal glands. The adrenal glands do not secrete their hormones at a constant level during the day. The highest amount is released in the morning and the lowest at night. This is obviously sensible as we are supposed to be ready to get going in the morning and are slowing down as we go the bed. Unfortunately, many people are in a constant state of stress and they have an abnormal rhythm of stress hormones. This can affect the body in many ways. Not having enough energy can be due to an abnormal adrenal rhythm, particularly if you find it difficult to get up in the morning. We are more prone to osteoporosis if the adrenal glands are overworking, because too high levels of cortisol (one of the hormones released by the adrenal glands) will prevent the proper build-up of bone. The reproductive system is especially susceptible to stress, and can cause your periods to stop or to become irregular. Your immune system and your thyroid function can also be compromised if the adrenal glands are not doing their job properly.

This test measures the rhythm of the adrenal glands by using four saliva samples over a day, which are collected at home and then sent to the lab for analysis.

For information on any of these tests, please contact me through 'Staying in Touch', page 507.

PART II

WOMEN'S HEALTH PROBLEMS

CHAPTER 5

The Menstrual Cycle

The menstrual cycle represents the heart of a woman's reproductive life. When she starts ovulating at around age 12, her periods should recur each and every month – except when pregnant or breast-feeding – until she reaches the menopause, the cessation of periods that marks the end of her reproductive years. But a number of things can go wrong with the cycle throughout the years, most of them hormonal, and most of which can be treated by methods other than drugs. You always have a choice.

PRE-MENSTRUAL SYNDROME (PMS)

Fifteen years ago, doctors claimed that PMS did not exist. Today, it's one of the most common conditions suffered by women, with symptoms that can be anything from mildly inconvenient to positively debilitating.

Admittedly, some women sail through their cycles without a mood swing or a hint of discomfort. But they are pretty rare: PMS is estimated to affect 70 to 90 per cent of women during their childbearing years. And 30 to 40 per cent of women are believed to have symptoms severe enough to interfere with their daily lives.

What is Pre-Menstrual Syndrome?

This is a term used to describe *any* symptoms that occur after the middle of your cycle (ovulation) and disappear almost as soon as your period arrives. The crucial point is not *what* symptoms you experience, but *when*.

Dr Katharina Dalton was the pioneering British doctor who first used the term pre-menstrual syndrome. Before this time, the problems associated with the second half of the cycle were called premenstrual tension (PMT). When Dr Dalton began publishing her work in 1953, she realised that tension was only one symptom among many that numerous women experienced in the weeks prior to their periods. A syndrome is simply a group of symptoms that characterise an illness, and its use was obviously appropriate in the case of pre-menstrual disturbances. Therefore, Dr Dalton changed the name from PMT to PMS, making it possible to include many more symptoms that occur at that time.

PMS became headline news in 1981 when a woman used the diagnosis of PMS as defence in a criminal case. After an argument, this woman had killed her boyfriend by running him over with her car. She said that 'she just snapped' and the diagnosis of PMS was accepted on the grounds of diminished responsibility. She was given a conditional discharge for 12 months and banned from driving for 12 months.

What are the Symptoms?

This is where things get complicated. Over 150 symptoms are now believed to form part of the syndrome, and these include:

- mood swings
- irritability
- anxiety and tension
- bloating
- breast tenderness and swelling
- water retention
- acne
- tiredness
- weight gain
- headaches/migraines
- crying spells
- depression
- sugar and food cravings
- constipation
- dizziness.

The personality changes associated with this time of the month can be very severe. Indeed, some women describe a 'Jekyll and Hyde' change, in which they literally become a different person pre-menstrually. Most interestingly, perhaps, the majority of women are aware that their feelings and the way they think are different – even irrational – but they have no control over those feelings. Other women see everything in a negative light and will often burst into tears for no real reason, while others will experience serious depression.

On the other hand, some women have commented on positive PMS symptoms. Many who work in creative fields, such as painting or writing, find that they work very differently in that pre-menstrual time – producing better and more original work. One woman commented to me that she didn't want to get rid of her PMS symptoms because that's when she took everything back to the shops to complain!

Types of PMS

In order to make the classification of PMS easier, an American doctor, Guy Abraham, devised a system of different categories for the different types of PMS symptoms:

Type A Anxiety

Type C Cravings

Type H Hyperhydration (too much water!)

Type D Depression

Type A – Anxiety

This category is very common in up to 80 per cent of women with PMS, and it includes symptoms such as mood swings, irritability, anxiety and tension.

Type C – Cravings

This group of symptoms includes cravings for sweets or chocolates, increased appetite, fatigue and headaches. Up to 60 per cent of women with PMS can experience these kinds of symptoms leading up to the period.

Type H – Hyperhydration

Type H includes symptoms such as water retention, breast tenderness and enlargement, abdominal bloating and weight gain. Up to 40 per cent of women with PMS experience these changes pre-menstrually.

Type D – Depression

Depression is the key symptom of this group, but others that fall into this category include confusion, forgetfulness, clumsiness, feeling withdrawn, lack of co-ordination and crying spells. Only 5 per cent of women with PMS experience these symptoms, but they can be very serious. It's not unknown for women with these symptoms to consider suicide.

It has been suggested that each group of symptoms is caused by its own hormone imbalance. Type A is believed to be an imbalance of oestrogen and progesterone, with the oestrogen levels being too high and progesterone too low. Type D, on the other hand, is linked with too little oestrogen and too much progesterone. The difficulty with this simple classification is that I have seen women with both Type A and Type D symptoms occurring in the same cycle, so it is hard to see logically how the hormone imbalances can fit that picture.

RISK FACTORS

There are a number of risk factors that can make you more likely to suffer from PMS. They include:

- being in your 30s or 40s
- having had two or more children
- having a mother who suffered from PMS
- having recently experienced a hormonal upheaval, such as having a baby, termination or miscarriage, being sterilised or coming off the Pill
- experiencing several pregnancies in quick succession.

Many women will get symptoms from each type during any one cycle. And for some women these symptoms can change from month to month, so they are not always experiencing exactly the same symptoms before each period.

What's the Cause?

From a conventional viewpoint, there is no answer to this question. In a nutshell, no one knows. There has been an enormous amount of research into PMS and an equally enormous amount of confusion in terms of its cause and treatment.

The first recorded cases of PMT (as it was called then) were in 1931 and yet, in 1995, the following quote appeared in a medical journal: 'PMS is a controversial and ill-defined phenomena, the aetiology *(cause)* of which remains an enigma, despite considerable research effort' (my italics).[1]

One of the main reasons for the confusion is that PMS is clearly a hormonal problem. It begins after ovulation and disappears once your period begins. But when scientists examine two groups of women, one with PMS and one without, in the second half of their cycles, no difference between the hormone profiles can be found. In other words, the women in the PMS group have similar hormone patterns to those in the non-PMS group. This is one reason why PMS needs to be viewed differently. If there is no hormone imbalance (there can't be a hormone imbalance if you can't measure it!), there has to be another cause. That cause is clearly being missed.

It is assumed that PMS has an effect on a woman's general health by giving her any number of 150 different symptoms. But what if the situation is really the other way round? In other words, what if your general health is what's causing PMS to manifest itself?

If you have not been eating well, maybe lacking in certain vitamins and minerals, not exercising, suffering from stress and generally feeling run down, it is very possible that your body's ability to produce the right balance of hormones and to utilise those hormones properly each cycle will be seriously compromised.

Katherine

Katherine was 34 when she came to see me. She already had two daughters, aged 5 and 6, but she wanted to have another child and didn't think that she would ever be well enough to contemplate becoming pregnant again.

She had breastfed both of her daughters, during which time she suffered night sweats. After the birth of her second daughter, she was put on the Pill. Two years later, she was put on a different Pill, which caused her to develop ovarian cysts that grew large and then burst. She then started to suffer from headaches and became very anxious. Her gynaecologist told her that it was a lack of oestrogen. The Pill was stopped and she was given oestrogen patches to use for two weeks in the month. She started to get dizzy spells, aches and pains, and pins and needles in her feet. She felt extremely tired and was spotting on days 14 and 15 of her cycle.

All of these symptoms fluctuated with her cycle (except the spotting), becoming worse in the second half. At this time, the anxiety was so severe that her doctor put her on Prozac. Her doctor claimed that she was clinically depressed, while her gynaecologist believed her problem to be a lack of oestrogen. By this time Katherine was at her wits' end and she had two young children to look after. When she came to see me she had stopped the Prozac and was back on the Pill. That month, she had been bleeding continuously since day ten of her cycle.

We discussed the fact that the ultimate aim was to get her back to optimum health. To do this we would ensure that she was eating well, and that any vitamin and mineral deficiencies were corrected. She mentioned that when she got anxious she would start to shake and then have a teaspoon of sugar. She had been tested for diabetes, but the test proved to be negative. I explained how blood sugar levels could affect what seemed like psychological symptoms, such as mood swings, anxiety and depression.

A hair mineral analysis showed that she was severely deficient in zinc and had high copper levels, which usually results from taking the Pill or any reproductive hormones. I put her on a programme to redress the zinc/copper imbalance, balance her blood sugar fluctuations and to support her adrenal glands. Katherine also decided to stop taking the Pill.

Katherine came back the following month to say that she had not any spotting for the first time in three-and-a-half years. She was also pleased to find that her bowel movements had become more regular, which had also not been the case for over ten years. Her energy had improved dramatically and she was starting to feel more like 'her old self'. That was two years ago. Katherine now has a daughter of eight months, whom she is still breastfeeding – with no night sweats!

How Do You Know If You Have PMS?

Doctors are taught at medical school to diagnose by symptoms. This is why PMS is often misdiagnosed. This is a condition that should be diagnosed by timing, not symptoms, and therein lies the problem from the conventional medical point of view.

The best way to know whether you have PMS is to keep a menstrual diary. Write down what symptoms you are experiencing and when you are experiencing them. What you are looking for is a pattern. At the beginning, ignore the type of symptom and just look at the timing.

Do different symptoms start in the week or so leading up to your period and then stop almost immediately when you bleed? If so, you have PMS.

You should have almost a week free of symptoms before they start again. This is a bit of an eye-opening exercise for many women. It becomes clear that you can suffer from PMS for two weeks, bleed for another week, and feel 'normal' for only one week out of every month. Work it out – you may only be feeling well for a quarter of every month. In fact, for a quarter of your life.

What Treatment Can You Be Offered By Your Doctor?

Because the symptoms can be predominantly psychological in some women, you may be prescribed tranquillisers or antidepressants. This means taking strong medication the whole month for a problem that occurs for about 7 to 14 days. A few years ago I actually saw a woman who had been institutionalised for PMS.

Other women have been just told to 'grin and bear it' or that it's part and parcel of being a woman. Still others have been faced with doctors who do not even believe that the condition exists – that 'it's all in the mind'.[2]

Furthermore, the confusion surrounding the cause of PMS has meant that approaches to treatment have been equally confused. The medical approach is to concentrate on the symptoms, by giving anti-depressants or diuretics, for example, or by manipulating the hormones in some way with drugs. But as the doctors do not know which way the hormones are out of balance, they cannot, therefore, really know which way to manipulate them.

What is important to remember when you are offered a drug approach is that not even one of the drugs currently used does anything to address the fundamental cause of PMS. When you stop taking the drugs, your symptoms will undoubtedly return.

Drugs

Drugs are mainly aimed at manipulating the cycle, to see whether there is an improvement in the symptoms or aimed at specific symptoms such as water retention or breast tenderness.

The Pill

The Pill has been used to treat PMS and for some women it is effective. Others find that it makes the problem worse. In fact, some women who do not normally suffer from PMS will experience symptoms for the first time when they start taking the Pill – an obvious reason to stop taking it straightaway.

More recently it has been suggested that if women are given the Pill continuously (in other words they do not stop the Pill to have a monthly bleed) their hormone cycles could be controlled.[3] This report also suggested that women should have the right to choose whether or not they have periods! If the Pill is taken continuously, you may end up eliminating your periods for ever. Some of the listed side-effects of the pill include nausea, vomiting, depression, weight changes, headache, thrombosis, changes in sex drive and depression. Many of these symptoms are the same as those experienced pre-menstrually, so it can make things much worse.

Danazol

Danazol is a synthetic weak male hormone that prevents ovulation and, in effect, shuts off ovarian function. This is turn stops your periods. The thinking behind this drug is that if you are not having periods, you are not likely to suffer from PMS. The side-effects can include severe mood swings, nausea, dizziness, rashes and headaches. Because danazol is a mild male hormone, other side-effects can include facial hair, acne, an increased sex drive, weight gain and deepening of the voice.

You'd have to weigh up which symptoms are worse – those caused by the drug or the PMS.

GnRH analogues

This type of medication also stops your normal cycle, and it plunges you into a temporary menopause. Unfortunately, the symptoms of the menopause (see page 402) such as hot flushes and night sweats can be as debilitating as PMS.

Bromocriptine

This drug works by reducing high levels of prolactin in your body. This is the hormone that is released in high quantities when women are breastfeeding. Because of this link with the breasts, bromocriptine has been prescribed for women whose main pre-menstrual symptom is breast pain. It has no effect on the other pre-menstrual symptoms and it is a powerful drug with side-effects that can include nausea, vomiting, headaches and dizziness. In my opinion, this is too strong a treatment for breast tenderness or pain when there are much more natural ways of dealing with the symptoms (see Chapter 9).

Mefenamic acid

This is a prostaglandin inhibitor – and certain prostaglandins will cause cramps and pain – so is usually used to treat painful periods and heavy menstrual flow (see pages 148 and 102). It has been used to treat pre-menstrual symptoms including headaches, mood swings and breast pain. The side-effects are centred on digestive symptoms and include indigestion, diarrhoea, nausea, abdominal cramps, constipation, bloating and flatulence.

Diuretics

These are often used to help with water retention and can increase the rate at which fluid is lost, but will also flush out important minerals. For example, potassium can be excreted in higher levels, which can be dangerous. One of the most important roles of potassium is to ensure that your heart functions correctly.

Oestrogen

Oestrogen patches have been shown to be effective in the treatment of PMS symptoms.[4] This is basically using hormone replacement therapy (HRT) to treat pre-menstrual symptoms. There are risks associated with the use of HRT (see page 403), and one of these is breast cancer. In my opinion, the risks of HRT do not outweigh the benefits if you are suffering from PMS.

Progesterone

Progesterone is the hormone that is released after ovulation and it makes sense that if symptoms are occurring in the second half of the cycle, then progesterone might be at the root.

The treatment of PMS with progesterone was pioneered by Dr Katharina Dalton and it is normally given in the form of vaginal pessaries because when progesterone is given by mouth, it is rapidly broken down by the liver. A vaginal cream is now also available.

Progesterone creams are also available for use on the skin but the doctors do not think that enough progesterone is absorbed this way.

Some women do well on progesterone pessaries, with a marked reduction in PMS symptoms. Other women experience no relief from their symptoms.

Progesterone in the form of pessaries and creams (either for the vagina or skin) are classed as being 'natural', as opposed to the progestogens that are synthetic forms of progesterone (see Dydrogesterone, below). But the word 'natural' used in front of progesterone is misleading. In this context, the word 'natural' means that the progesterone is chemically identical to that which you produce from your own ovaries. It is a hormone and it needs to be prescribed by a doctor. Some progesterone creams are made from wild yam and people have been confused because they thought they were taking a wild yam herbal product. They are not. Progesterone is synthesised from wild yam in a laboratory. Oestrogens can also be synthesised in a laboratory from wild yam or soya, which makes pharmaceutical companies think they have the right to call these products natural. Synthesising means making something that is chemically identical. It doesn't mean 'extracting' a natural substance. Furthermore, you must remember that progesterone is a drug, not a herbal product (see page 312).

Dydrogesterone
This is a synthetic progesterone (a progestogen) that has been used to treat PMS. It has been shown to be effective in some studies and not in others. Side-effects can include breakthrough bleeding.

Summing up the drug approach
The wealth of different drugs makes it fairly clear that there is a great deal of confusion about the approach to treating PMS. Some studies show that oestrogen works for PMS and others show that progesterone is the key. These are two completely different hormones that work very differently. It is virtually impossible that they could *both* work. Other studies state that neither oestrogen or progesterone has any effect on PMS.

One of the most interesting aspects of PMS research is that there is an enormously high placebo effect. What this means is that people taking 'dummy' tablets rather than a drug or anything else, often experience relief of symptoms. There are always some people in any study who will respond to the placebos, but in the case of PMS, it appears that this effect can take place in up to 94 per cent of the women studied![5]

Sometimes better results are obtained from the placebo than the actual medication being tested. Because of this placebo effect it is sometimes said that perhaps PMS is all in the mind, and doesn't really exist as a physical condition. But other researchers have suggested that the placebo effect is important and should be studied in some detail to understand how and why it is occurring.

There may be some truth in the idea that because women have been given an opportunity to talk and to have their symptoms taken seriously, their symptoms will improve whether they take drugs or a placebo. Too often symptoms are dismissed out of hand, and women may simply respond better to a different approach.

Surgical techniques

This is the most drastic treatment imaginable for PMS, but it is, from a medical point of view, a viable option. On page 471, I discussed a gynaecologist's address to a PMS seminar, which involved 'treating' PMS with a hysterectomy (with your ovaries removed; page 474). Don't even consider it. You would be plunged into a surgical menopause overnight, replacing PMS with menopause symptoms, and you would have the trauma of a serious operation to bear.

Natural Treatments

It seems that the scientists and doctors have been looking for a pre-menstrual 'Holy Grail' – in other words, one single mechanism that is responsible for the symptoms. However, as one scientist put it, 'Human behaviour cannot be understood within a single (hormone) frame of reference. Unravelling the pathogenesis *(the development of a disease)* of PMS requires a multidisciplinary approach' (my italics).[6]

This is why the holistic approach to PMS is so effective. In fact, this approach is so effective that the difference in symptoms can often be seen in the first month. Every woman is different, and so are her symptoms and the reasons why she has them.

The aim is not to look at all the different symptoms you might be experiencing and to work on treating them separately, but to work on your overall lifestyle to ensure optimum health and well-being. This means making sure that you are eating well, correcting any vitamin and mineral deficiencies, getting enough sleep, reducing stress levels and using any herbs that have been shown to help with PMS.

There are five stages to this treatment plan.

1. Improve your diet, using the hormone balancing diet outlined in Chapter 1.

2. Control fluctuating blood sugar levels by watching *when* you eat.

3. Use nutritional supplements that are known scientifically to help with PMS.

4. Use specific herbs that are known to help with pre-menstrual symptoms and balancing hormones in general.

5. Optimise the functioning of your liver so that any excess and 'old' hormones are excreted efficiently.

Penny

Fifty-year-old Penny came to see me, saying that my book *Natural Alternatives to HRT* (Kyle Cathie, 1997) 'had saved her'. Nine years earlier she had developed very extreme PMS. She became very aggressive and was in tears for nearly a fortnight each month. She was an infant teacher and was finding it very difficult to function professionally in her job. Penny was first prescribed a tranquilliser, with which she was not happy and then changed to progesterone given as pessaries. She was asked to use six a day every day of the month. She had been on progesterone for eight years, which had stopped her periods completely for the whole of that time. After being doubled up with pain for 14 hours, Penny saw her doctor, who took her off the progesterone. The pain stopped completely. A month later, Penny's periods came back and she had been regular ever since. After she stopped the progesterone, she realised that she had to do something else to stop the pre-menstrual symptoms from returning.

Penny read the dietary suggestions in my book and realised that she was a 'teapot', so she changed to herbal teas. She added in the herb *Agnus castus* and also took some supplements, including magnesium, which had been recommended in the book. By the time she came to see me, she said her PMS hardly even existed, although she was slightly irritable over the 24 hours before her period. She now wanted to make sure that she was not deficient in any nutrients and to prepare herself for the menopause. Her mineral analysis showed no deficiencies, but high levels of copper from taking the hormone progesterone over the eight years.

Dietary changes

What you eat is the foundation of your health and it is the most important aspect of preventing and treating PMS. There are many women who have eliminated their pre-menstrual symptoms simply by changing their diet. For this reason, it is extremely important that you follow the hormone balancing diet in Chapter 1.

Blood sugar

Of all the different dietary changes you can make, balancing your blood sugar is the most crucial one for eliminating PMS. In Chapter 1, there is an important section on balancing blood sugar, and the recommendations there will need to be followed carefully.

It has been found that the higher the sugar content of your diet, the more severe your pre-menstrual symptoms.[7] I would recommend that you eliminate sugar completely. That means not adding it to drinks or on your cereal, or to anything else. Avoid eating obviously sweet foods, such as chocolate, but look out for hidden sugars as well. Sugar is often found in many savoury foods, such as spaghetti sauces, soups, ketchup and even 'healthy' biscuits. A fruit yoghurt can contain up to eight teaspoons of sugar. Read the label – you might be surprised by what you see.

While changing your diet in order to control the pre-menstrual symptoms, you'll need to eliminate or drastically reduce your alcohol intake. First, it's important to give your liver a rest so that it can detoxify and excrete old hormones (see page 37) efficiently. Secondly, however, alcohol can cause blood sugar fluctuations, and this is one thing you need to keep under control.

It is also important to eat little and often, to help keep your blood sugar levels even. Choose foods that are rich in complex carbohydrates (not refined foods like white bread, biscuits or pastries, for example). The 'little and often' approach to eating prevents the blood sugar levels from dropping excessively and stops adrenaline being released. Adrenaline blocks the uptake (or utilisation) of progesterone in the second half of the cycle. The answer is to stabilise blood sugar levels by eating regularly, which stops the adrenaline interfering with the progesterone.

Not only do carbohydrates keep your blood sugar in balance, they also help to increase blood serotonin levels, the 'calming' brain chemical that helps to lift mood and curb appetite. One study showed that simply changing your evening meal to one that is carbohydrate-rich and protein-poor for the second half of the cycle can reduce PMS symptoms such as depression, tension, anger, confusion, sadness, fatigue, alertness and calmness.[8]

Caffeine

If breast tenderness is your main pre-menstrual symptom, you should avoid any drinks or foods that contain caffeine. Methylxanthines in caffeine have been proved to increase problems with painful, lumpy and tender breasts.[9] These methylxanthines are found in coffee, black tea, green tea, chocolate, cola and even decaffeinated coffee, as well as in medications that contain caffeine, such as headache remedies.

Unfortunately, it doesn't work simply to remove these substances in the second half of the cycle. They will have to be completely eliminated from your diet in order for you to see the benefits. Interestingly, cutting down doesn't seem to have any effect at all. You need to go the whole way on this one. Some women can drink five cups of coffee a day and experience no breast problems pre-menstrually. Others can drink just one cup and find that cutting out that single cup of coffee will make a dramatic difference to their breast symptoms. We are all unique and it really depends on how sensitive we are to these methylxanthines that makes the difference.

Supplements

Supplements are suggested to help get you back to optimum health. They ensure that your body has enough of the essential nutrients it needs to balance your hormones and everything else.

Vitamin B6

Vitamin B6 was first used for hormone imbalances in the 1970s, when it was used in the treatment of depression caused by the Pill.[10]

Since then there have been many studies showing the effectiveness of vitamin B6 on PMS with the latest review published in 1999 in the *British Medical Journal*.[11] Researchers found that daily doses of 100mg, or even 50mg of vitamin B6, were twice as effective as the placebo treatment. Some concerns had previously been raised about high doses of B6 causing tingling in the hands and feet, but the review in the *British Medical Journal* (which involved 940 women) found no evidence of any side-effects for doses of 100mg or less per day.

The majority of research has shown that vitamin B6 makes a substantial difference across the whole range of PMS symptoms, but some studies have shown no effects. It has been suggested that this could be due to the fact that vitamin B6 was given on its own.

We know that all the vitamins and minerals are 'synergistic', which means that they work together. No matter what other supplements you choose to take, you should always make a good multivitamin and mineral supplement the foundation of your programme.

In order for your body to convert B6 (as pyridoxine) into its active form (pyridoxal-5-phosphate), which your body can use, it needs other nutrients such as magnesium. So if you take B6 on its own, but have other (even small) nutritional deficiencies, your body may not be able to use that B6 properly. It is also possible to buy vitamin B6 in the form of pyridoxal-5-phosphate instead of pyridoxine, in the event that your body has any problems making the conversion to the active form.

Vitamin B6 plays a vital part in synthesising certain brain chemicals (neurotransmitters) that control your mood and behaviour. It is required as a co-enzyme in the production of dopamine, tryptophan and serotonin. When treating the depressive symptoms of PMS, it is important that nutrients known to affect serotonin production (such as B6) are taken in adequate quantities. Prozac, for example, is used in the treatment of depression and it is called a selective serotonin reuptake inhibitor (SSRI), because it optimises the use of serotonin.

Vitamin E

This vitamin has been shown to be helpful for breast symptoms associated with PMS, and also for mood swings and irritability.[12] It is interesting that women with PMS have not been found to be deficient in vitamin E,[13] and yet it seems to help the symptoms. At the moment, nobody is sure how it is working.

Magnesium

This is an important mineral in relation to PMS. It is classed as 'nature's tranquilliser' and is, therefore, vital in symptoms that relate to anxiety, tension or other emotional states.

Women with PMS have been found to have lower levels of red blood cell magnesium than women who don't suffer symptoms[14] and the supplementation of magnesium has been found to be extremely useful in alleviating many of the PMS symptoms and even more effective when taken with vitamin B6 at the same time.[15] Vitamin B6 and magnesium work together in many enzyme systems in the body and it is said that B6 works by helping to increase the amount of magnesium within cells. Without B6, magnesium cannot get inside the cells.

A magnesium deficiency can cause blood vessels to go into spasms, so if you suffer from menstrual migraines, magnesium can be useful in preventing these spasms.

Zinc

Zinc is an important mineral because it is a component of more than 200 enzymes. It helps the conversion of linoleic acid to gamma linolenic acid (GLA) (see pages 154–6), and it also plays a major part in the proper action of many of our hormones, including the sex hormones and insulin. Women with PMS have been found to have lower levels of zinc.[16]

Essential fatty acids (EFAs)

In Chapter 1 it was established that EFAs are essential for general health. They do, however, have an even bigger part to play in the treatment of PMS. The Omega 6 series of fatty acids (see page 155), linoleic acid, which is found in plants such as evening primrose, borage and starflower, is converted to GLA. Many women with PMS have been found to have a problem making this conversion to GLA.[17] There are a number of factors that can prevent the conversion of linoleic acid into GLA, including stress, a high-sugar diet, and deficiencies of B6, magnesium and zinc. Because of this problem with conversion it is important to supplement these EFAs in the form where the conversion has already taken place – in other words, in the form of GLA (once again, that's evening primrose oil, borage oil and starflower oil).

A number of studies have shown that evening primrose oil (EPO) was effective in reducing the symptoms of PMS,[18] whereas other studies have shown that EPO was no more effective than a placebo. The interesting point is that the best results with EPO occurred when women were also taking either B6 or a multivitamin at the same time,[19] which again confirms that supplements should not be taken in isolation.

Research has also shown that EPO may be most helpful to women whose main pre-menstrual symptom is breast tenderness or fibrocystic breast disease (see page 304).[20] Evening primrose oil needs to be taken for about three months to be effective, so don't give up.

Herbs

The aim with herbs is to help correct any hormone imbalances. As no one is sure with PMS exactly what hormones are out of balance, it is better to take herbs that have a general balancing effect. Also included are some herbs for water retention (which may be a particular problem), and herbs for the health of your liver, which helps to detoxify and excrete 'old' hormones.

Hormone-balancing herbs
Agnus castus (vitex/chastetree berry)
This is the most important herb in the treatment of PMS. It has been widely studied in relation to PMS and has been shown to be extremely helpful in re-establishing a normal balance of hormones.[21] *Agnus castus* works on the pituitary gland and has a balancing effect on the hormones, particularly in the second half of the cycle.

Black cohosh (Cimicifuga racemosa)
This herb was used by the Native North Americans. It is a good normaliser for the female reproductive system and can be useful for PMS. It has a generally calming effect on the nervous system and, as well as having a balancing effect on the hormones, it can be helpful when your main symptoms are anxiety, tension and depression. This would also be the herb to try if you get pre-menstrual headaches.

Skullcap (Scutellaria lateriflora)
Skullcap is a wonderful herb for the nervous system, so is especially helpful with the PMS symptoms of anxiety, tension, depression, irritability and insomnia.

Dong quai (Angelica sinensis)
This Chinese herb has been in use since ancient times. It is very popular for problems associated with the female reproductive system and it can be helpful for PMS symptoms because it promotes normal hormone balance. Dong quai also has muscle-relaxing qualities so it is particularly suggested for women who experience pre-menstrual pain and cramp.[22]

Herbs for Water Retention

As you change your eating patterns and approach optimum health, water retention will start to correct itself. You may, however, need some extra help at the beginning. Make sure that you reduce your intake of salt and salty foods. It's also important to drink more water. If you limit your intake of water your body will think there is a shortage and try to retain the water you have. Water is a natural diuretic.

*Dandelion (***Taraxacum officinale***)*

Dandelion is the herb of choice for water retention because it is a natural diuretic that allows fluid to be released without losing vital nutrients at the same time. It contains more vitamins and minerals than any other herb, and is one of the best sources of potassium. Dandelion also helps to improve liver function so it can be useful for general detoxification and elimination of hormones.

Liver function

Make sure that you follow the recommendations from Chapter 1 on liver function, so that this vital organ can help to eliminate 'old' hormones safely and efficiently during each cycle. When you are trying to keep your hormones in balance, you do not want 'old' circulating hormones adding to the problem.

If you suffer from pre-menstrual or menstrual migraines/headaches, it is even more important that your liver is functioning efficiently.

Exercise

Exercise is important for your general health but it is also important to eliminate PMS symptoms. Exercise releases brain chemicals called 'endorphins', which help us to feel happier, more alert and calmer. Exercise on its own has been shown to have a positive effect on people suffering from depression, stress and anxiety, many of the symptoms found in the pre-menstrual period.

Stress

This is an important factor in PMS because of the effects of adrenaline.

As you saw above, adrenaline is released when your blood sugar drops. It is, however, also released when you are under stress. Unfortunately, adrenaline prevents your body from being able to use progesterone properly in the second half of your cycle. When this occurs, you can end up with pre-menstrual symptoms because of stress. Certain nutrients, such as the B vitamins and magnesium can be extremely helpful when stress is a problem, but you do need to look beyond diet as well. Sit down and assess your lifestyle to see if there are ways to take off the pressure. Look into ways of helping you cope with stress, such as relaxation techniques or meditation. The herb Siberian ginseng (*Eleutherococcus senticosus*) can be particularly helpful if stress and blood sugar swings are a problem for you.

Natural Therapies

A number of different natural therapies could be useful alongside improving your nutrition and herbs. These could include acupuncure, homeopathy, aromatherapy and reflexology.

The Treatment Plan

Concentrate on applying the food recommendations from Chapter 1 and make sure that you follow the blood sugar suggestions on page 92. This is the most important aspect of controlling PMS symptoms, and you may find that you don't need any further treatment. Put the dietary changes in place first. It's simple and effective.

If your PMS is worse on the Pill, or started when you began taking the Pill, think seriously about using another form of contraception. You can still put the dietary advice in place, and take the vitamins and minerals recommended below, but you may just be fighting a losing battle. Your PMS may actually be *caused* by the hormones you are putting into your body. Don't take any of the herbs suggested in the sections above when you are on the Pill, unless you are under the supervision of a registered, experienced practitioner.

Follow this plan for three months, changing your diet, and taking the supplements and herbs. At the end of the three months, continue to eat sensibly. Obviously it is not necessary to be as strict, but if you go back to your original eating habits, the symptoms will probably return. Stop taking the herbs at the end of three months, and discontinue the supplements, apart from your multivitamin and mineral supplement.

There are some useful tests that can give you more information to help with PMS, such as testing for deficiencies and looking at your stress levels. These are described in Chapter 4.

The Integrated Approach

If you are suffering from PMS, you need to decide whether to take drugs or to try the natural approach. This is not one of those 'women's problems' where you can combine the conventional and natural. Even if you are on the Pill, you still need to eat well and keep yourself healthy, but the natural approach would not correct your PMS while you are taking it.

The natural approach to PMS is very successful so I recommend that you try it over a period of three months. Look at it this way – you have nothing to lose but the symptoms! If you have been given medication to help with PMS, you'll need to see your doctor before stopping. This is especially important if antidepressants have been prescribed.

My new book *Natural Solutions to PMS* will address this subject in much more detail.

Your Supplement Plan

- A good multivitamin and mineral supplement

- Vitamin B6 (as pyridoxal-5-phosphate at 50mg per day)

- Vitamin E (as d-alpha tocopherol, at 300iu per day)

- Magnesium citrate or amino acid chelate (200mg per day)

- Zinc citrate (15mg per day)

- GLA (150mg per day)

> **Note**
> Each nutrient represents the total intake for one day, so if your multivitamin and mineral contains 25mg of vitamin B6, you only need to add 25mg in a separate supplement form.

Herbs

- Use a tincture of equal parts *Agnus castus*, black cohosh, dong quai and skullcap, 1 teaspoon three times a day and stop when you have a period. Use this over three months.

- A separate tincture of dandelion can also be taken, 1 teaspoon three times a day, and stop when you bleed.

- Add a separate tincture of Siberian ginseng if stress is a major problem for you, 1 teaspoon three times a day, and stop when you bleed.

You can take any of the different tinctures at the same time mixed together.

To make this programme simpler, I have formulated the Natural Cycle Pack – PM Comfort, made by the Natural Health Practice, which contains the above nutrients and herbs. If you can't get this locally then call 01892 750511 and it can be posted to you.

In Summary

- Always investigate the cause of your symptoms before taking any drugs, or beginning a natural treatment programme.

- Keep a diary of symptoms, making a note of when they occur. If they always occur in the weeks before your period, but stop when your period begins, they are undoubtedly associated with PMS.

- Begin the hormone balancing diet (see page 16).

- Avoid caffeine, especially if you suffer from breast problems.

- Stop taking the Pill if your symptoms came on when you began taking it. Choose another form of contraception instead.

- Take steps to balance your blood sugar levels. This means giving up refined carbohydrate products in favour of wholegrain, wholemeal complex carbohydrates. Eat little and often.

- Have a complex-carbohydrate-rich, protein-poor evening meal.

- Include a good source of essential fatty acids (see page 27) in your diet.

- Take supplements for three months.

- Take herbs to help balance your hormones, for three months.

- Begin a regular exercise programme, which has a positive effect on PMS symptoms.

- Take care of your liver!

- Take steps to deal with any stress in your life.

HEAVY PERIODS (MENORRHAGIA)

Every woman's periods are different, and it can be difficult to assess whether or not your bleeding is heavier than it should be. Periods are obviously a personal subject, and most of us have no way of knowing if our bleeding is the same as that of our friends or anyone else. How do specialists gauge it? Well, thanks to a number of women who sent their sanitary towels and tampons to a lab for analysis, we now know what is considered to be 'normal'.

On average, we lose about 6–8 teaspoons (35ml), or about half an eggcup, over the course of a period. Some women lose more and others less, but this figure acts as a benchmark for an average woman in an average cycle.

Are Your Periods Heavy?

The easiest way to gauge whether your periods are unusually heavy is to work out how often you are changing whatever form of protection you are using. For example, if you have to change your tampon or pad every hour or sooner, or if you frequently leak in the night, chances are your periods are abnormally heavy.

For some women, symptoms are so extreme that they will actually flood to the point of haemorrhaging. I have had women describe flooding through their clothes and all over the car seat while driving. The blood may also contain clots that look like pieces of liver, which can be alarming. Some women have said that their flow has become so unpredictable and intense that they cannot stray far from a toilet. Many women reach the point where their lives are being planned around their periods.

When your period begins to affect the quality of your life and your ability to work, it's undoubtedly something that must be addressed.

Are There Other Symptoms?

Depending upon the cause of the heavy periods (also called menorrhagia), you may experience cramping or other symptoms. Heavy periods that cannot be medically explained (see page 104) often have no other symptoms.

What Can Cause You To Have Heavy Periods?

Heavy periods may have no obvious cause, in which case you will be suffering from something called 'dysfunctional bleeding'. This term simply means that you have nothing wrong with you from a gynaecological point of view, except for the fact that you bleed too much. You may be building up more womb lining than necessary, which needs to be shed every month. Furthermore, your womb, which functions as a muscle, may be poorly toned, causing more bleeding than normal.

The cause may be hormonal, in that excess oestrogen may be causing the womb lining to build up too much and therefore more blood has to be shed at your period. Excess oestrogen can be present if you are not ovulating, because there is no progesterone to balance the oestrogen. The other reason for heavy bleeding can be a prostaglandin imbalance. Prostaglandins are hormone-like substances that control blood clotting. Both a hormone and prostaglandin imbalance can be helped with a natural approach. Stress can cause heavy bleeding, so this would also need to be addressed.

There are other causes for heavy periods, and these include:

- fibroids (see Chapter 6)

- polyps (non-cancerous growths in the womb which are harmless, but very fragile structures that bleed easily)

- PID (pelvic inflammatory disease, see page 253) or another infection in the reproductive tract

- problems with the endometrium (the lining of the womb), including endometriosis (see Chapter 6), endometrial hyperplasia (an overgrowth of the lining of the womb) and, rarely, endometrial cancer

- hypothyroidism (an underproduction of the thyroid hormone) (see page 450) and other hormonal imbalances

- problems with your blood, including anaemia

- contraceptive devices, including the IUD and some injectable contraceptives, which can cause heavy bleeding

Finding Out If There is a Reason for Your Heavy Periods

All cases of excessive bleeding should be diagnosed by your doctor, who may refer you to see a gynaecologist. Getting a diagnosis is essential for all women, no matter how healthy you may otherwise feel. Although the condition is harmless in many women, it can be a symptom of something else that needs to be investigated.

A number of different tests will be undertaken to rule out the various causes of heavy bleeding. These can include an ultrasound scan, a hysteroscopy (a microscopic 'camera' inserted through the cervix to the inside of the womb), blood tests for thyroid function, blood clotting disorders and anaemia, and an infection screen (swabs taken to see if an infection is present).

When you have been given a diagnosis, you can then take appropriate steps to treat the condition. If, for example, you've been diagnosed with fibroids, turn to Chapter 6, to find out what choices you have.

You may also be told that there is no obvious cause, and that your tests have come back negative. This process of elimination is important; when you know that there is nothing more sinister afoot, you will have the confidence you need to try a natural approach. Any competent practitioner will suggest that you have a full medical investigation for heavy bleeding before offering natural treatment.

What Treatment Can You Be Offered By Your Doctor?

Your doctor may offer you a drug-based approach to dealing with heavy periods, even before any investigations are undertaken by a specialist. However, I feel that it is essential to have a proper checkup by a gynaecologist to see if there is any definite cause for the bleeding *before* you start taking drugs to control the flow. You could, for example, be offered the Pill to control your cycle, but this might mask a more serious problem that needs to be investigated.

Once you've been given the all-clear, you may be offered one of the following treatments.

Drugs

The contraceptive pill

This will control the flow because you will not actually have a cycle of your own. The monthly 'bleed' is not actually a real period, but your body's reaction to a drop in the level of hormones contained in the Pill. Your cycle will be regular and much lighter. Some of the side-effects of the Pill include nausea, vomiting, headache, thrombosis (blood clots), weight changes, lack of sex drive, depression and breast tenderness.

Progestogens

Progestogens are synthetic, or man made, progesterone. Progesterone is released naturally in the second half of the monthly cycle. Progestogens are often given regardless of whether or not a woman has a problem with progesterone production. It is taken for a number of days and when it is stopped, the womb lining is completely shed. Obviously, the hope is that bleeding will then return to normal. Side-effects can include nausea, acne, breast tenderness, bloating and mood changes. It's currently believed that progestogens are not very helpful for women with heavy bleeding and tranexamic acid (below) is the treatment of choice.

WHAT HAPPENS WHEN YOU STOP THE DRUGS?

The answer is simple: you are back where you started. Drugs only address the symptoms of heavy bleeding while you are taking them. They do not change the root cause of the problem. In other words, if you are having heavy periods because your womb lining builds up too much, once you stop the drugs that have been controlling the womb lining, it simply builds up again and the symptoms return.

The natural approach is different, and aims to do two things: to control the symptom of heavy bleeding, at the same time making a fundamental change in your biochemistry, which is causing you to bleed heavily in the first place. So that when you stop taking the herbs, for example, you are not back where you started, as your body and your health has changed.

Mefenamic acid

This drug works by controlling prostaglandins (see essential fatty acids, below), which are hormone-like substances that control the dilation of the blood vessels and the way blood clots. This type of drug is taken throughout your period, and controls the blood loss by up to 50 per cent. Side-effects can include drowsiness, diarrhoea and rashes.

Tranexamic acid

This drug is also taken during your period, and it works to reduce blood flow by improving clotting in the womb. This seems the most effective of the drug approaches for heavy periods. Side-effects can include vomiting, diarrhoea and nausea.

Danazol

Danazol is a synthetic weak male hormone that prevents ovulation, which in turn stops the womb lining from developing, in order to control the heavy bleeding. The side-effects can include severe mood swings, nausea, dizziness, rashes and headaches. Because danazol is a mild male hormone, other side-effects can include facial hair, acne, an increased sex drive, weight gain and deepening of the voice.

Gonadotrophin releasing hormone (GnRH) analogues

This drug works by putting you into a temporary but reversible menopause to stop you having a period altogether. These are synthetic hormones that can be given as an injection or a nasal spray. They work by preventing the pituitary gland from releasing both FSH (follicle stimulating hormone; see page 68) and LH (luteinizing hormone; see page 68). This prevents the ovaries from producing hormones, so oestrogen levels drop. One of the most common symptoms of this type of treatment is hot flushes, but other side-effects can include headaches, mood swings, vaginal dryness and insomnia (basically the symptoms of menopause!). Prolonged use (more than six months) can lead to osteoporosis.

Progestogen coil

This is a coil (IUD – intrauterine device) that can be used both as a contraceptive and to control heavy bleeding. The majority of IUDs can actually cause heavy bleeding, but this type of coil contains progestogen, which works to regulate the bleeding. Some women find that their periods stop completely when using this coil; others experience spotting between periods.

Surgical techniques

In some cases surgery will be recommended to deal with heavy periods. For some women, this can bring a welcome relief of symptoms, but in many cases (apart from the more permanent techniques, such as hysterectomy), the symptoms simply return. It's also important to bear in mind that surgery always holds some risk of complications, and you must take the time to discuss these fully with your specialist.

A surgical approach may be suggested when your bleeding is so severe that you are haemorrhaging, or when drugs have not been successful.

D&C (Dilatation and Curettage)

This procedure is commonly called a 'scrape', and it is performed under a general anaesthetic. The lining of the womb is literally 'scraped' away and discarded. Studies have shown that there is no real long-term benefit from a D&C in cases of inexplicable bleeding, but it can be a useful investigative tool. The lining can be sent to a laboratory for analysis, to rule out cancer, for example. A D&C is often combined with other diagnostic procedures, such as a hysteroscopy (see below), but it should not really be suggested as a treatment for heavy periods, because the womb lining will build up again within a couple of cycles. A D&C is performed under general anaesthetic, with all its risks (including infections and blood clots).

Endometrial resection and endometrial ablation

In endometrial resection the womb lining is examined using a hysteroscope, which is a thin telescope inserted through the cervix. The lining of the womb is 'stripped' off, using a hot wire loop (called a diathermy). The procedure takes place under a general anaesthetic.

The endometrial ablation uses much the same procedure as the resection, but this time a device is used to microwave or simply 'heat up' the lining of the womb. A general anaesthetic may not be necessary in this procedure. Sometimes a hot revolving metal ball called a rollerball is used to destroy the womb lining.

Drugs are often used before these procedures in order to thin the lining of the womb to make the technique easier. Periods will often stop or be extremely light after these techniques, but many women report an increase in period pains. With either of the above techniques, about 20 per cent of women will have to have a repeat operation around two years later, because the lining of the womb has built up again.

Which technique?
If you are given a choice between these two procedures, research has shown that the endometrial ablation is superior to the resection, in that it is more quickly performed and has fewer complications.[23]

Hysterectomy
This is the most extreme surgical procedure that could be recommended for heavy periods and it undoubtedly cures the problem – but only because you will no longer have *any* periods. Hysterectomy is a major operation and it can require up to three months off work (see page 471), and involve a number of quite serious side-effects (see page 472).

Hysterectomy is the most common major operation performed on women, and I firmly believe that it should only be offered to women whose lives are at stake if their wombs are not removed. However, with the enormous number of other choices available through both natural and conventional medicine, hysterectomy should always be an absolutely last resort.

Note
Chapter 1 contains important advice about using tampons (see pages 46–8).

What Natural Treatment Could Be Effective?

The natural approach focuses on working on a number of factors at the same time. Rather than simply alleviating the symptoms, or masking the problem using drugs, this treatment is aimed at curing the underlying problem – in other words, whatever is causing the heavy periods.

There are six stages involved in this treatment programme:

1. Improve your diet, based on the recommendations outlined in Chapter 1.

2. Use nutritional supplements that are known scientifically to help to control heavy periods.

3. Control excess oestrogens absorbed from your environment, and reduce high levels of oestrogens in your body (see page 40).

4. Control levels of 'bad' prostaglandins – which control blood flow and clotting – by altering what you eat, and by taking appropriate supplements.

5. Use specific herbs in the *long* term, in order to improve the general functioning of your womb and hormonal systems.

6. Use specific herbs in the *short* term, in order to get your blood flow under control while you are having a period.

Dietary changes

Begin by following the hormone balancing diet (see Chapter 1). One of the aims of the natural approach to heavy periods is to ensure that your hormones are balanced. If you have excess oestrogen, your womb lining can build up. Not only is the hormone balancing diet essential, but you will also need to make the following changes to your diet.

Coffee
Avoid coffee, which increases the menstrual flow.

Phytoestrogens
Foods that contains phytoestrogens (see page 20) are particularly important for heavy bleeding because they can help to keep oestrogen under control and prevent excessive build-up of the lining of the womb.

Alcohol
While you are working on alleviating heavy bleeding, watch your alcohol intake (see page 36), as it can compromise liver function and you need your liver to be working efficiently as your 'waste disposal unit'.

Dairy foods

While you are working on treating your heavy periods, eliminate all dairy produce. They have a high saturated fat content and will encourage the production of more oestrogen (see page 68). If you are concerned about your calcium intake, don't worry. There are many other foods that contain high levels of calcium, including sesame seeds, leafy green vegetables, nuts, fish (particularly with bones, such as tinned salmon) and seaweed. You will also get good levels from your multi-vitamin and mineral supplement.

Xenoestrogens

Do what you can to avoid excess oestrogens coming in from the environment (see page 40).

Supplements

The supplements are added to make the dietary changes more effective in a shorter period of time. Some are recommended because they have definitely been found to be deficient in women who have heavy periods, and others have been recommended because they can work on balancing hormones and hormone-like substances in your body, which may be causing the heavy bleeding.

Sandra

Sandra (40) came to see me because she had been experiencing periods that were so heavy, she was flooding with large clots. For four months before I saw her, she had been bleeding constantly with only three or four days in between each period. As always, I made sure that she'd had a check-up with her doctor to rule out anything serious. She had been told that she just had some small fibroids.

Sandra had been given ten iron injections over the previous few months, because not only was she anaemic, but also her iron stores (ferritin) were low as a result of the continual bleeding. She had been given medication for the bleeding, but it wasn't controlling it.

Her hair mineral analysis showed that she was deficient in zinc, chromium and selenium. I put her on a programme of supplements

---

to correct these deficiencies, and suggested herbs to help control the bleeding. We talked through her diet, and she mentioned that she regularly drank three cups of coffee early in the day, followed by three cups of tea later on. I explained that caffeine can actually make the bleeding worse, so she cut them out. I saw her two months later, and she reported that she was having regular cycles with no bleeding in between. However, her periods were still lasting ten days, and were heavy, with clotting. Two months after that she returned to say that the difference in her periods was 'remarkable'. She was no longer flooding and the clots had stopped.

Vitamin A

Vitamin A is an antioxidant that generally helps to protect your cells against damage. It helps cells reproduce normally and is also needed for red blood cell production. Vitamin A deficiency has been found in women with heavy periods.[24] One study showed that 92 per cent of women prescribed supplemental vitamin A found that their heavy bleeding was either cured or alleviated.

B vitamins

The B vitamins are particularly important for heavy periods for a number of reasons. First and foremost, they are needed by the liver to convert excess oestrogen into weaker and less dangerous forms. One of the B vitamins, B6, is needed for the production of beneficial prostaglandins, which help reduce abnormal blood flow.

The B vitamins are also crucial for the conversion of linoleic acid to GLA (gamma linolenic acid), which is necessary to produce these beneficial prostaglandins. The B vitamins are required to convert Omega 6 oils into a form that can be used by the body to produce the 'good' type prostaglandins. Without this conversion, your body will produce more of the 'bad' prostaglandins, which will increase the amount of bleeding at each period.

Vitamin C

Vitamin C and bioflavonoids (see page 214) help to strengthen the capillaries in the body, which can reduce heavy bleeding. Taken as a supplement, vitamin C has also produced excellent results for many women with heavy periods. One study showed that taking 200mg of vitamin C with bioflavonoids, three times daily, reduced bleeding in 87 per cent of the women tested.[25]

Zinc

This mineral is vital for the healthy functioning of the reproductive system and for hormone balance.

Iron

If you are bleeding very heavily, you may run the risk of becoming anaemic. Common symptoms of anaemia include fatigue, loss of appetite, constipation, irritability and pallor, among other things. If these symptoms seem familiar, see your doctor who will arrange tests. When you are tested for anaemia, the lab measures the level of iron available in your red blood cells (haemoglobin). However, iron is also stored as ferritin in other parts of the body, such as the spleen and liver. When your doctor orders tests, make sure that both your haemoglobin and ferritin are checked, as it is possible to be iron deficient even if your haemoglobin levels are normal.

Iron deficiency is a bit of a double-edged sword. If you bleed heavily throughout your periods, you will be more likely to be iron deficient. However, one of the symptoms of iron deficiency is also an increased risk of heavy bleeding. Iron helps the blood vessels to contract, which is necessary to slow down the flow during your periods.

If tests suggest that you are iron-deficient, take extra iron (as amino acid chelate or citrate) at 14mg per day. Vitamin C is essential for the body to absorb iron, so for maximum absorption take 1,000mg (1 gram) of vitamin C with your iron supplement on an empty stomach. Avoid taking the iron and vitamin C alongside any other supplements you may be taking.

Avoid taking iron in the form of ferrous sulphate (also called iron sulphate), which is less easily absorbed by the body. Only 2 to 10 per cent of the iron from this type of iron supplement is actually absorbed by your body, and even then, half is eliminated, causing blackening of your stools and constipation.

Ferrous sulphate is classed as an inorganic iron. Organic irons are much more easily absorbed and do not affect the bowels in the same way. Look for iron in the form of ascorbates, malates or amino acid chelates (it will say this on the label); otherwise, iron-rich herbal formulas such as Floradix can be purchased from your healthfood shop.

Try to avoid drinking Indian or regular black tea with your meals, which blocks the uptake of iron from your food. Similarly, phytates, found in raw grains, can prevent iron from being absorbed by the body. Herb teas and fruit juices are fine.

Essential Fatty Acids (EFAs)

EFAs are discussed in detail on pages 27 to 30, and they can be an important means of controlling heavy bleeding during periods.

One of the drugs used for menorrhagia, mefanamic acid, works by controlling 'bad' prostaglandins (see page 30), which can increase the flow of blood. It is possible to mimic the effects of this drug by making changes to your diet – in particular, to your intake of EFAs.

Both red meat and dairy produce contain something called arachidonic acid. This substance encourages the production of a 'bad' type of prostaglandin (called PGE2) that leads to increased blood flow, and a reduced blood–clotting ability. The result? Heavier periods. In fact, research has shown that women with menorrhagia have higher levels of arachidonic acid, causing more PGE2 to be made.[26]

What this means in practice is that women with heavy periods should ideally consume less arachidonic acid, which is found mainly in animal-based foods. The other goal is to increase levels of essential fatty acids, which create the 'good' type of prostaglandins. Beneficial prostaglandins help to reduce abnormal blood flow, and they are produced from certain unsaturated fats, called essential fatty acids. EFAs are found in nuts, seeds, some oils (linseed (flaxseed), for example) and oily fish (including mackerel and salmon).

Herbs

Herbs will be taken on either a short-term or long-term basis. Some may be taken throughout the month (long-term), and others will be used only when you are bleeding (short-term), in order to help control the flow.

Long-term herbal treatment

In the long term, these herbs will be used to improve the functioning of the womb, to help stop excessive blood flow, and to balance the hormones.

Dong quai (*Angelica sinensis*) can help to encourage the normal functioning of the womb, and it has also been found to regulate the production of unhealthy prostaglandins, which are responsible for increased blood flow. One of the key drugs used in menorrhagia (mefanamic acid) works in much the same way.[27]

Ladies' Mantle (*Alchemilla vulgaris*) helps to control heavy bleeding and has been used successfully in clinical trials. It is believed to increase the circulation to the reproductive organs, giving it a toning and nourishing effect. It is also believed to restore health to the blood vessels in the womb, and to the fragile capillaries throughout the body.[28]

For long-term treatment, combine equal parts of dong quai and ladies' mantle in tincture form.

Short-term herbal treatment

The majority of these herbs are astringent in nature, which means that they are used to help control blood loss.

Shepherd's purse (*Capsella bursa pastoris*) has been used in clinical trials to prevent heavy bleeding.[29]

Other herbs that can be used to control bleeding include:

- **cranesbill** (*Geranium maculatum*), which is an effective astringent widely used for diarrhoea, dysentery, haemorrhoids (piles) and menorrhagia

- **yarrow** (*Achillea millefolium*), which is believed to tone the blood vessels and is known for its astringent qualities

- **golden seal** (*Hydrastis canadensis*), which is both a tonic and an astringent, making it useful for many uterine conditions

For short-term treatment, blend equal quantities of shepherd's purse, cranesbill, yarrow and golden seal.

NATURAL MEDICINE

Both acupuncture and homeopathy can be extremely useful in conjunction with the dietary and herbal recommendations. Acupuncture can help to increase the energy flow to the pelvic area and stop any stagnation in the womb. It can also help to optimise liver function. The homeopathic remedies Lachesis and Sanguinaria are often used when there is excess bleeding.

The Treatment Plan

If you are taking the contraceptive pill or progestogen to control your periods, you will need to speak to your doctor before coming off. In fact, it is important to see your doctor before coming off any medication. The natural approach encourages your body to do the work, so if you are artificially controlling your cycle – for example, when taking the Pill – the herbs will not work.

If you have been taking either mefanamic or tranexamic acid, it is possible to use a combined approach. Many women are concerned that stopping these drugs will result in a virtual relapse, causing flooding and the problems accompanying that. If you are worried about the possibility of flooding, continue to take the drugs, but *only when you need them*. Both of these drugs are only required during the actual bleeding, and you can learn to use them only when necessary:

- Take the supplements and the long-term herbs throughout your cycle.

- Take the short-term herbs when you begin to bleed. If you can control the bleeding herbally, then do not take the drugs.

- If, however, the bleeding is unmanageable, then use the medication. Try to use a little less than usual, which should be adequate, given that the herbs will be undertaking much the same role in the body.

- Do the same each month and you should find that, after a few cycles, the herbs will control the blood flow and your need for medication will be reduced substantially. Eventually, you should not need the drugs *or* the herbs, as your body regains healthy cycles.

Your Supplement Plan

- A good multivitamin and mineral supplement

- Vitamin A as beta-carotene, not retinol (10,000iu per day)★

- Vitamin C with bioflavonoids (1,000mg per day)

- Vitamin B-complex (providing 50mg of most of the B vitamins per day)

- Zinc citrate (15mg) per day

* High doses of vitamin A are only a problem if you are planning a pregnancy. However, this caution applies only to vitamin A as retinol. Vitamin A as beta-carotene is safe.

Herbs

- Take a combination of the long-term herbs throughout the month, but *not* when you are actually having your period.

- As soon as your period starts, switch to the short-term herbs.

- When your bleeding becomes manageable during your period, stop the herbs.

- When your period is finished, start taking the long-term herbs again.

- Take the herbs for six months, and if there is no real improvement, see a registered practitioner.

To make this programme simpler, I have formulated the Natural Cycle Pack – Menstrual Light made by the Natural Health Practice, which contains the above nutrients and herbs. If you can't get this locally then call 01892 750511 and it can be posted to you.

In Summary

- Always investigate the cause of heavy periods before taking any drugs, or beginning a natural treatment programme.

- Don't give up your medication without consulting your doctor.

- Ask for tests to confirm whether or not you are anaemic.

- Begin the hormone balancing diet (see page 16).

- Avoid coffee, which increases the menstrual flow. Avoid drinking black tea and fizzy soft drinks with meals, which reduces the amount of iron that is absorbed.

- Take supplements (see page 115) throughout your entire cycle.

- Take short-term herbs only when you are bleeding, and alongside any drugs used to control the flow.

- Discontinue using the drugs gradually, as they are no longer required, and continue taking short-term herbs until bleeding is completely under control.

- Take long-term herbs for the remainder of the month.

IRREGULAR PERIODS

Suffering from irregular periods is a fairly clear indication that your cycles have become imbalanced. There are a variety of reasons for this, which will be discussed below, and also many ways to address the imbalance. Many women are unconcerned about having irregular cycles until they begin trying for a baby, but other women find it very difficult to plan their lives without knowing when their periods could appear.

What are Irregular Periods?

Irregular periods are simply those that are not regular. If you suffer from irregular periods, you simply will not know when your period is going to appear. Cycles can vary from 23 to 35 days, but they are classed as regular if your periods occur at roughly the same time each cycle. So, even if your periods are, say, 35 days apart instead of the usual 28, but they always appear at day 35, they would be classified as being 'normal'. Irregular periods can be extremely difficult or even impossible to track.

What Symptoms Could You Experience?

Minor cycle irregularities are common. For example, you may have your period on day 23 of one month and then the next month on day 35. If you are not happy with that level of unpredictability, follow the natural recommendations listed on pages 122 to 123 to make your cycles more regular.

You may, however, have a much more irregular cycle, in which case it is important that you have further investigations, so that other problems, such as polycystic ovary syndrome (see Chapter 7) can be ruled out. The following symptoms are characteristic of irregular periods, and you can experience a combination of any or all of these:

- large gaps with no periods

- some gaps and then periods coming too frequently for a while (for example, two in one month) followed by gaps again

- gaps of no periods and then bleeding continuously for a few weeks
- spotting in between periods

What Can Cause You to Have Irregular Periods?

Your cycle can change for a number of simple reasons and the odd slip in routine is not normally anything to worry about. Relatively routine aspects of life, including dieting, travel, stress, seasonal changes, exercise, post-pregnancy and pre-menopause can all have an effect on your cycle. But there are other reasons, some of which are more serious than others and it is for this reason that you should always investigate irregularities that last for longer than two or three cycles.

Causes may include:

- excessive build-up of the womb lining (endometrial hyperplasia)
- abnormalities of the cervix (see page 289)
- hormone imbalances (see page 129)
- polycystic ovaries (see page 232)
- womb cancer
- cervical cancer (see page 289)
- infection (see page 250)
- fibroids (see page 185)
- certain medications such as corticosteroids or drugs used for cancer treatment.

Finding Out If There is a Reason For Your Irregular Periods

Even if the irregularity of your cycle doesn't bother you, it is important to have any changes checked out by your doctor to rule out anything of a more serious nature. In many cases the reason can be easily pinpointed, and you can address the cause immediately. For example, if you have suddenly lost weight by crash dieting or exercising heavily, your periods can be affected. But don't dismiss the irregularities, even if you think you know the cause. By altering its cycles your body is giving you a message, letting you know that your lifestyle may be too extreme. Listen to your body.

Your body is very clever. If you do not have adequate fat stores, through dieting or exercise, your body will register that you are starving. Since it is not appropriate to become pregnant when food is short, your body is designed to 'turn off' the reproductive system. In real terms this means that ovulation or periods stop, or periods become irregular. As a case in point, it has been found that Bushmen women of Australia only ovulate at a certain time of year when food is plentiful.[30]

Furthermore, when your body is under stress, you can release the hormone prolactin, again in response to what your body sees as a 'crisis'. This hormone can affect ovulation and the regularity of your cycles, again as another protective mechanism. It appears to be nature's way of protecting women from pregnancy at times when they would find it difficult to cope. Studies show that women going through a bereavement or other kind of trauma, for example, can stop having periods altogether.[31]

Ultrasound investigation

This test involves using sound waves to examine the thickness of the womb lining and the condition of the ovaries. This information can help your doctor to come to a diagnosis of why your cycles are irregular. For example, they may pick up polycystic ovaries from the scan.

Endometrial biopsy

In this procedure, a small piece of womb lining is taken and sent to the lab for analysis. Although it sounds invasive, it is a quick and normally painless procedure that does not require anaesthetic of any nature. This is performed by a procedure called a hysteroscopy, where a hysteroscope (a lighted scope) is inserted through the cervix to allow doctors to see the inside of the womb. A small piece of womb lining is then extracted. This investigation helps to determine whether there is endometrial hyperplasia (overgrowth of the womb lining), infection or cancerous tissue.

Blood tests

A blood test can reveal problems with hormone balance and should include tests for thyroid function, prolactin (a hormone produced by the pituitary gland) and the reproductive hormones such as FSH (follicle stimulating hormone) and LH (luteinizing hormone). All of these hormones have to be within the correct range in order to have regular cycles. Problems with your thyroid can also cause irregular cycles, so this needs to be checked.

What Treatment Can You Be Offered By Your Doctor?

The treatment will obviously depend on what the investigations have pinpointed as the cause of the problem. However, treatment normally involves drugs and/or surgery, as described below.

Drugs

Your doctor may suggest using drugs to regulate your periods even before investigations have been undertaken. Avoid this approach if you can. Many of the drugs used will not actually be treating the cause of the problem, and the reason that you have irregular cycles (stress, or hormone imbalances, for example) can become worse if left untreated.

The contraceptive pill

You may be offered the Pill if your tests show that nothing is amiss, or as the first line of treatment *before* tests are offered. The Pill may appear to regulate your cycle because bleeding will occur at the same time each month. However, the reason for this is because you do not actually have a normal cycle at all. The bleeding that you experience is simply a 'withdrawal bleed' because of the way the drugs are given. The Pill will work to regulate 'periods' for as long as you take it, but as soon as you stop, symptoms will recur. When you come off the Pill, you are right back where you started.

Quite apart from the risks of masking a potentially more serious underlying cause, you should always be wary of taking the Pill over the age of 40. Always ask for full investigations before going down that route; studies show there is an increased risk of thickening of the womb lining (endometrial hyperplasia) after the age of 40. Some endometrial hyperplasias can progress to womb cancer so it is important that this is monitored or treated. Some of the listed side-effects of the Pill include nausea, vomiting, headache, thrombosis, lack of sex drive, weight changes, depression and breast tenderness.

Progestogens

Progestogens are synthetic, or man-made, progesterone-like drugs. Progestogens are used when the womb lining has thickened (endometrial hyperplasia) and needs to be cleared. They are given for a number of days and, when stopped, the womb lining is completely shed. Side-effects can include nausea, acne, breast tenderness, bloating and mood changes.

Surgical techniques

Surgery could be recommended if the womb looks very thick, indicating that it is not shedding properly every month. If it is left to build up, the cells could start to mutate and become cancerous.

Many of the treatments for removing excess womb lining are the same as those for heavy periods. D&C (see page 107) was once a popular procedure, but it is not favoured today, largely because it was not very successful.

Endometrial resection and endometrial ablation (see page 107) are also used when the womb lining is excessive (endometrial hyperplasia).

What Natural Treatments Could Be Effective?

The natural approach is designed to encourage your body to re-establish regular ovulation and to get your hormones back in balance. It will also help you to assess the different stresses in your life, to see what can be changed and to find other ways to cope.

There are a number of stages involved in this treatment programme:

1. Improve your diet, based on the recommendations outlined in Chapter 1.

2. Use nutritional supplements that are known scientifically to help to regulate your cycle.

3. Prevent womb cells from mutating if there is a tendency for your womb lining to be too thick.

4. Use specific herbs over a period of time to help regulate your cycle and address the underlying cause of why they became irregular in the first place.

5. Look at and address any lifestyle factors that may have caused your periods to become irregular.

Dietary changes

This is the foundation of your health and well being. The recommendations from Chapter 1 must be put into place before you will see any long-term benefits. In particular, adopt the 'hormone balancing diet' outlined on page 16. There are a number of additional remedies and supplements that can help to regulate your cycle, and these are listed below.

Linseeds
Linseeds contain both essential fatty acids (EFAs: Omega 3 and Omega 6) and also phytoestrogens (naturally occurring oestrogens found in plants). Research has shown that giving women 10g of ground linseeds per day increases the regularity of their cycle and improves ovulation.[32] Because linseeds have this phytoestrogenic effect, which means they are able to control excess oestrogen, they should be included in your diet, particularly if you have had treatment for thickening of the womb lining (endometrial hyperplasia) and are aiming to prevent your womb lining from building up again.

Other phytoestrogens
Irregular cycles may be caused by a hormone imbalance and the womb lining may also be thicker due to excess oestrogen. Adding other phytoestrogens into your diet can have a beneficial effect on regulating your periods.

The foods that contain phytoestrogens are explained in detail in Chapter 1 and include soya, chickpeas, lentils and garlic. These foods, which have a mild oestrogenic activity, can actually control levels of excess oestrogen by blocking oestrogen receptors in different parts of the body (such as the womb and breasts), thereby preventing more powerful oestrogens getting through.

Phytoestrogens have also been found to stimulate the production of sex hormone-binding globulin (SHBG).[33] SHBG is a protein produced by the liver that binds sex hormones such as oestrogen in order to control how much of them are circulating in the blood at any one time. Getting the right level of SHBG gives you a better chance of hormone balance and less excess oestrogen to build up the womb lining.

High saturated fat intake

Watch your intake of saturated fats – normally found in animal products, such as dairy and red meat. These fats can block your body's absorption of the essential fatty acids that are essential for hormone balance.

Fibre

The linseeds as mentioned above are often used successfully in the treatment of irregular periods. It may be that the essential fatty acids (EFAs) in the linseeds are beneficial, and/or it may be the fact that they are phytoestrogens (see page 20). Their beneficial effect on the bowels may also explain the reason why they seem to be so effective.

Fibre helps to eliminate excess hormones from the body because it optimises the transportation of waste products out of your system. Make sure that you are eating a good amount of fibre naturally occurring in your food. Include wholegrains such as brown rice, oats, rye and plenty of fresh fruit and vegetables.

Weight

Your weight is crucial for maintaining regular cycles – and overweight is as much a problem as underweight. Balance is the key here. If you crash diet or become anorexic, your periods may not stop completely, but they can also become irregular. You could also stop ovulating while having some periods, so periods are not always a sign that all is well.

Being overweight can also prevent ovulation, and you can suffer from irregular periods. Your womb lining could also start to build up because you are not producing progesterone in the second half of the cycle.

Research has shown that just losing weight can trigger back ovulation in overweight women who had stopped ovulating.[34]

Your liver

Your liver detoxifies harmful substances, such as toxins, waste products, drugs and alcohol. It also processes the hormones that your body produces and renders them harmless. It is supposed to deactivate oestrogen (this is explained more fully on page 37), but if your liver is not functioning efficiently, you can develop an accumulation of oestrogen because it is not being excreted properly. This could also encourage the growth of the womb lining.

Make sure that you have eliminated any substances that can compromise the functioning of your liver. Alcohol is the most important substance to eliminate.

Exercise

Exercise is great for overall health, and encourages the health of your heart and circulatory system. However, when taken to an extreme, exercise can cause your periods to become irregular and even stop. Check to see whether your exercise levels are appropriate.

Stress

Stress is an important factor in connection with irregular cycles but one that is often missed. If you are under stress, the normal messages between the different parts of your body (such as your hypothalamus and pituitary glands) can be affected. These messages determine whether or not your cycle is normal and regular. Furthermore, too much prolactin can be released when you are under stress (see page 44), which can prevent ovulation.

Eliminate any foods or drinks that can increase the production of adrenaline – the hormone that is released when you are under stress. In order to keep your blood sugar in balance (see page 39), eliminate all caffeine and sugar.

Find ways to help yourself cope with stress: use essential oils in your bath, have a massage, and learn relaxation techniques, such as breathing or meditation. Find out what works for you. Take the time to work out whether there are outside factors that can be changed. For example, is your job too stressful? Could you use some extra childcare or help around the house? Do you manage to get any time for yourself? Making changes can reduce demands that increase your stress levels.

Supplements

The supplements outlined below are designed to ensure that you are well nourished – in other words, your body has all the nutrients it needs. Given the right tools, your body has a remarkable ability to balance itself. Certain supplements are also included to help you to deal with stress, and as a protective measure to prevent cells undergoing any inappropriate changes. Suggested dosages will follow in the treatment plan (see page 128).

B Vitamins

These are often called the 'stress' vitamins because they can help you to cope with the pressures of everyday life. As stress can be such an important factor in causing irregular periods it is important that you have some help in dealing with it. Vitamins B2, B3 and B6 are also necessary for thyroid hormone production (see page 450) and B5 (pantothenic acid) is essential for optimum adrenal function. Both imbalances in thyroid function and stress can affect your cycle.

The easiest way to make sure you are getting a good supply of these vitamins is to take them in the form of a good B-complex supplement. B vitamins are synergistic, which means that they work together.

Antioxidants

Antioxidants are discussed in detail on page 17, and they are particularly relevant for irregular periods. It is believed that antioxidants have the ability to prevent cells from mutating. In other words, they prevent cells from becoming 'abnormal'. This is extremely important if you have been diagnosed with thickening of the womb lining (endometrial hyperplasia), because you don't want the cells to mutate (see below). Antioxidants include vitamins A, C and E and the mineral selenium. Their significance has been proven: women with womb tumours have been shown to have lower levels of both selenium and vitamin E than women without them,[35] so make sure you are getting enough of these valuable nutrients.

Magnesium

This mineral has been classed as 'nature's tranquilliser', so it is an essential inclusion in the diet of anyone suffering from irregular periods. In fact, anyone in today's hectic society will benefit from a magnesium supplement. Stress is often a factor in period irregularity, and this mineral will help to redress the balance of a stressful lifestyle.

Essential fatty acids (EFAs)

Linseeds, which contain good amounts of Omega 3 and some Omega 6 fatty acids, have been proven to encourage regularity of the cycle (see page 123) among other things. Even if hormonal imbalance is not at the root of your condition, it is worth adding these fatty acids to your diet (see page 27). There are many factors that are now known to affect the way the fatty acids are used by our bodies, including high adrenaline levels (in the case of stress), high alcohol consumption and high levels of cholesterol. If your body is not getting or using enough of the fatty acids consumed, your cycle can be affected. You can't lose by adding these supplements to your diet.

Ann

When Ann came to see me about her menopausal symptoms, she mentioned her daughter Elizabeth, who was 12. Elizabeth had started her periods ten months earlier, and from the very beginning they were irregular. She would have a period and then, 12 days later, start another one. She often bled for over two weeks. Elizabeth was very distressed about this situation, and Ann had taken her to see her GP, who had suggested the Pill. Neither Ann nor Elizabeth were very happy about this. They rightly realised that it was not going to address the actual problem. I suggested herbs to regulate the cycle, and within three months Elizabeth's periods were back to normal.

Herbs

Herbs have a long tradition of normalising irregular periods. Two herbs in particular (*Agnus castus* and false unicorn root) are extremely useful for balancing your cycle and they can be used effectively together.

Agnus castus (vitex/chastetree berry)

This herb stimulates and normalises the function of the pituitary gland, which in turn helps to balance hormone output from the ovaries and stimulate ovulation.[36] *Agnus castus* is also useful when there is an excess of prolactin which can be suppressing ovulation. Furthermore, it has been shown to reduce thickening of the lining of the womb (endometrial hyperplasia) and can be used on a preventative basis.[37]

False unicorn root (*Chamaelirium luteum*)

This is an excellent herb for regulating periods. It acts as a tonic to strengthen the reproductive system. It works across the whole cycle to ensure that balance is maintained, but its biggest impact is on the first half of the cycle, when it acts to regulate the action of the ovaries.

As well as using herbs to help normalise the cycle, they can also be used to help you control stress, which may be affecting your cycle. Herbs that are used specifically to cope with stress are known as 'nervines', and they act on the nervous system to relieve anxiety, tension and irritability. One of the best known nervines is valerian. It is most effective when combined with another herb, skullcap, which acts both to relax and tonify the nervous system.

Natural medicine

Both homeopathy and acupuncture can be very successful in the treatment of irregular periods and they can be used alongside the other recommendations.

The Treatment Plan

Before undertaking the treatment plan, you will need to have had full investigations to find out if there is a medical reason why you are having irregular periods.

Follow the plan below, depending on what diagnosis you have been given. In each section I have suggested how you can integrate this approach with recommendations from your doctor.

Tests show nothing wrong

If your tests are all clear, and that there is nothing unusual going on with your reproductive organs (your womb and ovaries, for example), go ahead and try the natural recommendations. Similarly, if the blood tests on the hormones are all normal, you can go straight on to the natural treatment plan.

Thickening of the womb (endometrial hyperplasia)

If you are told that your womb lining has thickened, you will need to take steps to address this immediately. Endometrial hyperplasia increases the risk factor for womb cancer. That's not to say you'll definitely suffer from cancer at some point in the future, but the risk is there, depending on the whether or not there have been cell changes. It has been estimated that between 1 and 4 per cent of women with mild hyperplasia develop womb cancer but more than 20 per cent of women develop cancer if the hyperplasia is in an advanced stage.[38]

Given the potential severity of the condition, I believe that it is essential to go for conventional treatment, followed by a natural approach to stop it recurring.

You need to get rid of that excess womb lining and your gynaecologist will recommend which approach would be most effective, depending on your particular situation and what has been seen on the ultrasound scans. So it may be suggested that you take drugs to shed the womb lining or have surgery to remove it.

While you wait for surgery or begin a course of drugs, begin taking nutritional supplements, but avoid the herbal treatments until after the excess womb lining has been removed. The aim of this treatment is to get you back into a regular cycle.

A follow-up scan would be useful six months after the start of treatment, to make sure that the natural approach is working and that your womb lining is not starting to build up again.

Hormone imbalance

If you are told that your irregular cycles are due to a problem with your endocrine (hormonal) system, there is a possibility that your condition could be related to your thyroid, pituitary, ovaries or the adrenal glands. In this situation, ask your doctor if the problem requires urgent medical attention and what would happen if you left it for six months. If the answer is that it is fine for you to adopt a 'wait and see approach', then embark on the natural recommendations immediately. The natural plan outlined below has proved to be one of the most successful ways to treat any problem associated with hormone imbalance.

Your Supplement Plan

- a good multivitamin and mineral supplement

- B-complex vitamin (containing 100mg of most of the B vitamins per day)

- magnesium (300mg per day)

- linseed oil (also known as flaxseed oil at 1,000mg per day)

- vitamin C (1,000mg per day)

- an antioxidant supplement, containing vitamin A and selenium)

> ### Note
> Each nutrient represents the total intake for one day, so if your multivitamin and mineral already contains 100mg of magnesium, for example, you only need to add in a separate magnesium supplement containing 200mg per day.

Herbs

Take a blend of equal parts of *Agnus castus* and false unicorn root. One teaspoon should be taken three times daily. Stop taking these herbs during your period, and start again after it has finished, to give your body a rest. These herbs can be taken over a period of six months to help regulate the cycle. If there is not sufficient improvement after six months, you need to see a qualified practitioner.

If you think that your problem is stress related, continue taking the above herbs, but add in another tincture containing equal parts of the herbs valerian and skullcap. Take these alongside the other herbs, and use them in the same way.

To make this programme simpler, I have formulated the Natural Cycle Pack – Menstrual Regular made by the Natural Health Practice, which contains the above nutrients and herbs. If you can't get this locally then call 01892 750511 and it can be posted to you.

> **Note**
> Chapter 1 contains important advice about using tampons (see pages 46–8).

In summary

- Always investigate the cause of irregular periods before taking any drugs, or beginning a natural treatment programme.

- Follow the hormone balancing diet on page 16.

- Take steps to reduce any stress in your life.

- Add linseeds to your daily diet for their phytoestrogen content.

- Ensure that you get plenty of the antioxidant vitamins and minerals, which can help to prevent womb cancer.

- Take supplements (see page 130) throughout your entire cycle.

- Take herbs between periods.

NO PERIODS (AMENORRHOEA)

Periods can be missed both at the beginning and end of our reproductive life. In the beginning, when we enter puberty, hormones can take a number of months to settle down into a proper rhythm. Much the same thing occurs as we move towards the menopause, and missing periods can be quite common. There are also natural reasons why we do not have periods – for example, during pregnancy and while breastfeeding. However, if you suffer from an absence of periods for more than six months, without any of these natural causes or at these normal times, you can be sure that what you are experiencing is not natural.

What is Amenorrhoea?

The term 'amenorrhoea' literally means 'the absence of periods'. It may seem like a fairly straightforward diagnosis – either you have periods, or you don't. However, amenorrhoea is not a diagnosed condition, but a symptom of another problem. There are a wide variety of reasons why you may not be having periods, and you must always take steps to find out what is causing your amenorrhoea.

It's not normal for women to have no periods, and there will be something at the root of the problem. I have come across many women whose periods have inexplicably stopped. When they visited their doctors, they were told that it was 'more convenient' to go without periods, and that there was no reason to look into it unless they wanted to conceive. Drugs could be then be offered at that time to stimulate ovulation.

There is no doubt that periods can be inconvenient, but the plain truth is that it is unnatural not to have them. Your body is designed to have menstrual cycles when you are not pregnant, and if you are not having periods there is something out of balance or unnatural happening in your body. This needs to be investigated and treated. For one thing, if you are not having periods, your risk of osteoporosis can be greatly increased.

Amenorrhoea is classified into two main groups: primary and secondary.

Primary amenorrhoea

Primary amenorrhoea occurs when your periods never start. Girls can normally expect to start their periods by the age of 12 in Western countries and at the same time various female characteristics mature, such as breast development and pubic hair growth.

The cause of primary amenorrhoea is often very different to that of secondary amenorrhoea (see below), where periods start normally but inexplicably cease for a number of months. One of the main causes of primary amenorrhoea is underweight. Fat is a 'factory' for making oestrogen, which is necessary for a menstrual cycle. It may be that weight is the root of your condition, but you will need to seek specialist advice so that detailed investigations can be undertaken.

It may be that your periods are simply much later than usual in coming. Late onset of menstruation tends to run in families, so if your mother didn't get her first period until she was 18, chances are that you won't either.

Secondary amenorrhoea

For the purposes of this book, we will concentrate on secondary amenorrhoea, which is more easily treated with a natural approach. In this type of amenorrhoea, your periods start normally but they stop for a period of at least six months. There are various causes, which will be discussed below.

What is the Cause?

If your periods stop for no apparent reason or you have come off the Pill and your periods have not come back, then you should ask to be referred to a gynaecologist. Many of the reasons why periods stop are not serious, but more serious health problems should always be ruled out before you decide upon a form of treatment.

A gynaecologist will normally organise an examination and a pelvic ultrasound scan to look at your reproductive organs. You will also be given a blood test, which will assess your hormone levels.

Common Causes of Amenorrhoea
and Conventional Treatments

Pregnancy

This may seem an obvious cause, but you'd be surprised at the number of women who have not considered this possibility. It's possible to be pregnant and still get monthly bleeding. Bleeding can occur when the newly fertilised embryo is implanting itself in the womb lining. This 'implantation bleed' can be lighter than a usual period. This can take place for about three months, around the same time that the normal period would occur. If you misinterpreted this bleeding as your usual period and didn't have intercourse the next month, you might assume that pregnancy was impossible! However, you were pregnant already!

Even if you are not having periods, it is important to use contraception if you are not planning a pregnancy. Some women become pregnant after months of having no periods because conception takes place during the first month of ovulation, in much the same way as it does with women who become pregnant while breastfeeding. Breastfeeding on demand can prevent ovulation for some time, but you may become pregnant during the first cycle that you ovulated, unaware that your periods were about to start again.

Polycystic ovary syndrome (PCOS)

PCOS can be one of the main reasons for periods to stop. This condition is diagnosed with a scan and blood tests, and the various treatments available are detailed in Chapter 7.

Coming off the Pill

This is a very common cause of no periods. Many of the women who have come to see me about period problems confirm that their periods were regular before they went on the Pill. After stopping, their menstrual cycles never resume. A pelvic ultrasound scan usually reveals that the ovaries look normal, but they are just not functioning.

Occasionally, taking the Pill can mask another problem, such as polycystic ovary syndrome (see page 232). The problem would not become apparent because the Pill gives women a regular 'bleed', unrelated to any natural cycle. Polycystic ovaries would show up on an ultrasound scan.

If the ovaries look normal, and all other medical checks are normal (for example, your hormone levels are within the normal ranges), then natural remedies can be enormously effective. The idea is to kick-start the body back into action. Long periods of time on the Pill mean that your body has gone without ovulating for some time. The ovaries often have to be triggered back into working again.

Unfortunately the usual medical 'treatment' for this problem is to put women back on the Pill so that you experience a cycle of some kind. You may trick your body into having a monthly bleed, but it is not a period. This approach does not address the problem and what tends to happen is that women continue on the Pill until they want to conceive, and then find that they need high levels of drugs to stimulate ovulation in order to do so.

High Prolactin Levels (Hyperprolactinaemia)

Prolactin is a hormone released by the pituitary gland, and in unnaturally high quantities, it can cause your periods to stop. It is the hormone that is released in high amounts when breastfeeding, and it can stop ovulation and menstruation. One of the symptoms of high prolactin levels is the secretion of breast milk, which can appear even in women who have not recently had a baby.

A blood test designed to check hormone levels will look out for high levels of prolactin. If they are found, further tests would be organised to rule out any factors that may be causing this overproduction. Possible causes of high prolactin levels include an underactive thyroid (hypothyroidism) or a tumour on the pituitary gland.

The usual treatment for this problem is the use of the drug bromocriptine or cabergoline. They do reduce prolactin levels, but there are some fairly debilitating side-effects, such as nausea, vomiting, headaches and dizziness.

It is also possible to suffer from high prolactin levels without any medical reason. One of the factors involved in raised levels that cannot be medically diagnosed includes stress (see below).

Premature menopause

Until recently, this problem has not received much attention and, as a result, was often missed as the diagnosis. Since then, an organisation called the Daisy Network (see Useful Addresses) has been set up to help support women who find out they have suffered a premature menopause.

It can be devastating for a young woman to discover that her periods have stopped due to an early menopause. Not only does it make having a baby much more difficult, if not impossible, but there are some difficult health issues to address, largely because the menopause is associated with so many symptoms, such as hot flushes, vaginal dryness and, even more dangerous for a young woman, osteoporosis.

Premature menopause is usually diagnosed with a combination of blood tests and scans. The hormone FSH (follicle stimulating hormone) rises as we get nearer to the menopause, and young women should have comparatively low levels. High levels are an instant indication that the menopause is on the horizon. This is one reason why it is essential that a battery of blood tests are undertaken at the same time. Your doctor will need a full picture of what is happening in your body, and early menopause is just one possibility that needs to be considered.

In my practice, I have seen some women experience premature menopause as early as 17 years of age. Periods start normally and then, after a couple of years, suddenly stop. For 70 per cent of women who experience a premature menopause, there is no medical reason why this has happened. For others it may have been caused by radiotherapy or surgery.

Any woman in this position will need medical help to become pregnant, and you will need to discuss the use of HRT (hormone replacement therapy). You may be surprised to hear me suggesting that HRT might be useful (one of my best-selling books is *Natural Alternatives to HRT*), but it is important to remember that premature menopause is not a natural menopause, which normally occurs around the age of 50. Premature menopause is a medical condition that means a young woman will be short of essential female hormones for as long as 30 to 40 years. These hormones are essential for her bones and for preventing many of the other symptoms that can occur around the menopause, such as vaginal dryness and hot flushes.

However, if there is no medical reason for your premature menopause and a scan indicates that your ovaries look healthy, it is well worth following the natural recommendations to get your periods back. From my experience, it seems that the sooner you do something about the problem, the greater the chance that the natural approach will work – in other words, if you start the treatment plan as soon as your periods stopped and your condition is diagnosed, you will have more chance of getting back your menstrual cycle.

Susan

Susan, a healthy 40-year-old woman, came to see because her periods had suddenly stopped. She had been to see her doctor and blood tests showed she was menopausal. She was getting hot flushes and was concerned because she felt she was a 'bit too young' to be going through the menopause. I asked her what had been happening around the time that her periods ceased, and she said that she had been made redundant and had also lost her father.

I explained that the aim would be to ensure that she was as healthy as possible, addressing any problems with her diet, checking out any vitamin and mineral deficiencies, working on her stress levels and using some herbs to help balance her hormones. She was happy with this approach because she felt that attaining optimum health would help her to feel much better, regardless of whether her periods came back. Within a couple of months, her periods returned and her doctor performed a further test that showed she was no longer 'menopausal'.

During times of stress, either physical (during weight loss, for example) or emotional (during bereavement), your body starts to shut down the reproductive system in order to give you the resources you need to cope with what is going on. Susan was able to address the cause of her amenorrhoea, and her body quickly kicked back into action.

Weight

Your periods can stop because you are either underweight or overweight. Nature is always striving for balance. It is just as unhealthy to have a low blood sugar problem as it is to have high blood sugar, and the same holds true with your weight. Women come in all different shapes and sizes, and there is a wide band to accommodate these variations. What is important is that you fall within this band (the normal range) for your height. Your hormone balance depends on your weight being right for your height.

The best guideline for assessing whether or not you fall within this normal band is to check your BMI (Body Mass Index), which is a measure of the ratio of your height to weight (see page 446).

It's obviously healthy not to be overweight, but being underweight can cause problems too.

Underweight

Your body is extremely clever. If you are going through a famine and food is in short supply, your body will shut down your reproductive system. The reproductive system is the only system you don't need in order to keep you alive. So, during times when your body believes that it could be on the brink of death, it channels its resources away from your reproductive organs to other areas of greater need. Another reason why this occurs is because your body throws into action a sort of natural birth control. It senses that there is not enough food to sustain both you and a baby, so it takes steps to prevent a pregnancy before it can happen.

If you lose 10–15 per cent of your body weight fairly quickly, your body will think there is a famine. It does not know you have lost weight deliberately (or even not deliberately!), it just registers the drop and causes your periods to stop.

Body fat is essential for reproduction and nature keeps fat stored on women's bodies just in case a pregnancy occurs. We now know, for example, that girls do not begin to menstruate until their bodies are composed of at least 17 per cent fat. We also know that over-weight young girls are more likely to menstruate early.

Crash dieting or simply being underweight in general can be the cause of your periods stopping, as can eating disorders such as anorexia.

Furthermore, if you have been restricting your food intake over time, it is likely that you will be deficient in certain nutrients. As well as looking at your diet, it is important to address any vitamin or mineral deficiencies.

In order to encourage your periods, you need to return to a normal BMI (see page 447). If you have anorexia, then you will undoubtedly need emotional support and psychological help because other, deeper issues will have to be resolved in order to resume a good pattern of eating (see Useful Addresses).

If being underweight is the reason for losing your periods, you will be reassured to know that this can be fairly easily redressed once you have started to nourish yourself properly, and have reached a weight that is natural for you.

Overweight

There are many reasons why being overweight can cause health problems. It's well known that it can increase the risk of heart attacks, high blood pressure, diabetes and more. What you may not know is that it can also cause menstrual disturbances. Your weight may the reason why your periods have stopped.

Overweight women have low levels of SHBG (sex hormone-binding globulin), which is a protein produced by the liver that binds sex hormones such as oestrogen and testosterone in order to control how much of them freely circulate in the blood at any one time. Body fat also manufactures oestrogen, so the more fat you have, the higher the levels of oestrogen you can have. While it may seem a good thing to be producing oestrogen, excess levels do, however, cause an imbalance between the hormones in your body. This can play havoc with normal egg development and ovulation.

It has been found that losing weight can make an enormous difference, by creating a normal hormone balance, making periods more regular and stimulating ovulation.[39] It is, therefore, very important to eat healthily and reach your natural BMI without dieting. If you would like additional help in order to lose weight, see page 458, or get a copy of my book, *Natural Alternatives to Dieting*.

If you are overweight and find it difficult to lose weight, consider the possibility that you may have a thyroid problem (see below).

Thyroid problems

Balance is the key word in health, and once again it is important that your thyroid hormones are balanced. Both an underactive thyroid (hypothyroidism) or an overactive thyroid (hyperthyroidism) can be at the root of your period problems.

An underactive thyroid causes lower levels of SHBG, a protein which binds circulating oestrogen and testosterone. If you do not have enough SHBG then you will have too much free circulating oestrogen and testosterone, which can stop your periods. An underactive thyroid is also connected with high levels of prolactin, which can prevent ovulation and cause your periods to stop. Prolactin is the hormone that is produced when you are breastfeeding.

An overactive thyroid is also problematic because it speeds up the metabolism and all the processes in the body. It can be the cause of periods stopping. Furthermore, most women suffering from an overactive thyroid are underweight, which brings its own problems (see page 138).

Levels of thyroid hormone in your body can be checked by a blood test, and suitable treatment will then be suggested (see pages 450–2).

Exercise

Your periods can stop if you exercise too often or too heavily. In much the same way that crash dieting can (see page 140), over-exercise reduces your body fat to a level where menstruation ceases. This is a common problem for female gymnasts and athletes, and it can even be the cause of primary amenorrhoea (where periods do not even begin), because the body fat ratio is so low. If you are suffering from any type of amenorrhoea, consider whether overexercise or training could be the cause. Try reducing the duration, frequency and intensity of your exercise programme to see if it makes a difference.

In some gyms, your body fat ratio can be measured, and you will be given an instant assessment which will tell you whether it is too low. In the case of a low ratio, you can work on decreasing exercise and putting on a little more weight to trigger the return of your periods.

It doesn't take very long or even much effort to encourage your periods to begin again. In one study scientists asked a 19-year-old runner who wasn't having periods to increase her calorie intake by a small amount a day and to reduce her training by one day a week. Within three months her periods were back to normal.

Stress

It is well known that emotional trauma, such as a bereavement or an accident, can cause your periods suddenly to stop. They can also stop when you are generally under stress from work pressures, relationship problems, financial concerns or anything else that places extra demands on your system.[40] Once again, it seems to be nature's way of protecting you from becoming pregnant at a time when you would find it hard to cope.

It is believed that stress interrupts the brain message GnRH (gonadotrophin-releasing hormone), which causes the pituitary gland to release the two hormones FSH (follicle-stimulating hormone) and LH (luteinizing hormone). These are needed to stimulate the ovaries to produce and release eggs. Stress can also increase levels of prolactin (see page 44), which again will prevent ovulation

Stress also affects your nutritional status. Adrenaline is a hormone that is released when you are under stress. It is meant to be released in a time of danger, and it is known as the 'fight or flight' hormone. When your body senses that it is under pressure or threat, it provokes an immediate and dramatic response. Your liver releases stored sugar into the bloodstream in the event that you may need instant energy. Blood is taken away from the skin and moved into muscles and internal organs. Your heart speeds up and the arteries tighten to raise your blood pressure in order to move the blood to where it is needed most. Your blood thickens, ready to clot, in case you are injured. Your digestion shuts down because all energy is diverted to the organs that need it most.

Unfortunately, this natural response to a stressful situation kicks into action all too often if your life is stressful. Where once it was designed to save a life when faced with real danger, it now comes into play on a regular basis for situations that are not life-threatening.

If you are living on adrenaline, your digestion will be compromised and you will not be absorbing nutrients properly from your food. Over time this can leave you malnourished, lacking vital vitamins and minerals.

Take a careful look at the stress in your life and consider whether you have unrealistic expectations or goals, are putting too much pressure on yourself, or whether there are other external factors with which you are forced to cope. You should look at what can be changed externally or whether you need to change your attitude to life in general. Relaxation techniques can also help you to cope with stress on a regular basis.

What Natural Treatments Can Be Effective?

If medical tests indicate that there is nothing seriously wrong, this section is for you. You may have been told 'to wait and see' or to go on the Pill as a form of treatment. In fact, this is one of those situations where the natural approach really comes into its own. By looking at your diet, correcting any vitamin and mineral deficiencies, and using herbs, it is possible to correct the underlying imbalance that is causing the loss of periods.

The programme is as follows:

1. Follow the hormone balancing diet from Chapter 1, which will ensure that your body is well nourished and that your hormones are working correctly.

2. Take the supplements to provide the nutrients your body needs to get itself back into optimum health, and add those nutrients that are important for the normal functioning of your reproductive system.

3. Use herbs in order to 'kick-start' your body back into having periods.

4. Look at your lifestyle to assess what you can do to alleviate stress levels, if this is a factor.

5. Aim to reach your natural weight, whether you are underweight or overweight.

Dietary changes

It is extremely important that you follow the hormone balancing diet detailed in Chapter 1. Your body needs to be well nourished in order to function normally and to encourage regular menstrual cycles.

You need to have a good variety of food. Do not restrict your diet to just a few food choices. The more variety you have, the more likely you are to get a good range of nutrients. Include grains, beans, vegetables, fruit, nuts, seeds and fish. Seaweed would also be a good food to eat because it contains significant amounts of the trace minerals zinc, manganese, chromium, selenium and cobalt, and the macro minerals calcium, magnesium, iron and iodine.

It is also important to look at your weight, to ensure that it falls within the normal range of BMI. Whether you are overweight or underweight, the effects on your cycle can be dramatic.

Stress, which causes adrenaline to be released, can be the product of outside pressures in your life. It can also, however, be caused by internal stress caused by demands placed upon your body. What you eat and drink can make a difference to how much adrenaline is surging round your body.

While you trying to get your periods back, cut out anything with caffeine and sugar, in order to keep your blood sugar in balance. If your blood sugar fluctuates, and you suffer from dips (hypoglycaemia), your body will automatically release adrenaline to encourage your liver to make more glucose in an attempt to bring up your blood sugar. You then experience surges of adrenaline during the day, when it really should only ever be released in response to danger. It's also a good idea to eat little and often, in order to keep blood sugar levels balanced (see page 39).

Also, watch your alcohol consumption. Alcohol puts enormous pressure on the liver, and this vital organ needs to be as healthy as possible in order to process hormones, toxins and waste products in the body.

If you have been dieting you are likely to be deficient in vital nutrients. The same applies if you have been under a lot of stress (see page 44).

Previous use of the Pill will also have upset your intake of nutrients. You may have low levels of the B vitamins, especially B2, B6, B12 and also folic acid.[41] It is also well known that the Pill upsets the balance of copper and zinc in your body. You can end up with too much copper and not enough zinc.[42] This imbalance can still exist even if it has been some time since you took the Pill regularly. Zinc is crucial for healthy functioning of your reproductive system (see below).

Supplements

B Vitamins
A B-complex supplement needs to be added to your diet on a daily basis. Choose one that contains good levels of all the B vitamins, including folic acid. Folic acid is absolutely crucial for your cells to multiply normally. When working on getting your periods back, it's important that your ovaries are able to produce eggs, and that the cells in those eggs are able to divide properly.

Zinc
Zinc is an important mineral for the normal functioning of your hormones. It plays a major part in the part in the normal function of many of our hormones, including the sex hormones and insulin. It is needed for normal egg production in the ovaries, and for your body

to attract and utilise your reproductive hormones, oestrogen and progesterone.[43] Zinc can be deficient if you have been using the Pill for a while.

Magnesium

This mineral has been classed as 'nature's tranquilliser', so it is essential that it is included at a good level when treating absent periods. Stress is often a major factor in amenorrhoea, and this mineral will help to redress the balance of a stressful lifestyle.

Essential fatty acids (EFAs)

In Chapter 1, I outlined the importance of essential fatty acids, and they are also essential for normal reproductive functioning. If you suffer from secondary amenorrhoea, it is likely that you are deficient in EFAs, and they will need to be included in your diet in supplement form. This is particularly important if you have been on a low-fat or no-fat diet.

Herbs

Herbal treatment is aimed at literally 'kick-starting' your reproductive system. This means that the right messages need to get to your brain so that the pituitary gland can send the correct message down to your ovaries to stimulate ovulation.

Agnus castus (vitex/chastetree berry)

Agnus castus is very much the herb of choice when trying to bring back periods. It works on the pituitary gland by balancing the levels of FSH (follicle-stimulating hormone) and LH (luteinizing hormone), which then sends a message to the ovaries. The result is that progesterone levels go up and your cycle kicks back into action. This can take between three and six months.

In one study, 10 out of 15 women's period had returned after using *Agnus castus* for a six-month period.[44]

Agnus castus is also helpful in reducing high prolactin levels, particularly those caused by stress.[45]

Other useful herbs

Agnus castus is the herb of choice and should be taken daily. However, it is a good idea to add in equal parts of two other herbs: black cohosh

(*Cimicifuga racemosa*) and false unicorn root (*Chamaelirium luteum*). Black cohosh helps to normalise imbalances in the female hormones and is used to restart periods. False unicorn root helps to improve the functioning of the ovary to encourage a normal cycle. This herb also has a balancing effect on the hormones.

If you suspect that stress may be playing a large part in your amenorrhoea, consider taking the herb Siberian ginseng (*Eleutherococcus senticosus*). This herb is classed as an adaptogen, which means that it works according to your body's need – providing energy when required, and helping to combat stress and fatigue when you are under pressure. It helps the adrenal glands, which will have been under extreme pressure if you have been stressed. Siberian ginseng is extremely useful when you have been under mental or physical stress and should be taken for around three months.

Natural medicine

Both acupuncture and homeopathy can be very useful in the treatment of amenorrhoea, and can be used successfully alongside the natural recommendations outlined above.

Joanne

Joanne came to see because she had stopped taking the Pill several years before our consultation, and her periods had still not returned. Her doctor suggested that she go back on the Pill, but she realised that this was no long-term solution. She was obviously concerned that her lack of periods would have an effect on her bones, but she wanted to address the problem naturally, because she felt that she would, otherwise, be on the Pill 'for ever'. An ultrasound scan had shown no abnormalities and that her ovaries were healthy. Nothing untoward showed up on the blood tests.

Joanne changed her way of eating and added in a number of supplements to correct deficiencies that were pinpointed by a mineral analysis. She also took some herbs to help 'kick-start' her reproductive system. Within three months, her regular cycle had returned. She discontinued the herbal treatment, but went on to a maintenance programme involving a series of supplements. She also continued to eat well and her periods have continued normally ever since.

Your Supplement Plan

- A good multivitamin and mineral supplement, eg The Healthy Woman by the Natural Health Practice
- B complex (providing 100mg of most of the B vitamins per day – including those supplied by your multivitamin supplement)
- Folic acid (800mcg per day – including those supplied by your B-complex supplement and your multivitamin)
- Zinc citrate (15mg per day)
- Magnesium (300mg per day)
- Linseed (flaxseed) oil (1000mg per day)

Note

Each nutrient represents the total intake for one day, so if your multivitamin and mineral already contains 100mg of magnesium, for example, you only need to add in a separate magnesium supplement containing 200mg per day.

Herbs

Have a tincture, which is an equal blend of *Agnus castus*, black cohosh and false unicorn herbs. Take 1 teaspoon three times daily. If you are under stress, add Siberian ginseng in tincture form (again, 1 teaspoon, three times daily).

Take these herbs for six months and, if your periods have not begun by then, see a qualified practitioner.

In Summary

- Always investigate the cause of your periods stopping before taking any drugs, or beginning a natural treatment programme. Remember that amenorrhoea is a symptom, not a condition in itself.

- Consider the possibility that you may be pregnant.

- Ensure that any blood tests involve checking for premature menopause, thyroid function and diabetes.

- Begin the hormone balancing diet (see page 16).

- Ensure that you are within the normal range of your BMI (see page 447), and that you address any overweight or underweight problems.

- Take steps to reduce the amount of stress in your life.

- Make sure you are not exercising too hard or too often.

- Take supplements (see page 143) for six months.

- Take herbs (see above) for six months.

- Do not take herbs if you are on the Pill, but begin the dietary recommendations and take the supplements (see page 143). When you stop taking the Pill, start taking the herbs (see page 144).

PAINFUL PERIODS (DYSMENORRHOEA)

It is estimated that between 50 and 70 per cent of women endure some degree of period pain and cramping. Of those, approximately 10 per cent experience contractions so extreme that they are one-and-a-half times more powerful than labour pains.

How Painful is Painful?

Every month many women suffer from pain around the time of their periods. For some women the pain can be so debilitating that they are forced to take time off work or can only get through their periods by dosing themselves with painkillers. Pain is normally considered to be a message from your body, telling you that something is wrong and that an investigation is in order. However, painful periods are viewed somewhat differently by the medical profession and many women who complain of period pains are advised to take a painkiller and to get on with it.

Every one of us has a different pain threshold, and it is impossible to imagine what another person might be experiencing. Only you know whether or not your period pains are unacceptably high for you, and if the pain is affecting the quality of your life, it's time to do something about it.

What Symptoms Could You Experience?

Obviously pain is the overriding symptom in dysmenorrhoea, but many women will experience other symptoms, including:

- nausea
- vomiting
- diarrhoea/constipation
- fainting
- light-headedness
- feeling dizzy
- headaches
- exhaustion and lethargy.

The pain itself can vary and women will often experience two types of pain:

- a constant, low, dull backache (congestive dysmenorrhoea) and/or
- cramping pains like contractions (spasmodic dysmenorrhoea)

Finding Out If There is a Reason For the Pain

Because pain is usually a warning signal from your body, it is important that the pain is investigated. But period pains can, however, be unusual in that there may actually be nothing medically wrong.

There are two categories of painful periods:

1. **Primary dysmenorrhoea** Primary dysmenorrhoea means that there is no specific problem or abnormality causing the pain.

2. **Secondary dysmenorrhoea** Secondary dysmenorrhoea means that the pain is caused by a specific condition, such as endometriosis, fibroids or an infection, etc.

You will need a full investigation in order to assess which of these two types of dysmenorrhoea you are suffering.

This section will concentrate on primary dysmenorrhoea – in other words, painful periods that do not have a diagnosable medical cause. If you are suffering from secondary dysmenorrhoea, you will need to address the cause of the pain, such as endometriosis or fibroids (see pages 165 and 185).

What Can Cause You to have Painful Periods?

Throughout the month, your womb contracts and relaxes on a regular basis. You will probably be entirely unaware that these contractions are taking place. However, around the time of your period, they become stronger. In order to squeeze out blood from the lining built up during your menstrual cycle, your womb has to contract. This should, theoretically, be a painless or only mildly painful occurrence, but for some women, the contractions are stronger than they need to be, causing enormous pain.

Cramping can also occur and this tends to be connected with

heavy periods (see page 102). The greater the build-up of womb lining, the more violent the contractions needed to get rid of the engorged blood.

There is also supposed to be a resting phase between contractions, but when the contractions are so strong, the womb does not relax properly in between. In this case, the blood flow and, consequently, the oxygen supply to the womb, is restricted, which can cause pain. This is the same principle as applies in the case of a tension headache – tense neck muscles constrict the oxygen supply to your brain and you experience pain as a result.

Prostaglandins

Another cause of painful periods can be the excess production and release of hormone-like substances called prostaglandins. Many of the prostaglandins are actually 'healthy', and have a beneficial effect on the body (see page 154). However, two types of 'bad' prostaglandins, known as PGF2 Alpha and PGE2, can be increased in some women. PGF2 Alpha is a vasoconstrictor, which means that it works to reduce the blood flow to the womb muscle, and PGE2 is a highly inflammatory substance that can trigger muscle contractions and increase the sensitivity of your nerve endings to pain.

Research has shown that women with primary dysmenorrhoea have significantly higher levels of both prostaglandins PGF2 Alpha and PGE2.[46]

Prostaglandins are present in every cell in your body. They tend to be low in the first half of the cycle and then rise sharply towards your period, and can cause a variety of other symptoms including headaches, nausea and fatigue.

The natural treatment section on page 155 explains how you can help your body to produce fewer of these 'bad' prostaglandins to alleviate your symptoms.

> **Note**
> Chapter 1 contains important advice about using tampons (see pages 46–8).

What Treatment Can You Be Offered By Your Doctor?

The usual medical approach would be to suggest using painkillers. If this is successful, you would take them as required during your cycle. If the pain is debilitating, you may be offered the Pill. The Pill produces a 'false' cycle, which means no real menstrual bleeding (only a withdrawal bleed) and therefore no pain.

Drugs

The Pill
The Pill works by suppressing ovulation, which gives you an artificial cycle. You will not really experience a period, just a monthly 'bleed' that occurs when you stop taking your tablet for a week each cycle. Some of the listed side-effects include nausea, vomiting, headache, thrombosis, changes in sex drive, depression and breast tenderness.

Mefenamic acid
This is a strong painkiller that blocks the production of prostaglandins (see above). It is available on prescription. Side-effects can include drowsiness, diarrhoea and rashes.

Ibuprofen
Painkillers, such as ibuprofen, can be more effective than aspirin because they not only kill pain, but they also act as a muscle-relaxant and an anti-inflammatory, and reduce the effect of 'bad' prostaglandins in the body. Side-effects can include gastrointestinal disturbances, nausea and diarrhoea.

WHAT HAPPENS WHEN YOU STOP TAKING THE DRUGS?

None of the drugs for painful periods do anything to reverse the imbalance at the root of the pain. For example, they do not address the underlying reason why you are producing too many of the prostaglandins that cause the womb to overcontract. They also do

---

nothing to treat the reason why you may be building up too much blood every month, or why your womb is unable to relax between contractions.

Furthermore, all drugs carry a risk of side-effects. Unfortunately those that reduce the production of prostaglandins (such as mefenamic acid and ibuprofen) have a wide range of side-effects and are particularly hard on the digestive system, causing nausea, diarrhoea, rashes and digestive discomfort.

Some of the drugs are only taken when there is pain (such as mefenamic acid and ibuprofen), which at least limits the potential damage done in your body. However, drugs like the Pill would be taken daily, which can have an effect on overall health when taken long term.

Surgical Techniques

The only surgical technique you would be offered is a hysterectomy. This should only be considered after you have tried everything else – an absolutely last resort. It is a drastic 'solution' to painful periods.

Hysterectomy

This is the most extreme form of medical 'treatment' for painful periods. The implications of having major surgery for painful periods would need to be considered; hysterectomy choices are discussed in Chapter 5. In order even to contemplate this 'treatment' you will have to have reached the stage where you felt you could not live with a period every month, and that no conventional or natural treatments have made the pain bearable.

What Natural Treatments Could Be Effective?

It is important to remember that the cause of primary dysmenorrhoea is simply an abnormal functioning of your body around the time of your period. This is pretty good news because it means that if you can get things back into balance, you'll not only get rid of the pain but you'll prevent it from returning. What the natural approach aims to do is to treat the condition, not simply mask the pain or 'turn off' your cycle. Furthermore, if you work to put your body back into balance, all aspects of your health and well-being will be improved. For example, if you sort out a prostaglandin imbalance, you will decrease the levels of 'bad' prostaglandins in your blood. These prostaglandins are the same ones that can make your blood clot inappropriately (stroke), raise blood pressure (heart attacks), increase inflammation and pain (which could lead to conditions like arthritis) and lower your immune function (which leaves you susceptible to many other problems).

So, in the short term, the aim is to get rid of the pain, but by following the recommendations below you'll also achieve optimum health.

There are five stages involved in this treatment programme:

1. Improve your diet, based on the recommendations outlined in Chapter 1.

2. Use nutritional supplements that are known scientifically to help with painful periods.

3. Control high levels of 'bad' prostaglandins, which can increase the pain, by what you eat and by taking appropriate supplements.

4. Use specific herbs in the *long* term, in order to improve the general functioning of your womb, so that it does not overcontract.

5. Use specific herbs in the *short* term, in order to help control the pain while you are having a period.

Dietary changes

In Chapter 1 we established the concept that what you eat is the foundation of your health. Taking that one step further, diet is also extremely important – even critical – to the treatment of painful periods. Why? Because the substances (prostaglandins) that are normally at the root of the pain are increased or decreased according to what you eat.

As you have seen, there are both 'good' and 'bad' prostaglandins. PGE2 is classed as a 'bad' prostaglandin because it increases the womb contractions and increases the pain. PGE1 is classed as a 'good' prostaglandin because, among other things, it also does the following:

- relaxes and widens blood vessels, which improves blood flow

- prevents inflammation

- improves the way your body gets rid of sodium (salt, which is connected to water retention and bloating)

- regulates the immune system

PGE3 can also be classed as a 'good' prostaglandin because it helps to reduce inflammation and abnormal blood clotting.

It's fairly obvious that you need more of these 'good' prostaglandins if you are suffering from period pains, but your body has to produce them in order for them to be there to have an effect.

How are prostaglandins produced?

Essential fatty acids (EFAs) in your diet provide the raw materials for the production of prostaglandins. So the starting point is the amount and quality of essential fatty acids (oils) that you eat. The essential fatty acids are discussed in detail in Chapter 1 and below you will see how your body makes the choice between producing 'good' or 'bad' prostaglandins.

What you need to do as a starting point is to adjust your diet so that you are increasing those foods that begin the process of producing beneficial prostaglandins (PGE1 and PGE3) and reduce the foods that cause your body to produce too many of the negatives ones (PGE2), which increase contractions and inflammation. As well as providing your body with the right foods to kick-start the beneficial prostaglandin process, you also need to make sure that there is nothing in your diet or your lifestyle that will prevent your body from converting the right foods into healthy prostaglandins.

The best way to get to grips with this system is to imagine that there are two trains (Omega 3 and Omega 6) running along a number of tracks. The Omega 3 train needs to reach the PGE3 station and the Omega 6 train needs to reach the PGE1 station. If there are any obstacles on the Omega 6 track, the train will be redirected towards the PGE2 station.

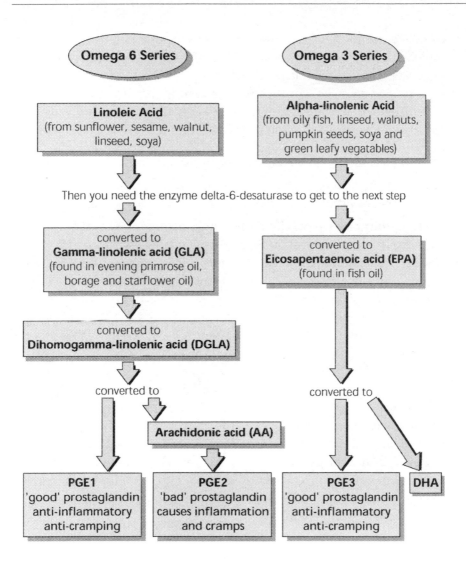

The production of good and bad prostaglandins

Foods that encourage the production of 'bad' prostaglandins (PGE2)

As you can see from the chart above, it is very important that you avoid all of those foods that are high in arachidonic acid (AA). Your body produces PGE2 from AA, of which the main sources are dairy products. This means eliminating or at least reducing dairy in any form, including milk, cheese, cottage cheese, yoghurt, butter and even dairy ice–cream. AA is also present in red meat and although the saturated fat content of red meat is higher than in the white meats, AA is higher in chicken and turkey than in red meat.

You may then be concerned about your calcium intake without dairy produce in your diet, but there are many other good sources of calcium, including leafy green vegetables and even sesame seeds (see page 176). If you want to be extra sure, take a multivitamin and mineral supplement that contains good levels of calcium as well as other nutrients for your bones.

Factors that can block the conversion of essential fats

In order to start the ball rolling, your body has got to convert the Omega 6 series, linoleic acid (LA) into GLA (gamma–linolenic acid). It has been discovered that many women have an inherent (naturally occurring) problem in their bodies, which means that there is some difficulty converting the essential fatty acids to GLA.[47]

If you are one of these women, and you are also a big dairy food eater, you will undoubtedly end up with very little PGE1 (good) and too much PGE2 (bad). Obviously when the balance is tipped in that direction, you'll be much more likely to suffer some nasty symptoms, and one of those can be severe period pains.

There are a number of other factors that can hamper the conversion of linoleic acid to GLA and these include stress, a diet that is high in sugar, and deficiencies of vitamin B6, magnesium and zinc. An enzyme called delta–6–desaturase helps your body make this conversion (see chart, page 157) and this enzyme needs B6, magnesium and zinc in order to do its job.

If you are suffering from painful periods, it is important that you take nutritional supplements for between three and six months, to ensure that the nutrients required for the conversion are present in adequate levels.

Supplements

Vitamin B6

Vitamin B6 is needed to help produce 'good' prostaglandins, so it is worth taking a good B-complex supplement. This vitamin has been shown significantly to reduce the intensity and duration of period pains.[48]

Vitamin B1

This B vitamin is very effective in helping with period pain. In one study, it was given to 556 women (aged 12 to 21 years), who had moderate to severe dysmenorrhoea. Some of the women were given the B1 first for 90 days and then changed to a placebo. Others were given the placebo first for 90 days and the B1 next. A full 87 per cent of the women were completely cured after starting the B1 treatment. This effect remained for at least two months after the B1 was stopped.[49]

Vitamin B12

Because both vitamins B1 and B6 are helpful with treating period pains, the best approach is to take a vitamin B complex. This will also give you vitamin B12, and it has been found that a combination of fish oil and B12 is actually more effective than just fish oil on its own for relieving dysmenorrhoea.[50] The scientists could not explain why the B12 made the treatment more effective.

Vitamin E

Up to 70 per cent of women have found the supplementation of vitamin E to be useful in treating painful periods.[51] The reasons for this effect are unclear, but it may be that vitamin E's antioxidant properties help with the pain, or control the levels of prostaglandins.

Vitamin C and bioflavonoids

Bioflavonoids are helpful with period pain because they help to relax smooth muscle and reduce inflammation. Bilberry is one of the best bioflavonoids for this, but other bioflavonoids can be helpful. Include berries of any kind (including blackberries, blackcurrants, raspberries and even grapes) in your diet.[52]

Magnesium

Magnesium acts as a muscle relaxant and it has been shown to have a beneficial effect on painful periods and lower back pain,[53] so it is worth taking as a supplement. Magnesium also has the ability to lower the 'bad' prostaglandins that may be causing the womb to over-contract.[54]

Finally, along with vitamin B6, magnesium is required by your body to help convert the essential fats into beneficial prostaglandins. Try always to take them together.

Zinc

This mineral is important for eliminating period pains because it is needed for the proper conversion of LA to GLA.

Essential fatty acids (EFAs)

Taking EFAs in supplement form is extremely important in the treatment of painful periods. Research has shown that women with low intakes of Omega 3 fatty acids (the ones that come from fish, linseed and walnuts), have more painful periods than women who have a good intake. The study that found this link also discovered that the extent of the pain was connected to the ratio or balance of the Omega 3 and Omega 6 fats. The women with the worst period pains ate a much lower ratio of Omega 3 fats in relation to Omega 6 fats – a one to four ratio.[55]

I would suggest adding either fish (EPA) or linseed oil capsules in order to keep the 'bad' prostaglandins (PGE2) under control.

Bromelain

This is an enzyme contained in pineapples and it has been found to be extremely useful for treating painful periods. It has anti-inflammatory properties and helps as a natural blood thinner. Bromelain also acts as a smooth muscle relaxant and is thought to decrease PGE2 and increase PGE1 (the 'good' prostaglandins).[56]

Herbs

Herbs can have a tremendously beneficial impact on painful periods when used alongside the dietary recommendations.

Herbal treatment has two aims:

1. In the long term, to help your womb 'behave' normally. In other words, it ensures that your womb does not overcontract to squeeze out the lining and that the blood supply to the womb is not restricted.

2. In the short term, to relieve the pain you are experiencing during your period.

Long-term herbal treatment

There are two herbs that are particularly useful in helping your womb to function normally. I would suggest that you use an equal blend of each. This mixture would be taken during the month, and then you would switch to the short-term treatment below just before or as your period starts. Once the pain stops for that cycle, stop the short-term treatment, wait until your period stops and then go back to the long-term blend.

Dong quai (Angelica sinensis)

This herb is classed as 'woman's tonic', and has a particular affinity to the womb. There has been a great deal of research into this herb. In 2000, the American Pharmaceutical Association published a review of the herbs that are of special interest to women, and dong quai featured as the main herb of choice for period pains.[57]

Dong quai helps to encourage the normal functioning of the womb by changing the rhythm of the contractions and by improving the circulation to the womb. By making sure the blood supply to the womb is optimum, it helps to ensure that enough oxygen reaches the tissues, which acts to minimise pain and cramping. Quite apart from all of this, dong quai acts as a natural painkiller.

Studies have also shown that dong quai helps to regulate the production of prostaglandins, which is an important factor in the treatment of painful periods.[58]

Black cohosh (Cimicifuga racemosa)

This is another herb with a relaxant effect on the womb.[59] It has been used for centuries by Native North Americans and has a normalising effect on the female reproductive system.

Short-term herbal treatment

A good mix to alleviate the pain is equal parts of crampbark, skullcap, black haw and black cohosh at a dosage of 5ml (one teaspoon) three times a day, when needed.

Crampbark (Viburnum opulus)

The name of this herb conveys its prime properties: it works as an anti-spasmodic and muscle relaxant.[60]

Black haw (Viburnum prunifolium)

This herb has also been shown to be effective in the treatment of period pains. Studies show that it may contain a number of active constituents that help the womb to relax.[61]

Skullcap (Scutellaria laterifolia)

This is an anti-spasmodic herb, and it combines well with the other herbs suggested above. Skullcap helps to stop the womb from over-contracting.

Black cohosh (Cimicifuga racemosa)

Not only is this an excellent long-term herbal treatment (see above), but it can be very useful in the short term to help ease the pain of periods. Take in combination with the other herbs mentioned.

Exercise

Exercise is also highly beneficial as it can help alleviate period pains by increasing circulation to the pelvic region.[62] Exercise can also reduce stress and it is well known that it encourages the release of brain chemicals called endorphins, which help us to feel happier, more alert and calmer.

Relaxation

Learning techniques to help you relax and cope with stress have been proved useful in the treatment of period pains.[63]

Natural medicine

Aromatherapy can be an excellent way to encourage relaxation, and specific oils can also be used to help with painful periods, such as chamomile, marjoram and rosemary.

Homeopathy and acupuncture are also both effective in the treatment of painful periods, and they can be used successfully alongside the other recommendations above.

The Treatment Plan

Your main aim will be to eliminate those foods that may be making your period pains worse. You'll also take supplements and herbs to rectify the cause of the problem.

The Integrated Approach

The best plan is to use a combination of treatments. Begin by changing your diet and taking nutritional supplements. Alongside, take the 'long-term' herbs throughout your cycle, stopping when your period is due. Then switch to the 'short-term' herbs when your period is due, or as soon as the pain begins. For the first few months you may also need to take your regular painkiller when you have your period. Try to use the painkillers only as needed because you will find that, as the months pass, you will need increasingly smaller amounts.

In the long term, when you are completely free of period pains, you can stop taking both types of herbs.

Your Supplement Plan

- A good multivitamin and mineral supplement
- Vitamin B complex (100mg of most of the B vitamin per day; including what you get from your multivitamin and mineral supplement)
- Magnesium (300mg per day)
- Vitamin E (300iu per day) as d-alpha tocopherol
- Zinc citrate (15mg per day)
- Vitamin C with bioflavonoids (1,000mg twice per day)
- Linseed (flaxseed) oil (1,000mg per day)
- Bromelain (500mg, three times a day between meals)

> **Note**
> Each nutrient represents the total intake for one day, so if your multivitamin and mineral already contains 100mg of magnesium, for example, you only need to add in a separate magnesium supplement containing 200mg per day.

Herbs

- Take a combination of the long-term herbs throughout the month, but stop when the pain starts (1 teaspoon, three times a day)

- As soon as your period (or the pain) starts, switch to the short-term herbs (1 teaspoon, three times a day)

- When your pain is manageable, stop taking the short-term herbs

- When your period is finished, start taking the long-term herbs again

- If there is no improvement at all after three months, see a qualified practitioner

To make this programme simpler, I have formulated the Natural Cycle Pack – Menstrual Relief, made by the Natural Health Practice, which contains the above nutrients and herbs. If you can't get this locally then call 01892 750511 and it can be posted to you.

In Summary

- Always investigate the cause of period pains before taking any drugs, or beginning a natural treatment programme.

- Begin the hormone balancing diet (see page 16).

- Watch your intake of essential fatty acids, which can prevent the production of 'bad' prostaglandins.

- Avoid foods that are high in arachidonic acid (AA).

- Take steps to reduce stress in your lifestyle, which can affect period pains and discourage the production of healthy prostaglandins.

- Make sure you get plenty of exercise, which has been proven to help with dysmenorrhoea.

- Ensure that you get plenty of the key nutrients: vitamin C, bioflavonoids, magnesium, the B-vitamins, EFAs, vitamin E and zinc in your diet, and supplement throughout the treatment programme.

- Take supplements (see page 61) throughout your entire cycle.

- Take short-term herbs only when you are menstruating, or in pain, and alongside any drugs used to ease the pain.

- Discontinue using the drugs gradually, as they are no longer required, and continue taking short-term herbs until the pain is completely under control.

- Take long-term herbs until you have your period. Stop and resume when your period is finished.

CHAPTER 6

The Womb

The physical position of the womb or uterus is low in the pelvis, and it is connected to the vagina by the cervix. It is of prime importance in the reproductive cycle, in that it serves as the receptacle and nursery for the fertilised egg that will become a baby. When a woman's reproductive years are over, some doctors believe that the role of the womb is over and that a hysterectomy would 'tidy things up'. But where there are problems with the womb, for example, cancer (which is beyond the scope of this book), a hysterectomy may be necessary.

ENDOMETRIOSIS

Endometriosis is a very common gynaecological condition, which can affect up to 15 per cent of all women. Half of all women with endometriosis will be infertile. After fibroids (see page 185), endometriosis is the most common gynaecological problem. The National Endometriosis Society (see Useful Addresses) estimates that between 1.5 and 2 million women in Britain have endometriosis. In the US that number is closer to 5 million.

Endometriosis is more common in childless women over the age of 30. It is now believed that endometriosis is sensitive to oestrogen; therefore, women who have had more cycles, without a break for pregnancy, will have had more exposure to the female hormones. Today, with more and more women putting off having children until their later years, the incidence of endometriosis-linked infertility is increasing.

HOW DOES ENDOMETRIOSIS CAUSE INFERTILITY?

Endometriosis is more common in older, childless women, and it can cause scarring that can block the Fallopian tubes so severely they are unable to pick up an egg at ovulation. Furthermore, the ovaries themselves may become scarred, which means that ovulation may occur but the egg becomes entrapped in scar tissue.

What is Endometriosis?

Endometriosis is a condition in which the lining of the womb (the endometrium) implants and grows outside the womb itself. These endometrial implants can grow in the pelvis, Fallopian tubes, ovaries, bowel and bladder. More uncommonly, they can also crop up in the lung, heart, eye, armpit or knee.

Wherever it grows, the womb lining responds to the natural hormone cycle and bleeds every time a period occurs. When women bleed normally throughout menstruation, blood leaves the body through the vagina. However, in the case of endometriosis, the blood has no outlet and becomes trapped in the tissue, causing pain, inflammation, cysts and scar tissue. You may find blood in your stools or urine during your period, or experience pain in diverse areas of your body. Some of my patients experience nosebleeds during their periods because they have endometrial patches in the nasal passages.

Endometrial implants can all look different, depending upon where they are found in the body. For example, on the ovaries they form cysts that are often known as 'chocolate cysts' because they are filled with brownish, old blood. In other places, they take the form of lesions, which are tiny, pinpoint areas of bleeding. Over time, fibrous tissues can grow around these lesions and then scar tissue (called adhesions) can form, causing the organs to stick together within the pelvic cavity, or to the abdominal wall.

ENDOMETRIOSIS, THE MENOPAUSE AND HRT

Because endometriosis is sensitive to oestrogen, treatment is aimed at shutting down the female hormones (see page 171). As we age, our oestrogen levels naturally fall to a lower point by the time we reach the menopause. Therefore, sufferers of endometriosis should naturally find relief from the condition around this time. During the menopause there are no monthly hormone cycles to stimulate the growth of endometrial tissue. However, if a woman with a history of endometriosis takes HRT, this *may* reactivate the condition, causing a recurrence of exactly the same symptoms. What's the answer? Endometriosis sufferers are not usually suitable candidates for HRT, and should try to manage their menopause in a more natural way (see Chapter 11).

What are the Symptoms?

The symptoms vary between women. In some women, endometriosis can cause extremely painful periods and painful sex, but some women experience no symptoms whatsoever.

Symptoms can occur at any time of the month – during a bowel movement, or when urinating, for example. The most severe pain can start between five and seven days before a period and last for two to three days during the period itself. Painful sex (called dyspareunia) is a feature of the condition in up to 59 per cent of all women with endometriosis, and acts as a keynote symptom – something that alerts doctors to a possible diagnosis.

Symptoms often improve dramatically after pregnancy, and it is believed that having a break from the monthly cycle actually 'quietens down' the disease in some sufferers.

Women have talked about how the endometriosis takes over their lives. Holidays are planned to avoid periods and social arrangements are cancelled at the last minute when the pain becomes intense. Many women are forced to take days off work each month in order to cope with the condition and some women have had to give up work altogether because employers cannot cope with their frequent absences.

COMMON SYMPTOMS OF ENDOMETRIOSIS

- painful periods (dysmenorrhoea)
- heavy or irregular periods
- painful sex (dyspareunia)
- back pain
- nausea
- fatigue
- gastrointestinal problems, including diarrhoea, bloating and painful defecation
- infertility
- general pain in the pelvic area

What's the Cause?

Nobody knows! There are plenty of theories and not a lot of agreement within the medical profession about the cause of endometriosis. Some have suggested that it is due to migration of the endometrial tissue up the Fallopian tubes and into the abdomen (retrograde or 'backwards' menstruation). According to this theory, muscle spasms during a period force the blood back up the tubes. There is a gap between the Fallopian tubes and the ovaries (see page 63), and during ovulation the Fallopian tubes have to 'catch' the egg as it is released. If blood is pushed back up the Fallopian tubes it can spill out of the end of the tubes and into the abdomen. The difficulty with this theory is that some women who have been sterilised by having their tubes tied or cut will still get endometriosis. It also fails to explain how endometrial patches can end up in the lungs or the nasal passages.

Another theory suggests that the disease first occurs during foetal development. It is believed that young endometrial cells are displaced and only begin to grow when a woman reaches puberty. This might explain why endometriosis seems to run in families. Scientists are also looking for a genetic cause, because it is believed that some 15 per cent of all cases could be inherited.

One more theory is based on the idea that endometrial tissue is transported from the womb to other parts of the body through the lymphatic system (which runs parallel to the circulatory system and comprises part of the immune system), or that the sufferer has some sort of immune deficiency. Scientists have discovered that women with endometriosis do not have strong immune systems. They also found that natural killer cells do not function as well as they should and so endometrial cells that should be treated as 'foreign' in areas where they do not belong are not being destroyed.[1] At the end of each cycle, these natural killer cells, which are part of our immune systems, should 'mop up' all the endometrial debris. If this doesn't happen then endometrial cells can migrate to other parts of the body and form lesions that provoke an inflammatory reaction because the immune system does not have the right defences to remove these cells.

Yet another theory (metaplasia theory) suggests that cells in the body can change into endometrial cells by exposure to hormones, chemicals, infection and other hostile environmental or physical substances. This theory has been supported by the fact that endometrial patches were found in the bladders of men who were given oestrogenic drugs for the treatment of prostate cancer.[2]

The bottom line is that nobody is sure what causes endometriosis and, sadly, the medical treatments are not very reliable either because of the extremely high incidence of recurrence after treatment.

How Do You Know If You Have Endometriosis?

Research has shown that it can take up to ten years for some women to get a diagnosis of endometriosis.[3]

Many women have visited their doctors repeatedly, suffering from painful periods and other symptoms, but too often the response is that 'painful, heavy periods are common' and that it is possible to 'cope'. Some women end up relying on strong painkillers when they have their periods.

If you are in a similar situation, and recognise that your symptoms are not the same as those of anyone else you know, don't be dismissed. One important research paper was entitled: 'Women with endometriosis: dismissed, devalued and ignored'. Don't fall into that category. Your symptoms may be put down to stress, and you may be told that you need to relax. Interestingly, endometriosis was once considered to be a disease of successful, career women and yet it was described in the medical texts dating back some 300 years.[4]

Don't be afraid to demand tests if you are in this situation. And remember that endometriosis is notoriously under-diagnosed.

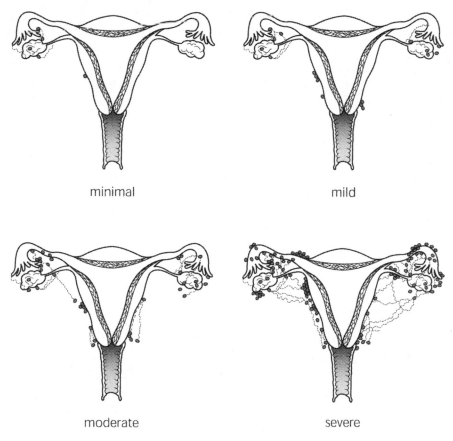

minimal   mild

moderate   severe

Degrees of endometriosis

Laparoscopy

Diagnosis is made by laparoscopy, where a laparoscope (a small fibre-optic viewing tube with a light) is inserted into the abdomen via a small incision just below the navel. It is performed under a general anaesthetic and allows a good view of the womb, Fallopian tubes and ovaries. It is normally a quick operation lasting around 20 minutes, during which carbon dioxide gas is pumped into the abdomen so that the surgeon can see the internal organs more easily. The carbon dioxide is released afterwards, but some women do complain of shoulder pains after a laparoscopy, because some gas can become trapped under the diaphragm (the sheet of muscle between the abdomen and the chest).

Not all endometrial patches will be visible from the laparoscopy because some may be hidden from view, particularly if organs are joined together by adhesions. Furthermore, implants in other organs – the bowel, for example – will not be visible from a laparoscope.

Some doctors suggest that a laparoscopy is performed just before your period, at a time when the problem will be most active. This is not easy to arrange on the NHS (or any other busy health service), so it may be worth while arranging it privately, especially if you have been told that a previous laparoscopic examination was negative and you are still suffering from excruciating pain.

It is interesting to note that some women were only diagnosed with endometriosis when examinations by laparoscopy were made to ascertain a cause for infertility. The other anomaly is that many mild cases of endometriosis cause debilitating symptoms, while some women suffering from widespread patches can have much milder symptoms.

Ultrasound

This involves using very high frequency sound waves to obtain images of structures within the body. It can create an image of your pelvic cavity through a device that can be placed on your abdomen and/or in your vagina. Ultrasound can be extremely helpful as a first screening test because it can show cysts, adhesions and adenomysis, which is endometriosis in the wall of the womb, and this will give a clue that there could be endometriosis elsewhere and that a laparoscopy is needed.

What Treatment Can You Be Offered By Your Doctor?

Treatment normally involves using drugs or surgery.

Drugs

Because endometriosis is influenced by the menstrual cycle, drug treatment involves shutting down the female hormone output so that periods do not occur. Endometriosis is oestrogen-dependent, so the aim is to reduce the amount of oestrogen in the body.

The contraceptive pill

Birth control pills work as a contraceptive because they trick your body into believing it is pregnant. Therefore, ovulation does not occur and the monthly 'bleed' is not a real period, merely your body's reaction to a drop in the level of hormones contained in the pill. The contraceptive pill has been used, with some success, to treat endometriosis but in order for the treatment to be effective all bleeding has to stop. This usually requires high doses, which can result in unpleasant side-effects, including nausea, vomiting, headache, thrombosis (blood clots), changes in sex drive, depression and breast tenderness.

Progestogen-only pills

Birth control pills contain a combination of both oestrogen and progestogen, but it is also possible to use progestogen-only pills, such as those containing norethisterone and dydrogesterone, which put the body into a state of 'pseudo-pregnancy'. Side-effects can include tender breasts, irritability, nausea and bloating.

Danazol

The main drug treatment for endometriosis is danazol. This is a synthetic weak male hormone that prevents ovulation, which in turn stops the womb lining from developing. Again, as with any drug, it comes with side-effects, which some women can tolerate and others can't. These can include severe mood swings, nausea, dizziness, rashes and headaches. Because danazol is a mild male hormone, other side-effects can include facial hair, acne, an increased sex drive and weight gain.

Danazol vaginal ring

In the treatment of endometriosis, danazol is normally administered orally, but recent research has shown that it can be administered using a vaginal ring containing the drug.[5] According to a 1998 study, the ring significantly relieved period pains and did not have the usual side-effects associated with oral danazol.

Gonadotrophin releasing hormone (GnRH) analogues

These are synthetic hormones that can be given as an injection or a nasal spray. This drug works by preventing the pituitary gland from releasing both FSH (follicle stimulating hormone) and LH (luteinizing hormone), and this in turn stops the ovaries from producing hormones, thereby lowering oestrogen levels in the blood. In a nutshell, these drugs put you into a temporary menopause, which causes the endometriosis patches to shrink. Not surprisingly, one of the most common symptoms is one that is traditionally associated with menopause: hot flushes. Other side-effects can include headaches, mood swings, vaginal dryness and insomnia.

Goserelin

This is also a GnRH analogue (see above), but is given as an implant under the skin once per month. The idea is to achieve the same effect on the hormone system as the injection or nasal spray. Side-effects can be similar to those you might expect from GnRH.

Surgical techniques

Surgery using diathermy or laser

Patches of endometriosis can be burned off with diathermy (the use of intense heat) or laser. If a large chocolate cyst (see above) has taken over an ovary, a surgeon can use a laser to open the cyst, to allow the old blood to drain out. Adhesions (scar tissue) can also be removed during the same procedure, but unfortunately there is a risk of new scar tissue being created. To prevent this from happening, some surgeons use protective membranes to separate the organs, leaving them in place following the procedure to stop them from sticking together again.

Drugs (see above) are occasionally used for several months prior to surgery, to help minimise the extent of the endometrial patches, and to make them easier to remove.

Helica thermal coagulator

This procedure was developed fairly recently at the Heriot Watt University in Scotland, and it involves using helium jets to destroy the endometriosis. Basically, a helium beam is used to heat the surface of the endometrial tissues, causing them to dry out. The dry tissue is then reabsorbed into the system without forming a scab. The ionised helium beam heats the surface of the tissue to dry it out and the remaining dry tissue is reabsorbed into the system without forming a scab. Unlike diathermy or laser treatment, helica thermal coagulator treatment is not penetrative or cutting.

THE LIMITS OF CONVENTIONAL MEDICINE

Because the actual cause of endometriosis is not addressed by conventional treatment, it almost always recurs. Women who are trying to get pregnant are advised to try to conceive as soon as possible after treatment, before the endometriosis grows back.

Hysterectomy

This is the most extreme treatment offered for endometriosis, but it is all too commonly used. In Chapter 14 I discuss the different types of hysterectomy, some of which are more radical than others. In the case of endometriosis, usually only a hysterectomy that also removes the ovaries will be advised. Even if patches are found only on the womb, you will need to have your ovaries removed because they will continue to produce oestrogen even without the womb in place. Patches can occasionally crop up elsewhere in the body, or they can form on the ovaries themselves, which can be very painful.

After a hysterectomy with the ovaries removed, you will literally enter the menopause overnight, and you will immediately begin to experience one or more of the symptoms that accompany the menopause, including hot flushes, vaginal dryness, irritability and more (see page 402). Remember that a natural menopause is a gradual process in the body, where hormone levels slowly decline. In most women, the lead up to the menopause can take some ten years, so a surgical menopause is a shock to the system of any woman.

Furthermore, the sudden loss of oestrogen can be a risk factor in developing osteoporosis (brittle bones). What's the answer? If you are showing signs of osteoporosis, chances are that you will be offered HRT, and if you begin to take HRT, any other endometrial patches in your body (in your bowels, for example), can begin to grow and bleed again. Some experts recommend waiting for between six and nine months before taking HRT following a hysterectomy, to allow endometrial patches elsewhere in the body to shrink.

Jane

Jane, who was 45, came to see me after having a total hysterectomy plus ovaries removed for endometriosis. Following the operation she had been given HRT to manage the menopausal symptoms. The effect of the hormones she was taking was devastating, and all of her original symptoms returned. When she came to me she was unsure whether she should put up with the symptoms of the menopause, which had been fairly debilitating, or to accept that the endometriosis was part and parcel of taking HRT to alleviate the symptoms of the menopause. She had been led to believe that having a hysterectomy was the answer to her problems, and she had not been advised that taking HRT following the procedure would exacerbate the patches of endometriosis elsewhere in her body. Not surprisingly, she felt that she had gone through a serious surgical procedure for nothing.

What Natural Treatment Could Be Effective?

Treating endometriosis naturally involves taking a dramatically different approach to the condition, and it is aimed at altering the underlying problems that trigger the endometriosis to grow. At the same time, symptoms will be controlled. Your goal will be to get yourself into optimum health and, in the process, alleviating or even completely eliminating your endometriosis in the process.

A multi-factorial approach is the quickest way to achieve this aim, as endometriosis can be triggered by a combination of factors, including hormone imbalances, stress and nutritional deficiencies.

There are five main stages to the treatment programme, as follows:

1. Improve your diet, based on the recommendations outlined in Chapter 1, and particular issues, listed below.

2. Use supplements and other natural remedies to help control the pain while you are working on the underlying cause.

3. Control levels of excess oestrogen that your body may be producing, or taking in from your environment. Endometriosis grows in the presence of oestrogen, which is why drug treatments are aimed at shutting down the normal female cycle, or using male hormones to help the endometriosis to shrink. But can you reduce your oestrogen levels in a more natural way? The answer is yes.

4. Improve the function of your liver. Your liver is responsible for ridding your body of excess oestrogen.

5. Boost your immune system so your body becomes capable of recognising endometrial patches outside the womb as being 'invaders', and subsequently destroys them.

Dietary changes

The first and most important step is to adopt the hormone balancing diet (see Chapter 1). However, in the case of endometriosis, you will need to take things a step further. Your main aim will be to keep your diet low in any foods that encourage the production of oestrogen, focusing instead on those foods that can help your body get rid of excess oestrogen.

Other factors

- **Alcohol**: You will need to avoid alcohol completely for a couple of months and then limit your intake to only one or two units a week. Your liver helps control the excretion of your hormones and if you want it to work efficiently it is better not to have alcohol, which causes your liver to work overtime.

- **Saturated fats**: Dairy produce and red meat should also be avoided for a few months because they contain a substance called 'arachidonic acid', which encourages the production of hormone-like substances called prostaglandins. The prostaglandin that is produced from saturated fats is PGE2, a highly inflammatory substance that can cause swelling and pain and, in some cases, thicken the blood itself. It can also trigger muscle contractions and constriction in the blood vessels, which can increase period pains, endometriosis-related cramps and the spread of endometrial tissue. The high saturated fat content of both dairy and red meat is also a factor in producing more oestrogen. If you can, drop them from your diet completely.

- **Caffeine**: As well as having a diuretic effect on the body, which depletes valuable stores of vitamins and minerals that are essential to healthy hormone balance, intake in excess of two cups of coffee a day has been linked to endometriosis.[6]

WHAT ABOUT CALCIUM?

You may be concerned that a diet low in dairy produce will be deficient in calcium. Don't worry. There are many other equally good and, indeed, better sources of calcium in foods such as broccoli and other leafy green vegetables, seafood, almonds, asparagus, oats and sesame seeds, to name just a few. Furthermore, most good vitamin and mineral supplements contain useful levels of calcium and other important nutrients for your bones.

Boost your immune system

When you suffer from endometriosis, it is important to ensure that your immune system is functioning at optimum level. It is believed that women who do not suffer from endometriosis have immune systems with an ability to mop up the endometrial debris after each period. This cleaning process should take place naturally every month. Women with endometriosis do not seem to have this ability to 'mop up', and the debris lies around, which gives it an opportunity to take hold.

Follow the dietary recommendations given in Chapter 1. A good diet not only balances your hormones, but also provides the nutrients that your immune system needs to function at its best. Furthermore, you'll be avoiding foods that compromise your immune function, such as sugar.

Take the supplements listed below to ensure that your body has adequate levels of all of the key nutrients.

ARE YOU OVERWEIGHT?

Oestrogen is stored in fat, so it is particularly important that you find and stick to your natural weight (see Chapter 13). Studies also show that women who are overweight generally have more oestrogen in circulation because fat is also an oestrogen-manufacturing plant.

If you are overweight, try the treatment plan described on page 464.

Supplements

I have recommended particular supplements not only to strengthen your immune system, but also for their unique ability to address certain health conditions, including hormone imbalance. The idea is to address all possible known causes of endometriosis, while at the same time ensuring that you reach optimum health, where your body can start to fight its own battles. Suggested dosages will follow in the treatment plan (see page 458).

The B vitamins

The B vitamins are particularly important for endometriosis sufferers for a number of reasons. First and foremost, they are needed by the

---

Jennifer

Thirty-one-year-old Jennifer had been diagnosed with endometriosis eight years earlier. It was giving her four days of intense pain during her period, and even painkillers failed to 'touch it'. She felt that her periods were getting worse – both heavier, and with more clotting.

I gave her a programme of supplements to follow for three months, which included a linseed oil supplement, because essential fatty acids are crucial for period pains. We talked about her diet and I also gave her herbs to help with the endometriosis. When I saw her three months later, she had had three periods without any pain at all. It often takes a couple of months for the natural approach to take effect, but Jennifer had noticed a difference in the first month. Her mood swings disappeared, and only the first two days of her periods were heavy. Over time, these became lighter as well.

liver to convert excess oestrogen into weaker and less carcinogenic forms. One of the B vitamins, B6, has been shown to significantly reduce the intensity and duration of period pains, which will help many sufferers.[7]

The B vitamins are also crucial for the conversion of linoleic acid to GLA (gamma linolenic acid), which is necessary to produce beneficial prostaglandins (hormone-like substances that have a relaxing effect on the womb muscles and anti-inflammatory properties). This might sound confusing, but it's a crucial concept. Linoleic acid is an essential fatty acid (EFA), and it is found in foods such as corn oil, fresh nuts and seeds, and sunflower oil. It's also known as an 'Omega 6' oil. The B vitamins are required to convert this essential oil into a form that can be used by the body to produce a 'good' type of prostaglandin. Without this conversion, our bodies would produce more of the 'bad' prostaglandins, which can increase the period pains and set up inflammation from the endometrial patches.

Vitamin E
This is an important vitamin in endometriosis because it has been shown to relieve menstrual cramps in 70 per cent of women within two menstrual cycles.[8]

Vitamin C and bioflavonoids
Vitamin C is one of the most important vitamins for immune function, and it is crucial that your immune system is operating at optimum level so that your body can recognise and destroy endometrial patches as they occur. Bioflavonoids are helpful with pain occurring around the time of your period because they help to relax smooth muscle and to prevent inflammation.[9]

Magnesium
Magnesium acts as a muscle relaxant and has been shown to have a beneficial effect on painful periods and lower back pain,[10] so it is worth taking as a supplement.

Essential fatty acids (EFAs)
Your body produces beneficial prostaglandins from essential fatty acids (see page 27), which help to reduce period pains. They also have an anti-inflammatory response, which is particularly beneficial to endometriosis sufferers.

The minerals zinc and vitamin B6 are also important for the correct metabolism of fatty acids and their conversion to beneficial prosta-glandins (PGE1 and PGE3). Certain prostaglandins (PGE2; see page 150) can be negative in high amounts. In particular, PGE2 is a highly inflammatory substance that can cause swelling and pain and also thicken the blood, which can then cause congestion and stagnation in the pelvic area.

In 1998, an interesting study reported in a highly regarded medical journal, *Fertility and Sterility*, considered the effects of making dietary changes.[11] Women with endometriosis were asked to eliminate caffeine, to control their blood sugar by eating little and often, eliminate foods containing sugar, and supplement with essential fatty acids. Doctors found that by making these simple changes, women taking part in the study experienced a significant decrease in the symptoms of endo-metriosis.

Herbs

Herbs can have a tremendous impact on helping with the period pains while you are working on your diet. The approach is two-fold, using diet and herbs to work on normalising hormone balance, and then taking different herbs to help you to cope with the worst symptoms. At the beginning you may require both painkillers and herbs to deal with the pain; however, gradually your dependence upon the painkillers will be reduced to the point where they are unnecessary. Eventually it will also be possible to stop taking herbs.

Hormone balance

Agnus castus (vitex/chastetree berry) is one of the most important herbs for female hormone problems, and it works to stimulate and normalise the function of the pituitary gland. This gland controls and balances the hormones in our body. *Agnus castus* works by restoring balance, whether your hormone levels are too high or too low.

Milk thistle (*Silybum marianum*) is an excellent herb for the liver, which needs to work efficiently to balance the hormones. A number of studies have shown that its use can result in an increase of new liver cells to replace old damaged ones.[12] This beneficial effect is due to something called 'silymarin', which is the collective name for the substances in milk thistle that have therapeutic benefits on liver tissue.

Dandelion root (*Taraxacum officinale*) also helps cleanse the liver, the major organ of detoxification, and it gets rid of accumulated 'old' female hormones.

Echinacea (*Echinacea purpurea* or *Echinacea angustifolia*) is the herb of choice for the immune system and it helps to increase the white blood cell count. It seems to be more effective when taken on and off. I suggest ten days on, three days off, ten days on etc. for maximum immune system benefits.

Period pains

Crampbark (*Viburnum opulus*), whose name appropriately describes its action, works as an anti-spasmodic and muscle relaxant.

It's helpful to blend herbs when addressing painful periods, and I have found that the following work well together in equal parts: crampbark, skullcap, blackhaw and black cohosh at a dosage of 5ml (1 teaspoon) three times a day when needed.

EXERCISE

Exercise is highly beneficial for endometriosis sufferers as it can help to alleviate period pains by increasing circulation to the pelvic region. It also helps to control excess oestrogen (see page 42). Exercise can also reduce stress, which can exacerbate the problem in some women. Finally, exercise releases brain chemicals called endorphins (the body's natural painkillers) into the body, and they also help us to feel happier, more alert and calmer.

Controlling excess oestrogen

One of the key ways to control excess oestrogen in your body is to avoid environmental oestrogens, also known as 'xenoestrogens'. In Chapter 1 the problems associated with xenoestrogens are examined in some detail. However, sufferers of endometriosis will be interested to learn of another link between environmental factors and the condition. Researchers have found a connection between dioxins (a class of xenoestrogens from pesticides) and the development of endometriosis. They found that 79 per cent of female rhesus monkeys spontaneously developed endometriosis after being fed food containing dioxin. The severity of the endometriosis was dose related, so the more exposure to dioxin, the more severe the endometriosis.[13]

Dioxins can be found almost everywhere, not only in the food we eat but also in many products we use on a daily basis, such as the material used to make tea bags and some sanitary products. Use unbleached sanitary towels if you have endometriosis and avoid tampons unless absolutely necessary. If you must use them choose unbleached brands. The chemical content of tampons is bad enough, but they also act as a sort of 'dam' to soak up the blood and it is much healthier to allow blood to flow naturally during periods (see Chapter 1).

The Integrated Treatment Plan

Choose from the categories below to choose the most appropriate treatment plan for your individual needs.

You will see that the treatment suggestions are different, depending on your age and whether or not you want to conceive. If you want to try the natural approach, you will need to stop any medication that is controlling your hormones (such as the Pill or Goserelin); although this should be cleared with your doctor first. Then use painkillers each month as needed, but reduce the dose as the natural approach starts to take effect.

If you are under 35 and not planning to get pregnant

Follow the natural supplement plan (below) and use painkillers as needed when you have your period. As the pain lessens each month, take fewer painkillers until you get to the point where you do not need them.

If you are under 35 and planning to get pregnant

If you have been told that the endometriosis is probably preventing conception, follow the natural supplement plan (below) for six months, while increasing your intake of key nutrients such as folic acid (see page 375).

After this time arrange for a laparoscopy to see if the endometriosis has receded to any significant degree, and if any of the patches could still be preventing you from becoming pregnant. You may need surgery to remove the patches. If you choose this route, begin trying to conceive as soon as possible after the procedure. When you are trying to conceive, you should continue to follow the nutritional recommendations, but avoid taking any herbs during this period.

If surgery is considered to be unnecessary, follow the natural treatment plan for six months, adding the preconceptual treatment plan (see page 349) alongside for the last three months. If, at the end of this time, you get the all clear, then you are healthy and ready to conceive.

If you are over 35 and not planning to get pregnant

Follow the same recommendations as for under-35s.

If you are over 35 and planning to get pregnant

Time is of the essence, since fertility declines with age. You should follow the recommendations for a woman under the age of 35 but only for *three* rather than *six* months. After *three* months, ask for further investigations to see how the endometriosis is responding to treatment. If surgery is necessary, start trying to conceive as soon as possible after the procedure, but continue with the nutritional recommendations. What you will be aiming to do is to prevent further patches from occurring in other parts of the body.

Anyone who wishes to become pregnant

It's essential that you follow a good preconception plan (see page 349).

Your Supplement Plan

- A good multivitamin and mineral supplement, eg The Healthy Woman by the Natural Health Practice

- Vitamin B complex (100mg of most of the B vitamins per day; take into consideration how much is in your multivitamin supplement)

- Magnesium (300mg per day)

- Vitamin E (300iu per day)

- Zinc citrate (15mg per day)

- Vitamin C with bioflavonoids (1,000 mg twice per day)

- Linseed oil (flaxseed oil) (1,000 mg per day)

> **Note**
> Each nutrient represents the total intake for one day, so if your multivitamin and mineral already contains 100mg of magnesium, for example, you only need to add in a separate magnesium supplement containing 200mg per day.

Herbs

The herbs should be taken as follows. Take a tincture made up of half *Agnus castus*, one-quarter milk thistle and one-quarter dandelion, one teaspoon three times a day, for three to six months. Have a separate tincture of echinacea, taken ten days on, three days off, etc. If there is no improvement, see a qualified practitioner. During periods, stop the *Agnus castus* mix and take equal parts of crampbark, skullcap, blackhaw and black cohosh, one teaspoon three times a day when the pain is bad. When the period is finished, stop the crampbark mix and start back on the *Agnus castus* formula.

In Summary

- Avoid foods that are high in saturated fats; choose foods rich in unsaturated fats, such as oils, nuts, seeds and oily fish.

- Eat organic foods wherever possible, to avoid ingesting high levels of xenoestrogens and other unacceptable chemicals used in the growing process.

- Avoid caffeine, including that found in tea, colas, coffee and chocolate.

- Watch your weight. Excess weight can lead to higher oestrogen levels.

- Avoid high levels of alcohol: do not drink every night and have no more than a couple of glasses a night at the weekend.

- Avoid using tampons, which could contain dioxins, and which hamper the natural flow of blood. Use unbleached towels instead.

- Avoid HRT if you suffer from endometriosis; it can encourage the growth of endometrial patches.

- Try to get plenty of regular exercise, which can decrease pain.

- Continue to take painkillers alongside the natural programme, but after a couple of months gently ease off.

FIBROIDS

What are Fibroids?

Fibroids (also called myomas) are non-cancerous growths in or on the muscular wall of the womb (the myometrium). They can vary in number and size, according to the individual. Doctors will refer to the size of a fibroid in terms of a developing baby that size – such as 12 weeks. Some fibroids can be as small as a pea, but others can be as large as an eight-month-old foetus.

Fibroids are given different names depending on where and how they grow:

- **submucosal fibroids** grow on the inside of the womb and extend into the uterine cavity

- **intramural fibroids** grow within the uterine wall (the wall of the womb)

- **subserol fibroids** grow on the outside of the womb, on the lining between the uterus and the pelvic cavity

- **pedunculated fibroids** can be attached either to the inside or outside wall of the womb, and they are characterised by a stalk

Fibroids are very common and can affect 20 per cent of women over the age of 30. They are not common in women under the age of 20, except Afro-Caribbean women who are more susceptible to fibroid growths, even in their teens. Fibroids seem to run in families, but it is not certain at present whether this is a genuinely genetic predisposition, or whether lifestyle and diet play a role in some families.

Can Fibroids Become Cancerous?

Although fibroids are called growths and tumours, fibroids are almost always benign (non-cancerous). In fact, less than 1 in 1,000 cases will be malignant (cancerous). To put that into perspective, the mortality rate (risk of death) from having a hysterectomy is about 1 in 1,000. So, chances are your fibroids will not be life-threatening.

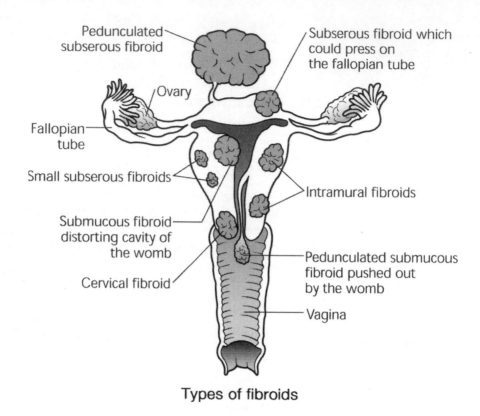

Pedunculated subserous fibroid

Subserous fibroid which could press on the fallopian tube

Ovary

Fallopian tube

Small subserous fibroids

Intramural fibroids

Submucous fibroid distorting cavity of the womb

Cervical fibroid

Pedunculated submucous fibroid pushed out by the womb

Vagina

Types of fibroids

What are the Symptoms?

- The main symptom of fibroids is heavy periods. When fibroids grow inside the womb (submucosal or intramural), the mechanism that operates menstrual flow may not work properly. The heavy bleeding can be a result of the fibroids making the womb bigger (creating a larger surface of womb lining that has to bleed every month), or the pressure of the fibroids may disrupt the normal blood flow. As a result many women with fibroids will have heavy periods, but experience no pain.

- Some women *do* experience pain with fibroids – not necessarily intense period pains, but a feeling of pressure and a dragging sensation in the abdomen.

- If fibroids are on stalks (pedunculated), they can twist, causing extreme pain.

- In some cases, the bleeding can be so severe that sufferers develop anaemia.

- During menstruation, some women lose clots of blood that resemble pieces of liver. If the blood flow is heavy, the anti-clotting factors that are normally present in the menstrual blood may not be able to keep the blood flowing smoothly, hence the pieces of clotted blood.

- Other women can experience periods that go on for weeks, sometimes with no real break between one period and the next.

- In many cases, fibroids can be symptomless. If they grow in a way that doesn't cause pressure on the neighbouring organs, you can live with even large fibroids for many years without requiring any medical help. In most cases, they shrink in the menopause and post-menopause years.

- In some cases the first indication that there may be fibroids is when there is trouble conceiving (infertility) or maintaining a pregnancy (miscarriage).

- Many women will never know they have fibroids, as they can give no symptoms. Significantly large fibroids can enlarge and distort the womb, making it impossible for a fertilised egg to implant. Many women who have been treated for infertility may have perfectly normal cycles. They will not have even known that they were pregnant, because the fertilised egg would have been unable to attach itself to the lining of the uterus with fibroids there.

- If fibroids press on other organs, such as the bladder or bowel, you may experience frequent urination, constipation or even backache.

- There may be pain or discomfort during intercourse.

- Most women do experience some abdominal swelling, although it may be minor. In other women, the lower abdomen can look as though they are in the early stages of pregnancy.

What's the Cause?

Although fibroids are very common, their exact cause is not known. We do know that fibroids are sensitive to oestrogen. So, if you already have fibroids and you suddenly have increased levels of oestrogen in your body (taking HRT during the menopause, for example), your fibroids can grow. Similarly, during the menopause, when levels of oestrogen naturally decline, fibroids can shrink.

This points to the idea that an excess of oestrogen may trigger the growth of fibroids in the first place. As we age, or during times of emotional stress, it is possible to have cycles where there is no ovulation. During those cycles, oestrogen will be produced without progesterone (which is only released after ovulation) to counterbalance it. In this case, you end up with an oestrogen dominance (excess oestrogen), because the other necessary hormone (progesterone) is not there to balance it.

Women with anovulatory cycles (no ovulation) can also suffer from fibroids because they have the same problem (excess oestrogen and no progesterone).

ARE YOU ANAEMIC?

If you bleed excessively during periods, ask your doctor for a blood test to check that you have not become anaemic. Heavy blood flow is very often the cause of anaemia in women of reproductive age.

Symptoms of anaemia can include:

- exhaustion
- shortness of breath
- dizziness
- sore tongue
- headaches

How Do You Find Out If You Have A Fibroid?

Fibroids can be diagnosed in several ways. Often they are picked up by a simple internal examination. If the fibroids are small, then a pelvic ultrasound can be used. This method is often done to confirm the diagnosis from the internal examination.

What Treatment Can You Be Offered By Your Doctor?

There are various treatments available and the ones offered will depend on the size of your fibroids, where they are situated, how many there are and whether they are causing symptoms, such as infertility, miscarriages and heavy periods.

Drugs

The best thing to do is to obtain a full diagnosis, and advice, from a gynaecologist, who is experienced in dealing with fibroids. After that, you can weigh up the treatment options available and decide upon the best form of treatment for you. On pages 193 to 198, I'll discuss the natural approach to treating fibroids, and you can use this on its own or in combination with the best that the conventional system has to offer.

Mefenamic acid and tranexamic acid

If your main symptom is heavy bleeding, your doctor will probably suggest the same medication used to treat heavy periods (see page 102), *without* offering a diagnosis first. These drugs will control bleeding by up to 50 per cent, but they will do nothing to address the cause of the bleeding – in this case, fibroids. Furthermore, without a thorough investigation by a gynaecologist, usually involving an ultrasound scan, you will never know for sure if your bleeding is due to fibroids. The two main drugs used to control bleeding are mefenamic acid and tranexamic acid, which can give side-effects such as drowsiness, diarrhoea, rashes and nausea.

GnRH analogues

GnRH analogues – drugs that bring on a temporary menopause (see page 106) – can be used. As mentioned earlier, oestrogen levels fall during menopause, which means that fibroids are more likely to shrink or even disappear. However, research has shown that when drug treatment is ceased, fibroids grow back to their original size within four to six months. Sometimes doctors suggest using GnRH analogues for two to three months prior to surgery (see below) in order to shrink large fibroids to make them easier to remove. These drugs can also reduce bleeding during surgery. Side-effects can include severe mood swings, nausea, dizziness, rashes and headaches.

Progestogen

Progestogen, which is synthetic progesterone, can also be used to control heavy bleeding but it can cause side-effects such as nausea, mood swings and bloating.

Progesterone

If fibroids are stimulated by excess oestrogen, it's logical that adding in progesterone could be helpful. Remember that progesterone is a drug – it doesn't matter whether it has the word 'natural' in front of it. The 'natural' just means that it is chemically identical to the progesterone you produce from your ovaries. It is not used as part of conventional treatment and its use has only become popular with the suggestion that progesterone may be useful at the menopause (see page 408). As yet there is no real data to show that it is effective and side-effects can include acne, fluid retention, weight changes, gastrointestinal disturbances, changes in libido, breast discomfort and menstrual irregularities.

Surgical techniques

Some women are told that their only surgical option is to have a hysterectomy (see page 471). Indeed, many doctors are of the opinion that a hysterectomy is the best way to deal with fibroids. Other doctors will have specialist expertise in removing fibroids (the operation is called a myomectomy), where the womb is left intact, and you may need to do some research to find a good surgeon near to where you live. Many women are told that if they are past childbearing years, or if they have completed their families, a hysterectomy is the best option. There is no doubt that it is easier for a surgeon to remove the whole lot than to remove individual fibroids. Removing fibroids takes much longer, and requires a great deal of skill, and a botched operation can lead to blood loss requiring a full hysterectomy anyway. Hysterectomy is *not* the only way to cope with fibroids. Talk to other women with the same problem – in most cases your gynaecologist can put you in touch with a good self-help group – and ask for a referral to a doctor who doesn't depend on full-scale removal of the womb.

Myomectomy

In this procedure fibroids are removed surgically, leaving the womb intact. If your fibroids are not too large, but they are preventing pregnancy and/or increasing the risk of miscarriage, this is a treatment option. As with any surgery, complications can arise; the main complications for myomectomy include excessive blood loss and the development of adhesions (scar tissue) which can, paradoxically, lead to infertility. There are now many different surgical tools used to help minimise these complications, and lasers have helped to reduce both the bleeding and the number and extent of the adhesions.

A myomectomy can be performed in a number of ways, and the choice of the technique will depend upon the size and position of the fibroids.

Hysteroscopic myomectomy

This technique is used when the fibroids are relatively small (about 2.5cm/1in) or less and of the submucosal type (which means that they are growing on the inside of the womb). Under a general anaesthetic, the neck of the womb (the cervix) is widened and a hysteroscope (tiny camera) is inserted into the womb. The fibroids can then be destroyed by laser or any other surgical instrument. If the fibroid is pedunculated (on a stalk), then the stalk is cut.

Abdominal myomectomy

When the fibroids are growing on the outside of the womb or within the uterine wall then an abdominal myomectomy is usually performed. This operation is also used for fibroids growing in other parts of the abdominal cavity. Under a general anaesthetic, an incision is made in the abdomen and the fibroids are removed or 'scooped out'.

Laparoscopic myomectomy

This is similar to abdominal myomectomy, but the surgery is done with a laparoscope. A laparoscope is a narrow instrument with a telescopic lens. In this case, it is inserted through a small incision below the navel.

Uterine artery embolisation

This is a fairly new technique that works on the theory that fibroids have their own blood supply. If that blood supply is cut off, then the fibroids will stop growing and may even shrink. This technique is performed by a radiologist (a specialist whose expertise is X-rays and radiation) rather than a gynaecologist. A small catheter (flexible tube) is placed into an artery in the groin to identify the two major arteries to the womb. Tiny 'plugs' of polyvinyl alcohol are injected through the catheter to block these arteries. The fibroids that depend upon these arteries should shrink and die. The shrinkage rate of fibroids treated with this technique varies from between 40 to 70 per cent.[14] There can, however, be severe pain after the procedure and strong painkillers are needed. Complications can arise, ranging from infection requiring a hysterectomy to death from septicaemia (blood poisoning).[15]

This is a relatively new technique for treating fibroids, and we do not yet have adequate scientific data available about the risks and success rate.

Myolysis (laser ablation)

This is also a new technique that is based on a process called 'necrotic coagulation', where the centre of the fibroid is destroyed by laser. The fibroid is then reabsorbed into the body over the following weeks and months. A small scar may be left in the centre of the fibroid.

An MRI (magnetic resonance imaging) scan is used to guide the insertion of lasers in order to 'zap' the middle of the fibroid and also to watch the destruction of the fibroid during the procedure. Dr Penny Law at St Mary's Hospital, Paddington in London has pioneered this approach and it is estimated that fibroids can shrink by up to 40 per cent with this technique.[16]

This procedure is carried out under a local anaesthetic on an outpatient basis and ultrasound scans are used to follow up progress at six weeks and then again at three months after surgery. The procedure can also be repeated later on, particularly if the original fibroid was very large.

CAN FIBROIDS RE-GROW?

The answer is yes. You have about a one in four chance of your fibroids re-growing after a myomectomy. If you make no changes to your diet or lifestyle, there is a pretty good chance that your fibroids will grow again. If all the factors that encouraged their growth in the first place remain, they are more likely to grow again. If you do decide to go for the surgical approach, make sure that you take steps to alter your diet and lifestyle to prevent recurrence in the future.

Another factor affecting fibroid re-growth is your age. If you are nearing the menopause (over 45 years old in the majority of women),

---

the likelihood that they will recur is much lower. As you move towards menopause, your oestrogen levels will naturally decline. Since fibroids are oestrogen sensitive, they'll be much less likely to re-grow.

Endometrial ablation and resection

In these procedures, the womb lining can be destroyed by the use of a hot wire loop diathermy (endometrial resection) and/or a hot revolving metal rollerball (endometrial ablation) to burn away the tissue. If you suffer from submucosal fibroids (growing inside the womb), this technique should be able to remove the fibroids and ease heavy periods. It is not appropriate when fibroids are growing outside the womb.

Your periods stop completely because the womb lining is destroyed and therefore no bleeding occurs at the time a period would be expected. This is not a practical solution for women who want to conceive and sometimes sterilisation is offered at the same time.

Hysterectomy

This is the most invasive and extreme form of treatment for fibroids. Hysterectomy, which involves removing the womb alone, or with the ovaries, Fallopian tubes and cervix (see page 473) is the one of the most commonly performed operations today. In my opinion it should only be considered as a last resort. In many cases hysterectomy can be totally unnecessary, particularly when there are so many conventional and natural treatments available, which can make a big difference to your overall health.

The general consensus among many medical professionals is that the womb is unnecessary in women who have completed their families, or are over the age of about 40. Don't listen if anyone tells you this! There are few reasons why a hysterectomy is absolutely necessary, and in the majority of cases you have a choice (for more on this, see Chapter 14).

What Natural Treatments Could Be Effective?

Natural treatment will enable you to work on a number of factors at the same time:

1. Improve your diet, based on the recommendations in Chapter 1 (see page 16).

2. Use nutritional supplements that are known scientifically to control heavy periods, thereby alleviating the main symptoms of fibroids. This treatment is done alongside secondary treatment to help shrink the fibroids naturally.

3. Control excess oestrogens from environmental sources, and reduce your own levels of oestrogen, which 'feed' the fibroids.

4. Control levels of unhealthy prostaglandins, which control blood flow and clotting, by adjusting your diet and taking supplements.

5. Use herbs in the long term to help shrink the fibroids.

6. Use herbs in the short term to control blood flow during periods.

Dietary changes

Begin by following the hormone balancing diet (see Chapter 1). This diet works because it helps to control excess levels of oestrogen that can encourage fibroids to grow. And if you need to have surgical treatment because a fibroid is preventing conception, for example, then it is crucial that you start the hormone balancing diet as soon as can, even before the surgery, in order to prevent a fibroid from re-growing after it has been removed.

All of the recommendations in Chapter 1 are important, but particular attention should also be paid to the following.

Coffee

Avoid coffee, which increases the menstrual flow. Instant coffee has been shown to increase the likelihood of developing fibroids in mice.[17]

High saturated fat intake

Watch your intake of saturated fats (mainly found in animal products, such as dairy and meat). They will contribute to weight gain, which can be particularly problematic for someone suffering from fibroids, because body fat is a manufacturing plant for oestrogen and you must keep your oestrogen levels balanced.

Saturated fats can also block your body's absorption of the essential fatty acids which are essential for helping with fibroids.

Weight

Watch your weight (see Chapter 13). We have seen that fat is a manufacturing plant for oestrogen so it is important that your weight is kept under control. Any excess oestrogen will increase the size of fibroids, and possibly contribute to their growth.

Your liver

Your liver detoxifies harmful substances, such as toxins, waste products, drugs and alcohol. It also processes the hormones that your body produces and renders them harmless. It is supposed to deactivate oestrogen (this is explained more fully on page 37), but if your liver is not functioning efficiently you can develop an accumulation of oestrogen because it is not being excreted properly. Again, this will encourage the growth of a fibroid.

Make sure that you have eliminated any substances that can compromise the functioning of your liver. Alcohol is the most important thing to eliminate, but cut out caffeine and a diet high in saturated fats.

Fibre

Ensure that you get plenty of fibre from your diet (see page 34). It helps to reduce excess oestrogen levels by helping to eliminate them efficiently from your body. Include whole grains, such as brown rice, oats, rye, and plenty of fresh fruit and vegetables.

You can also use foods containing fibre to help constipation. It is important that you are not constipated when you have fibroids because your bowels will help to excrete toxins, waste products and hormones. Do not use bran as your source of fibre (see page 436), as it can block the uptake of valuable nutrients.

Phytoestrogens

Certain foods are high in phytoestrogens (naturally occurring oestrogens; see page 20), and if you suffer from fibroids you could be forgiven for thinking that these should be eliminated from your diet. However, they can be very beneficial.

These foods are discussed in detail on page 20, but they include such things as soya, chickpeas, lentils and garlic. Because these foods have mild oestrogenic activity, they can actually control levels of excess oestrogen by blocking oestrogen receptors in different parts of the body (such as the womb and breasts), preventing the more powerful oestrogens from getting through.

Phytoestrogens have also been found to stimulate the production of sex hormone-binding globulin (SHBG).[18] SHBG is a protein produced by the liver that binds sex hormones such as oestrogen in order to control how much of them are circulating in the blood at any one time. The fewer hormones that are circulating the less there is available to stimulate the fibroid to grow.

Brenda

Brenda was 52 when she came to see me. She had been diagnosed 3 years earlier with a fibroid, which she was told was the size of a 20-week pregnancy. She was desperate to avoid a hysterectomy, but had been advised that there was no option. Brenda had been on HRT for three years, but had stopped four months before I saw her. Brenda was not experiencing any difficult symptoms from the fibroid, except that she needed to pass urine more often.

Her hair mineral analysis showed that she was deficient in zinc, chromium and selenium and had above-average levels of lead and mercury. I talked through her diet and recommended a programme of supplements for her to follow for three months (see page 201). I then asked for her to be tested again.

We discussed the possible sources of exposure to lead and mercury, and I gave her antioxidants to help remove them from her system. I also gave her herbs to help with the fibroid. Brenda had a repeat scan ten months later and the fibroid had shrunk enough to avoid the need for a hysterectomy. She had arranged with her gynaecologist to be scanned once a year to keep an eye on the fibroid.

XENOESTROGENS

Because fibroids are dependent on oestrogen it is important that all sources of excess (unnecessary) oestrogen are controlled. This includes those foreign oestrogens (xenoestrogens) that come from environmental sources. In Chapter 1, I list a host of ways to control xenoestrogens. Make sure that you take steps to do so in every aspect of your daily life. Fibroids have been found to contain larger amounts of the pesticide DDT than any other tissue in the womb.[19] Although DDT is banned in the UK, it is still used in some developing countries and can therefore enter our food chain through imported goods. Buying organic produce is even more important when you are suffering from fibroids. It's not clear why this is significant, but DDT is a foreign oestrogen, and because fibroids grow in the presence of oestrogen, there might be some affinity.

Essential fatty acids

The drug, mefenamic acid, works to regulate heavy bleeding, which is the main symptom of a fibroid, by controlling prostaglandins, which can increase blood flow. But you can also help to control these prostaglandins through dietary measures.

Both red meat and dairy contain arachidonic acid (AA), which encourages the production of PGE2 (the prostaglandin that leads to increased blood flow and blood clotting). The result is heavier periods. Women who suffer from heavy blood flow have higher levels of available arachidonic acid and more PGE2.[20]

So reduce your intake of saturated fats by cutting down on animal foods (not fish). The reason for this is that you want to increase the production of 'good' prostaglandins, which help to reduce abnormal blood clotting. These beneficial prostaglandins are produced from foods that contain certain unsaturated fats that are classed as essential fatty acids, and they are contained in nuts, seeds, oils and oily fish.

Supplements

The approach for controlling the excess bleeding from fibroids involves undertaking the same programme suggested for menorrhagia (heavy periods; see page 102). The idea is to use vitamins, minerals and essential fatty acids to control the main symptoms (heavy bleeding), while you use herbs and dietary changes to help control the growth of the fibroids

Herbs

The herbs suggested here are broken down into those used on a short-term basis, and those used on a long-term basis. In principle, this means that certain herbs will be used throughout the month (long term) to help control the growth of the fibroids, while others will only be used when you are bleeding, to help control the flow.

Long-term herbal treatment

The aim of the long-term herbal treatment is to regulate any oestrogen imbalance (in this case, excess oestrogen) that may be promoting the growth of your fibroids.

Agnus castus (vitex/chastetree berry) is best known as a female hormone balancer, and it helps to regulate the oestrogen and progesterone balance so that progesterone levels are optimum. This in turn reduces any oestrogen dominance that could be stimulating the fibroid growth.

Milk thistle (*Silymarin marianum*) is an important herb for the liver – working to encourage the detoxification process, which can help to excrete excess oestrogen out of the body, and prevent 'old' oestrogens from recirculating. Oestrogen should be deactivated by the liver and then excreted. If the liver does not work efficiently, there is an accumulation of hormones – what is normally produced during the cycle, plus 'old' oestrogen from other cycles, which have not been excreted.

Peony (*Paeonia lactiflora*) is a traditional Chinese herb that helps to balance oestrogen levels in the body, and research shows that it may have a dramatic effect. In 1992, a herbal formula containing peony was used in a trial on women with fibroids. Ninety per cent of the women given the herb experienced an improvement in their symptoms and 60 per cent experienced a reduction in the size of the fibroid.[21]

Short-term herbal treatment

The short-term herbs are to be used while you are having a period in order to help control excess blood loss. Shepherd's purse (*Capsella bursa pastoris*) is an excellent herb for the main symptom of fibroids because it is astringent in nature. Shepherd's purse has been used in clinical trials to prevent heavy bleeding.[22]

Other herbs that are helpful to control the bleeding are cranesbill (*Geranium maculatum*), yarrow (*Achillea millefolium*).

Integrated Treatment Plan

First and foremost, get a proper diagnosis from a gynaecologist, preferably with an ultrasound scan so that any other problems (such as ovarian tumours) can be ruled out.

In the end, however, the decision you make about treating your fibroids will be based on a number of issues, including the severity of your symptoms, your age and whether the fibroids are causing other problems that are affecting your life – your fertility, for example.

Wait and see approach

Before deciding on any treatment, you need to ask yourself what difference it will make to your life and your lifestyle. Fibroids are not life-threatening and you may decide to work on a natural approach instead of going for a conventional solution straightaway. There is no reason why you can't have a scan in, say, six months' time, to monitor the situation. If you find that they are the same size, or getting smaller, and you aren't suffering unduly from any associated symptoms, you may wish to continue using the natural approach for another six months. Remember, it normally takes at least six months for natural remedies to kick in. So, this is not a quick-fix solution, but it will have long-term effects.

Follow the dietary recommendations, and take the suggested supplements and herbs. If you have been using either mefenamic or tranexamic acid, then it is possible to use a combined approach. Your fear may be that if you stop either of these two drugs, you will end up flooding again and not be able to go out. So the best way is to use the medication as needed, because both of these drugs are only used when you bleed. The supplements are used all the time and so are the long-term herbs. The short-term herbs are used when you have your period so you can incorporate a tandem approach. As you start to bleed use the short-term herbs. If the bleeding is unmanageable then use the medication, but you may not need as much as usual. Do the same each month and you should find that, after a few cycles, you do not need the medication because the herbs are controlling the blood flow. Eventually you should not even need the herbs.

Pregnancy issues

If you have been told that your fibroids are preventing conception, or playing a part in recurrent miscarriages, you will need to consider treatments that will enhance your fertility and act quickly.

Removal of the fibroids is probably your key concern, and you will want to act swiftly. In these circumstances, your best option is a myomectomy. Other treatments, such as myolysis and embolisation, do not remove fibroids. They either destroy them slowly or shut off the blood supply to the fibroids. Neither of these would be recommended if you were trying to conceive.

Talk to your doctor about the most appropriate type of myomectomy. The decision will be made according to the size of the fibroids and where they are growing. Ask for and expect the least invasive technique.

The natural approach is extremely effective, but it is necessarily slower. When you want to conceive, I suggest going for the myomectomy and then using the natural recommendations to help prevent your fibroids from recurring.

Age

If you are over 45, I would definitely suggest the 'wait and see' approach, using the natural treatment programme alongside. As long as you are able to cope with the symptoms until the natural treatment 'kicks in', this is your best course of action.

Remember that fibroids grow in the presence of oestrogen, and as you near the menopause, your oestrogen levels will naturally reduce, encouraging the fibroids to shrink on their own. Ironically, however, fibroids can also delay the onset of the menopause (see page 400) because you have higher levels of oestrogen for longer. However, if you can get to the menopause, your symptoms will reduce dramatically.

Not wanting to conceive

If you do not want to get pregnant, are younger than 45 and your fibroids are causing you problems such as excessively heavy bleeding or pressing on the bowel or bladder, you may choose a more immediate treatment.

NATURAL MEDICINE

Both acupuncture and homeopathy can be extremely useful in conjunction with the dietary and herbal recommendations. Acupuncture can help to increase the energy flow to the pelvic area and stop any stagnation in the womb. It can also help to optimise liver function. The homeopathic remedies used in treating fibroids will be tailored to the symptoms and any emotional symptoms will be taken into account as well. The homeopathic remedies Lachesis and Sanguinaria are often used when there is excess bleeding.

At the moment, with the medical choices available, the best choice would seem to be myolysis using an MRI scan to target the fibroids. At the same time, use the natural approach to augment the myolysis treatment, and to prevent any re-growth.

Your Supplement Plan

- A good multivitamin and mineral supplement, e.g. The Healthy Woman by the Natural Health Practice
- Vitamin A★ as beta-carotene, not retinol; (10,000iu per day)
- Vitamin C with bioflavonoids (1,000mg per day)
- Linseed oil (1,000mg per day)
- Vitamin B complex (providing 50mg of most of the B vitamins per day)
- Zinc citrate (15mg per day)

★ High doses of vitamin A as retinol are only problematic if you are planning a pregnancy (see pages 375–6). If so, keep vitamin A to 2,500iu per day.

Note
Each nutrient represents the total intake for one day, so if your multivitamin and mineral already contains 5mg of zinc, for

---

example, you only need to add in a separate zinc supplement containing 10mg per day.

Herbs

Use an equal mix of the long-term herbs (*Agnus castus*, milk thistle and peony, 1 teaspoon three times a day) when you are not having a period and then switch to an equal mix of the short-term herbs (shepherd's purse, cranesbill and yarrow, 1 teaspoon three times a day) once your periods begin. When your bleeding becomes manageable during your period, stop taking the herbs. When your period is finished completely, start back on the long-term herbs.

Follow this treatment programme over six months. If your menstrual bleeding becomes manageable before the six months are up, you can stop the short-term herbs. Keep the long-term herbs going and arrange for a scan to see what is happening to the fibroid.

If you think that the bleeding is not progressively improving over the first three months then see a qualified natural practitioner to get some individual help.

In Summary

- Always investigate the cause of heavy periods before taking any drugs, or beginning the natural treatment programme. Ensure that you have a diagnosis of fibroids, and an idea of their size and position within the body before deciding on a treatment.

- Consider your age, lifestyle and whether you want children before deciding on a form of treatment.

- Don't give up your medication without consulting your doctor.

- Begin the hormone balancing diet (see page 16).

- Avoid coffee, which increases the menstrual flow.

- Eat organic food whenever possible.

- Take supplements (see page 201) throughout your entire cycle.

- Take short-term herbs only when you are bleeding, and alongside any drugs to control the flow.

- Discontinue the drugs gradually, as they are no longer required, and continue taking short-term herbs until the bleeding is completely under control.

- Take long-term herbs throughout the month, but change to short-term herbs when your period arrives.

PROLAPSE

Prolapse is a common condition and it occurs when the structures designed to keep organs in place weaken or stretch, causing them literally to 'prolapse'. There are many causes for prolapse, but the two main causes, gravity and childbirth, can affect us all, so it's important that you keep an eye out for symptoms. A prolapse can be fairly mild but it can also become serious, and once the damage is done, it's virtually impossible to undo it.

What is a Prolapse?

Prolapse literally means 'to fall' or 'slip out of place', and the term can relate to different organs in the body. It is possible to have a rectal (prolapse of the rectum), bladder, vaginal or womb (uterine) prolapse and some of these can occur at the same time.

Womb prolapse

The womb is held in place by the pelvic floor muscles and supporting ligaments. When these muscles start to weaken and/or the supporting ligaments lose their elasticity, the womb starts to drop down into the vagina. It is also called a 'dropped' womb and refers to the sagging of the womb into the vagina or even out of the body.

A prolapse of the womb can also be common around the menopause because the muscle support often becomes thinner when the hormone levels – in particular oestrogen – are reduced.

Vaginal prolapse

The front and back walls of the vagina can become weakened, and it begins to move downwards, often turning itself inside out. Normally, as the womb prolapses, the vagina will also drop. Unfortunately, the biggest risk of vaginal prolapse is after a hysterectomy (where the womb is removed), sometimes years later, because the vagina may have become weakened during surgery.

Prolapse of the bladder (cystocele)

The bladder normally sits directly above the vagina but if there any weakness at the top of the vagina, this can cause the bladder to drop down, where it begins to bulge into the vagina itself. This is called a cystocele. This type of prolapse can lead to recurrent urinary tract infections in some women, while others will experience stress incontinence (see page 209). Again, some women will experience no symptoms at all.

Prolapse of the urethra (urethrocele)

This type of prolapse differs from that of a cystocele in that only the urethra, the tube that leads from the bladder to the outside of the body, drops down. In this case, the bladder itself normally remains in position. A urethrocele can cause stress incontinence (see page 209), particularly if you are suffering from both a cystocele and urethrocele. In this condition, there is an increased risk of urinary tract infections and pain on intercourse.

Prolapse of the rectum (rectocele)

If the lower part of the vagina, which is normally tight, is weakened, then the rectum (which is the last part of the colon before the anus) can bulge into the vagina. Some women can remain unaware that they are suffering from a prolapsed rectum, while others will experience severe constipation, as stools become 'trapped' in the pouch formed by the bulge, making it difficult to defecate.

What Symptoms Could You Experience?

The symptoms for all of the different types of prolapse can be similar. Some women experience few if any symptoms, but others can find a prolapse debilitating. Some of the most common symptoms include:

- lower back pain

- a dragging sensation or feeling of 'something falling out'

- stress incontinence (where small amounts of urine are passed while sneezing, coughing or exercising; see page 209)

- constipation

- difficult or painful sex.

What Causes a Prolapse?

Here we will concentrate on a prolapse of the womb, as this is the most common.

The two major causes of womb (uterine) prolapse are long labours and extremely hard physical work, particularly when pregnant. Given that these two causes no longer pose such a threat (intervention can prevent over-long labours, and women are advised and normally heed the advice to take it easy during pregnancy), this type of prolapse is, thankfully, becoming less common.

Although the physical causes of prolapse are now well understood, there are women who suffer from this condition without having any of the predisposing factors. For example, some women have never had children, or a weight problem, but can experience prolapse of one or more organs. It's now believed that prolapse is largely due to the effects of ageing, and while it can be made worse by some of the causes below, there is no doubt that being an 'upright' species, with the continual pull of gravity, will eventually take its toll. Some experts also believe that prolapse runs in families, perhaps due to a genetic weakness of the muscles in the pelvic area.

Prolapse can be caused or exacerbated by the following.

- **Having children** – The risk increases according to the number you've had, and how quickly you had them. If you had four children, well spaced out, you could be at less risk than a woman who had three with only a year between each.

- **Giving birth** – It is believed that inducing labour can increase the risk, as the womb may be forced to contract abnormally. Long and intense labours can also be a problem because there is an increased risk of injury to the pelvic muscles. The current advice is to give birth in an upright position. This allows the pull of gravity to speed up the process, and it helps to prevent an unnatural strain on the womb itself during labour.

- **Episiotomy** – Incorrectly performed episiotomies, which involve cutting the vaginal wall during birth, can cause future problems by damaging the supporting muscles. When these muscles become damaged, the cervix can, over time, begin to push through the vagina. This may be diagnosed as a prolapse of the womb, and hysterectomy may be suggested. In this case, corrective surgery would be more appropriate.

- **Constipation** – Straining to pass faeces can put unnecessary pressure on the womb.

- **Overweight** – Being overweight is a risk factor because abdominal fat presses down on the organs and other structures in the pelvic area, putting pressure on the womb and the bowel, among other things. The heavier you are, the higher the risks.

- **Coughing** – A chronic cough (including asthma) can put pressure on the pelvic floor, weakening muscles required to hold the abdominal organs and other structures in place.

- **Menopause** – See page 400.

How Do You Know You Have a Prolapse?

If you have any of the symptoms mentioned on pages 205 and 206, you should see your doctor. Diagnosis may be possible by internal examination, or you will be referred to a gynaecologist who can arrange a scan to confirm the diagnosis by ultrasound.

What Treatment Can You Be Offered By Your Doctor?

The main focus of conventional treatment would be surgery, particularly if the prolapse is quite far advanced. There are also non-surgical measures available, and these will normally be suggested as a first line of treatment.

Non-surgical approaches

Pessaries
A pessary is a plastic or rubber ring that fits around the cervix and holds back the womb. This device is used in the case of prolapse of

the womb. The pessary does not actually treat the prolapse, but it can help to limit symptoms, such as stress incontinence caused by exercising and lower back pain. A pessary can be inserted as and when it is required – for example, just before exercising – and taken out afterwards.

Vaginal cones

These cones are literally small weights that are used to help strengthen the pelvic floor and vaginal muscles. When these muscles are weak, prolapse is more common, as is stress incontinence (see page 209). A small plastic vaginal cone is inserted into the vagina in the same way as you would insert a tampon. The cone is hollow and it unscrews so that weights can be placed inside.

In the same way that weights at the gym strengthen muscles in your body, these cones work on the muscles of the pelvic area. The effects build up over time, and as your pelvic muscles become stronger, you can increase the weight of the cone.

The cone is first inserted with a small weight inside, and you will be instructed to keep it in place for about 15 minutes a day, while standing upright. You can expect to see a difference between 8 and 12 weeks.[23] Once you have achieved the desired result (normally gauged by an improvement in the prolapse itself, your symptoms and any stress incontinence), you can maintain the muscle tone by using the cones two or three times a week.

Some women find the cones easier to use than practising pelvic floor exercises (see page 209), partly because they are fairly effortless, but also, and more importantly, because they automatically work the right muscles in the pelvic area. Pelvic floor exercises are only effective if they are done properly.

Note
The vaginal cones should not be used if you are pregnant, during your period, or if you are suffering from a urinary tract infection or thrush.

If you have trouble obtaining the cones, contact me directly (see Staying in Touch, page 507).

Pelvic floor exercises

These exercises were designed by Dr Arnold Kegel in the 1940s to help strengthen the muscles in the pelvic area. Most women are encouraged to practise pelvic floor exercises during pregnancy, and it is suggested that you continue to practise them after the birth on a regular basis.

Some women find it difficult to locate the correct muscles, and there are two groups that need to be worked. To locate the muscles, try to stop your urine flow in midstream, using the relevant muscles in the vaginal area. Don't do this on a regular basis, however: it can push urine back up into the bladder and lead to infections and bladder weakness.

There are two types of muscles that need to be worked, and two types of exercises to work them. First of all, slowly bring up your pelvic floor by contracting the muscles. Hold for a count of five and then gently let it down again. Work at this, several times a day, until you can hold the count for 15. You may find that you lose control part way through the count. Start again, and make sure that you can feel the muscles being released as you 'let down' your pelvic floor.

The second type of exercise involves quick tightening and releasing of the muscles in the pelvic floor. As quickly as you can, tighten and then release the muscles. Do this about 30 times, and then take a break.

Each session should comprise two sets of the 'slow' exercises and two sets of the 'fast' exercises. Take a minute's break in between. Some women find it easier to practise these exercises while sitting on a kitchen chair because you can actually feel the muscles as they rise and fall against the chair. In the beginning it may also help to perform the sets while lying down, because the pressure of gravity is reduced.

Pelvic floor exercises can also be combined with the use of the vaginal cones in order to give faster results.

STRESS INCONTINENCE

Stress incontinence is a common condition, and it is caused by a variety of factors, including most of those that can lead to prolapse (see page 204). Many women first experience stress incontinence during pregnancy, when the weight of the baby presses down on the pelvic floor, weakening bladder control. Following the birth, the pelvic floor muscles can be weakened so that normal control is not resumed for several months (or even years), unless pelvic floor exercises are regularly practised.

Common symptoms of stress incontinence include leaking when you cough, laugh or sneeze, leaking when you are exercising or lifting, having little warning of the need to pass water, which means that you may not reach the toilet in time, and occasionally an increased urgency or need to pass water. Some women may find that they dribble urine without even realising it.

DEALING WITH STRESS INCONTINENCE

Stress incontinence can occur simply because your pelvic floor muscles have become weakened (through pregnancy and childbirth or during the menopause, for example), and this weakening can result in a lack of control over the bladder. You can also suffer from stress incontinence because of a prolapse. If leaking is your most troublesome symptom and other aspects of the prolapse are not causing you problems, then it is worth exploring other options (such as cones, pessaries and pelvic floor exercises) to help the leakage.

SURGERY

There are two main types of surgical techniques for stress incontinence:

- **Colposuspension** – This technique involves 'hitching' up the bladder neck to the pubic bone ligament. This can be done through keyhole surgery. This is normally performed before a sling operation.

- **Sling operation** – This is usually the 'last resort' approach to stress incontinence. It involves placing a strip of tissue in the vagina, under the bladder, to act like a hammock to support it. The procedure is successful in some women, but there have been many cases where the problem has remained.

Collagen Bladder Neck Injections

This technique is usually used where incontinence is caused by a weak valve or where previous surgery has been ineffective or only partially successful. Collagen (a fibrous connective tissue) is injected around the outlet of the bladder. This narrows the outlet and tightens up the valve. The procedure usually takes about five minutes and is performed in hospital (usually under general anaesthetic). The success rate is about 60 to 70 per cent, with few side-effects. Following the operation you may notice some stinging on passing urine, or perhaps a little blood in your urine. This treatment is designed specifically for stress incontinence.

Fluid intake

Keep fluid intake to a reasonable level to ensure that your bladder doesn't become overfull. Keep a diary and make a note of how many times you go the toilet, when you need to go, and how often you have leaked. Then compare this against the amount of fluid you have taken. Try varying your fluid intake to see if it makes a difference. For example, the number of times you get up in the night to urinate may depend on how late you drink water, so make a note of anything that seems relevant. You are aiming to see what amount of liquid works best for you.

An important change to make to your diet is cutting out any drinks that have a diuretic effect. The main diuretic is caffeine, so cut out or at least reduce by a great deal your intake of colas, tea and coffee.

Cranberry juice

Unsweetened cranberry juice has been enormously successful in the treatment of urinary tract infections and cystitis (see page 276), but what you may not know is that it can encourage bladder function and help to prevent incontinence. Try a glass a day.

Exercises

Pelvic floor exercises (see page 209) and vaginal cones (see page 208) are an excellent way to tighten up the floor of your pelvis and many women experience complete relief of symptoms after several months of regular practice. Make sure you exercise your pelvis daily to prevent the condition from deteriorating, and to work towards toning the pelvic area.

Herbs

Ladies' mantle (*Alchemilla vulgaris*) and horsetail (*Equisetum arvense*; see page 216) are specifically indicated for stress incontinence. All of the herbs and supplements suggested for prolapse (see page 215) are relevant for stress incontinence because they are all aimed at strengthening collagen.

Surgical techniques

Hysterectomy

This is one of the most common solutions offered for a prolapse of the womb but I would suggest that you explore other options before agreeing to this radical technique. Hysterectomy should be a last resort only (see page 471).

Paradoxically, hysterectomy can solve the problem of a prolapse of the womb (because afterwards there is no womb to prolapse), but it can lead to a vaginal prolapse because other supporting structures (such as the cervix) have been removed during the hysterectomy. If you are showing signs of weak vaginal walls, or already have a vaginal prolapse, you should think very carefully about alternatives to hysterectomy. Chances are you'll end up requiring another procedure to address the vaginal prolapse.

You could opt for a sub-total hysterectomy (see page 474), where the cervix is left intact. This reduces the chances of the vagina dropping down.

Repair operation

It is possible to re-suspend the womb back into its normal position, thus avoiding the need for a hysterectomy. You will need to be referred to a good gynaecologist who specialises in this procedure, but it certainly is a viable alternative to hysterectomy. Dr Vicki Hufnagel is the eminent US gynaecologist who pioneered female reconstructive surgery to help women avoid hysterectomy, and she has written an interesting book entitled *No More Hysterectomies* (Thorsons). If you are faced with making a decision about hysterectomy, it's worth investing in a copy.

It is also possible to have surgery to correct a cystocele and rectocele, so again it is worth contacting an expert in this area.

What Natural Treatments Could Be Effective?

Dealing with a prolapse requires a completely different approach to the majority of conditions outlined in this book, largely because it is a structural problem rather than one of hormone imbalance or nutritional deficiency. However, many of the recommendations below are aimed at strengthening the ligaments and tendons in the pelvic area, ensuring their integrity and elasticity. Many of the treatments are aimed at tonifying the uterus and other organs in the area. Depending on the severity of your condition, however, you may need to undertake these recommendations alongside conventional treatment.

There are three stages involved in this treatment programme:

1. Improve your diet, based on the recommendations outlined in Chapter 1.

2. Use nutritional supplements that can help to control the condition, and to prevent symptoms and further problems.

3. Use specific herbs in the long term, to improve the overall functioning of the organs and structures in the pelvis.

Dietary changes

No matter what health problems you may suffer from, taking steps to improve your diet will encourage all parts of your body to function better. Although prolapse is not a strictly hormonal condition, there is no question that it can become worse or even begin during the menopause, when hormone levels start to dip. Therefore, the recommendations from Chapter 1, will help to ensure that hormone levels are stabilised, thereby preventing the condition from becoming worse. In particular, adopt the hormone balancing diet outlined on page 16. There are a number of additional remedies and supplements that can help to address both the problems associated with prolapse and overall health.

Fluid intake

Although it is important to drink plenty of water to flush toxins from the body and encourage optimum health, it is just as important, in the case of prolapse, not to overdo it. A full bladder can put additional strain on the pelvic muscles, and too much fluid intake can exacerbate stress incontinence (see page 209). The more liquid you drink on a regular basis, the more likely your bladder is to lose its elasticity, as it becomes stretched over and over again. If you do drink a lot, ensure that you empty your bladder frequently – even before you feel the urge to urinate.

> **BREASTFEEDING**
>
> Breastfeeding can help to prevent prolapse because it encourages the womb to contract back to its pre-pregnant state more quickly.

Fibre

Fibre is essential for regular bowel movements, and ensuring that you have plenty in your diet can help to prevent constipation, which can exacerbate or even cause a prolapse because straining to go to the toilet is going to put extra pressure on the womb. To get your bowels working naturally, increase your intake of fresh fruit and vegetables to at least five per day. If you need more help, sprinkle 15ml (1 tablespoon) of linseeds on to your breakfast cereal in the morning or soak 15ml (1 tablespoon) of linseeds in water and then swallow.

Normal laxatives work by stimulating or increasing the number of bowel movements or by encouraging a softer or bulkier stool. Unfortunately, they do not address the cause of the problem, which is likely to be a lack of fibre. It's also possible to become dependent upon laxatives: the more you take, the less your body has to do for itself. Ultimately the bowel can lose its tone and muscle action, and then cannot function.

Herbal laxatives, which can include butternut, blue flag and psyllium, are generally more gentle. Their effects are two-fold: first, they create a healthy and frequent bowel movement; and second they tone the bowel to encourage its own natural function.

Flavonoids

When you are suffering from a prolapse, you need to use any measure that will help to strengthen the muscles and ligaments, and to tone the pelvic area. Collagen is a protein that is in abundant supply in the body. It maintains the integrity of ligaments, tendons and bone, and gives skin its elasticity. For this reason, it is important that you maintain good levels of collagen in your body, and one of the best ways to do this is to up your intake of flavonoids.

- **Bioflavonoids** help to preserve the collagen matrix, which can be damaged by free radicals (see page 17). These bioflavonoids are closely associated with vitamin C and eating good amounts of them can help to preserve the collagen inside the vagina and also maintain the elasticity of the urinary tract (thereby preventing stress incontinence; see page 209). These flavonoids are found in many foods, such as citrus fruits, onions, parsley, legumes (such as lentils) and green tea.

- **Proanthocyanidins** are another type of flavonoids and like bioflavonoids they also help to strengthen the collagen matrix and prevent the destruction of collagen. They are excellent 'free radical scavengers', which can help to slow down the degenerative effects of ageing. These flavonoids give the deep colour to many berries such as blackberries, blueberries, cranberries and raspberries, and are also found in grapes. Make sure you get plenty of these in your daily diet.

Supplements

Suggested dosages will follow in the treatment plan (see page 217).

Vitamin C with bioflavonoids
We know that vitamin C and also bioflavonoids help with the formation of collagen,[24] so it is important that you take these nutrients in supplement form if you are suffering from either prolapse or stress incontinence, or both.

Vitamin A
This vitamin is known to help the body produce collagen, and can also encourage the strength of your cartilage (which is required to keep the organs and other structures in the pelvic area in position). Make sure you get plenty in your daily diet, and take vitamin A as a supplement.

Manganese
This mineral is needed for healthy bones, cartilage and skin. There is usually enough in a good multivitamin and mineral to cover any deficiency that might be at the root of your pelvic weakness.

Herbs

In herbal medicine uterine tonics are used for prolapse of the womb as listed below.

True unicorn root (*Aletris farinosa*)

This herb is especially indicated for prolapse because it helps when there is a sense of heaviness and 'falling out'. It is classed herbally as a tonic for the womb and is especially useful for any weaknesses connected with the pelvic floor.

Ladies' mantle (*Alchemilla vulgaris*)

This herb is often used for a prolapsed womb and is, interestingly, the herb used for urinary incontinence. It is, therefore, particularly useful in the case of prolapse, even if you are not experiencing stress incontinence. Conversely, take also for stress incontinence to help ensure the integrity of the reproductive organs. Ladies' mantle contains flavonoids (see page 214), which can help to protect connective tissue and to retain elasticity.

Dong quai (*Angelica sinensis*)

This herb is the best tonic for women in traditional Chinese medicine. It helps with congestion in the pelvic area and increases circulation there.

Red raspberry leaf (*Rubus idaeus*)

This herb – which is well known for its beneficial effects in the last months of pregnancy – is excellent for toning the womb in those who are not pregnant. It also strengthens the pelvic muscles.

False unicorn root (*Chamaelirium luteum*)

This herb is an excellent choice when there is any weakness in the womb, so it is ideally suited for treating prolapse. It is specifically indicated when there are dragging sensations.

Horsetail (*Equisetum arvense*)

This herb is not classed as a uterine tonic, but as an astringent, and it is particularly useful for stress incontinence. It is beneficial for prolapse because it contains flavonoids and helps to strengthen connective tissue.

Acupuncture and homeopathy

Both these natural therapies could be helpful for treating a prolapse. And I would suggest that you explore either of these along with the nutrition and herbs.

The Integrated Treatment Plan

Before undertaking the treatment plan, you will need to have had full investigations to assess the severity of your prolapse. Follow the plan below on the basis of your diagnosis.

If your prolapse is so severe that structures are starting to protrude from your body, natural treatments can be helpful but they will need to be used alongside surgery in order to get the problem back to a manageable position. If you opt for repair surgery rather than a hysterectomy, the aim will be to use natural treatments to try to prevent the problem recurring.

If your prolapse is mild rather than severe, it is worth putting into place the dietary and herbal recommendations listed below, as well as using some of the physical therapies, such as pelvic floor exercises and vaginal cones in order to correct the problem and to prevent it from becoming worse. The idea is to keep the prolapse manageable in order to avoid surgery. Surgery should really only be considered when your prolapse is so severe that it is affecting your daily life, causing pain or discomfort, or making sexual relations difficult.

Whether you opt for surgery or physical therapy (such as cones), you should begin the dietary changes immediately, as well as taking the supplements and herbs.

Nutritional supplements should be taken throughout your cycle, for six months. Herbs should be taken throughout your cycle, until your period arrives, at which point stop taking them. Start again when your period is over. Continue with the treatment for six months. After this time, a good diet and programme of pelvic floor exercises should keep the problem at bay.

Your Supplement Plan

- A good multivitamin and mineral supplement, e.g. The Healthy Woman by the Natural Health Practice
- Vitamin C with bioflavonoids (1,000mg twice a day)
- Vitamin A (as beta-carotene at 25,000iu per day)
- Proanthocyanidins (50mg per day)
- Manganese (5mg per day)
- Cranberry supplement (only for stress incontinence)

> **Note**
> Each nutrient represents the total intake for one day, so if your multivitamin and mineral already contains 5mg of manganese, you do not need to add in a separate manganese supplement.

Herbs

Take a combination of true unicorn root, dong quai, red raspberry leaf, ladies' mantle, false unicorn root and horsetail. Take 1 teaspoon a day over a period of six months.

In Summary

- See your doctor if you are suffering from symptoms of prolapse or stress incontinence, to work out how severe the problem might be.
- Follow the hormone balancing diet on page 16, which will help to keep levels of hormones that affect the integrity of the ligaments balanced.
- Practise pelvic floor exercises at least twice daily (see page 209), and consider using vaginal cones to enhance the effect.
- If the problem is severe, you may need to consider surgery, but the natural recommendations should be followed alongside any conventional treatment.
- Watch your fluid intake and, if you are suffering from incontinence, cut out caffeine.
- Ensure that you have plenty of fibre in your diet, which can help to prevent constipation.
- Add flavonoids to your diet, to help strengthen the muscles and ligaments, and to tone the pelvic area.
- Take supplements (see page 215) throughout your entire cycle.
- Take herbs throughout your cycle, taking a break when your period comes, and then starting again afterwards. The herbs should be taken for six months.

CHAPTER 7

The Ovaries

The ovaries, small organs positioned just below the Fallopian tubes on each side of the womb, are the egg producers of a woman's reproductive cycle. Each month, from a few years after the beginning of a girl's menstrual cycle until the menopause, the ovaries will release eggs. The ovaries also produce hormones, including oestrogen and progesterone. A number of problems – including cancer, which I do not discuss in this book – can affect the ovaries.

OVARIAN CYSTS

Many women develop growths, known as 'cysts', in or on their ovaries. These cysts are fluid-(water) filled sacs (rather like a blister). In some women cysts are completely harmless, requiring little or no treatment. These cysts are 'benign', or non-cancerous. Other cysts, however, can be cancerous, which is why a diagnosis is extremely important when ovarian cysts are suspected. Cysts can vary in size. They are normally small, which means that you may not even know you have one until a routine examination picks it up. However, some are large enough to cause menstrual irregularities or discomfort.

What Are Ovarian Cysts?

There are two main types of ovarian cysts: functional and abnormal. These are then broken down into several further types, depending on the characteristics and cause.

POLYCYSTIC OVARIES

Many women experience a large number of small cysts in the ovaries, often accompanied by hormonal imbalance. This condition is called 'polycystic' (see Polycystic Ovary Syndrome, page 232), although technically they are not cysts, but very small egg follicles.

Functional cysts

These are the most common type of ovarian cysts. Many ovarian cysts are due to abnormal cell growth, but functional cysts are different, caused mainly by a slight alteration in the normal functioning of the ovary.

There are two types of functional cysts: follicular and luteal, named according to the half of the cycle at which they appear. Follicular cysts appear in the first half; luteal cysts appear in the second half.

Follicular cysts

Each month the egg-making follicle of your ovary releases an egg. However, in the case of follicular cysts, the egg is not released and the follicle continues to grow, becoming enlarged and filled with fluid. These cysts can cause few if any symptoms and may only be diagnosed when you are seeing your doctor for other reasons. Normally ultrasound is the form of diagnosis.

Luteal cysts

This type of cyst develops in the second half of the cycle after the egg has been released (at ovulation). As soon as ovulation has taken place in a normal cycle, the ruptured follicle then develops into the corpus luteum, which produces progesterone in anticipation of a pregnancy. If the egg is not fertilised, the corpus luteum withers, progesterone levels fall and a period occurs. A luteal cyst is formed when the corpus luteum fails to wither when it should, and fills with blood instead.

Pain or spotting at ovulation (called mittelschmerz) can be caused by the release of blood from the corpus luteum when there is a slight drop in oestrogen at ovulation.

Abnormal cysts

These are very different from functional cysts because they are the result of abnormal cell growth. This does not, however, mean that they are cancerous. Many cysts are simply benign growths. No one knows for sure what causes this abnormal cell growth. The cysts can remain for ever, without causing any problems, or they may burst, requiring emergency surgery. Different kinds of abnormal cysts include the following.

Cystadenoma cysts

These cysts develop from cells on the outer surface of the ovaries. They can grow to a large size and are sometimes attached to the ovary by a stem. The cysts themselves may not cause any remarkable symptoms, but they can twist on their stems and then rupture, which can be extremely painful, and require emergency surgery.

Endometrial cysts

Endometriosis is a condition in which the lining of the womb (endometrium) begins to grow in parts of the body other than the womb (see page 168). These endometrial patches can form on the ovaries, creating cysts known as 'chocolate cysts' because they are filled with old blood.

Every month during your period these endometrial patches of tissues that have become encapsulated in a cyst will bleed. Because there is no outlet for the bleeding, the cyst becomes larger. Even small chocolate cysts can rupture, although they may grow very large causing severe pain.

Dermoid cysts (teratomas)

Dermoid cysts are a very bizarre phenomenon, and are classed as tumours rather than simply cysts. Every one of your eggs has the potential to create another human being, and dermoid cysts are effectively structures that are filled with pieces of bone, teeth, hair and skin. One theory is that an unfertilised egg begins to produce various body tissues. Alternatively, it has been suggested that we are effectively carrying a 'twin' inside. It is unknown how or why these kinds of tumours grow. They are solid structures, which means that they are not, technically, cysts, but they can become malignant (cancerous).

Are There Any Symptoms?

The simple answer is not always. Some women develop cysts and experience no symptoms whatsoever. Others notice changes in their monthly cycles that indicate potential problems. Still others experience pain and obvious symptoms, such as the following:
• irregular periods
• pain, dull aching or cramping in the abdomen
• pain during intercourse
• breakthrough bleeding
• swelling in the abdomen

What Can Cause You To Have Ovarian Cysts?

Functional cysts are often easier to explain. The more menstrual cycles you have without interruption, the more likely you are to develop functional ovarian cysts. This is because your body effectively produces cysts in the process of ovulation every month. The egg should be released, but if it isn't, it can continue to grow (see pages 63–7). Therefore, menopausal women who do not have a menstrual cycle cannot develop functional cysts.

Functional cysts are also impossible to develop if you are on the birth control pill because this form of contraception prevents ovulation, which is when the cysts are formed. As a result, the Pill is often used as a form of treatment for women who regularly develop functional cysts.

Ovarian cysts can develop during fertility treatment because the ovaries are being stimulated to mature more than one egg.

Our modern lifestyle may also be to blame for the increasing incidence of ovarian cysts. In previous generations and in traditional cultures, women began having babies earlier and tended to have many more children. Breastfeeding usually lasted for up to two years or even more, often followed by a pregnancy immediately after a baby was weaned. The result was (and is) of course that women had much fewer menstrual cycles over the course of a lifetime. Today, childbearing is often delayed until a woman is in her late 30s, and then only one or two children are normally conceived. As a result, women ovulate many more times than was previously the norm and there is a strong possibility that this 'interference' with the natural order sets the stage for problems, such as cysts.

You are more likely to develop ovarian cysts if:

- you are between the ages of 20 and 35

- childbearing is delayed

- you smoke. Women who smoke or who have in the past smoked are 1.5 times more likely to get ovarian cysts than non-smokers.[1]

Getting a Diagnosis

If you have any of the symptoms listed above it is important that you see your doctor to arrange a check-up. Your doctor will normally perform a number of diagnostic procedures, usually in the following order.

Pelvic examination

Some cysts can be felt by examining the abdomen and feeling the size of your ovaries. This can involve both an internal and external examination. Depending on the results from this examination you could be sent for further investigations. The next step would be to have an ultrasound scan.

Ultrasound scan

This involves using sound waves to create an image of your pelvic cavity through a device that can be placed on your abdomen and/or in your vagina. Functional cysts can be easily identified by ultrasound. If a cyst does appear on the screen during the scan, and there is any doubt about its type, you may be advised to have a laparoscopy.

In some clinics newer techniques are available using colour doppler ultrasound, which can help exclude cancerous cysts, especially if combined with blood tests that look at tumour markers.

Laparoscopy

This procedure is performed under a general anaesthetic and it involves inserting a narrow tube with a telescopic lens into the abdomen via a small incision below the navel. Through the lens, your doctor can clearly see all structures in the abdomen.

What Treatment Can You Be Offered By Your Doctor?

The treatment offered by your doctor will depend on the type of ovarian cyst you have.

The 'wait and see' approach may be used for both follicular and luteal cysts, as functional cysts are often reabsorbed without any further problems.

Drugs

If you have recurrent functional cysts, you may be offered the Pill to prevent the cysts from forming. This is the treatment of choice for functional ovarian cysts.

The contraceptive pill

The Pill has a very high success rate (some 80 to 90 per cent) in preventing ovarian cysts,[2] because it stops you from ovulating, which means that the cysts cannot develop. However, it does not do anything to address the root cause of the problem. As soon as you stop taking the Pill, you are likely to begin forming cysts again. Some of the listed side-effects of the Pill are nausea, vomiting, headache, thrombosis, weight changes, changes in sex drive, depression and breast tenderness.

The surgical approach

Aspiration

If your doctor has tried the 'wait and see' approach, but your functional cyst proves to be persistent (it is not reabsorbed), surgery may be required. During a laparosocopy (see page 224), which is performed under general anaesthetic, the fluid in the cyst can be suctioned off (aspirated) and the cyst will collapse like a balloon when the air is released.

Surgical removal

Any type of cyst other than functional will need to be removed. All other types of cysts are the result of abnormal cell growth, and there can be a risk of further problems, such as cancer. Surgery is performed under a general anaesthetic. If your cyst is fairly large, a cut will be made in your abdomen in order to remove it. The cyst would then be sent off to the lab to check that it was not malignant.

If you do need surgery, find a gynaecologist who will try to remove the cyst while leaving your ovary intact. This may not always be possible, depending on the size and the type of cyst. It is obviously easier for a doctor to take out the ovary and cyst together (see page 235), but this will be much more traumatic for you. It may be that half of the ovary can be left in place, and this is still better than total removal.

Your doctor will probably not be able to confirm what he or she intends to do until surgery has begun. But it is essential that you make clear your choices in advance, both in discussions with your doctor, and on your consent form (see page 479).

What Natural Treatments Could Be Effective?

Before you embark on any natural approach to ovarian cysts it is essential that you have a firm diagnosis. You need to know what type of cyst you have, and its size. Not every health condition can be sorted out with natural remedies, and if you have a cyst that is potentially cancerous, or causing serious problems in your pelvic area, it is sensible to follow conventional advice until such time as the problem is manageable. But consider carefully the medical advice you are given.

You may, for example, discover that you have a cyst that has been in there for years without presenting any symptoms. In these circumstances, you may wish to leave things as they are, particularly if you have been given confirmation that the cyst is not malignant. If you are, at any stage, unhappy with either the diagnosis or the proposed form of treatment, get a second medical opinion. It is important to say here that a hysterectomy with the ovaries removed is often the proposed form of surgical treatment and, in the large majority of cases, this approach is unnecessary.

Natural treatment is aimed at prevention. A functional cyst may disappear by itself, or you may have been advised to have it aspirated. In either case, the goal is to prevent it from recurring. It's clear, in the case of functional cysts, that something is awry with your cycle and hormones. Either an egg has failed to be released, and the follicle fills with fluid, or an egg is released and the cyst forms later. In either case, you will need to get your hormones back into balance to stop it from happening again. Herbs and nutrition can help to do this. Furthermore, you will need to work on the health of your liver, to ensure that any excess hormones are excreted.

If you have had an abnormal cyst removed, you will also need to prevent a recurrence. The underlying problem here is not a simple hormonal imbalance, but abnormal cell growth. The approach in this instance is to ensure that your immune system is functioning properly, so that abnormal cells can be engulfed and destroyed. You'll also need to optimise the function of your liver, which plays a part in the destruction of abnormal cells and foreign substances before they reach the bloodstream.

Overall, for either type of cyst, you will need to get yourself into optimum health, so that your body functions well.

Dietary changes

- Follow the hormone balancing diet from Chapter 1. This is especially important if you're prone to functional cysts, but it can also be an excellent way to control abnormal cell growth by cleansing the body, helping you to detoxify wastes and toxins.

- For both types of cysts, you will need to eliminate sugar, coffee, cigarettes and alcohol. One reason is that they can affect hormonal balance, but secondly, they are all 'toxins' to the body, which can affect liver function. Alcohol is one of the worst, as far as the liver is concerned, so ensure that you cut it out completely.

- Drink plenty of water in order to flush the toxins from your system.

- Take steps to ensure that you are not constipated. Your body needs to work efficiently to ensure that toxins contained in the stools are passed out of the body before they can be reabsorbed into your system. Your bowels can also help to eliminate excess hormones from your body. Include plenty of wholegrains in your diet, such as brown rice, oats and rye, and lots of fresh fruits and vegetables – organic, if possible.

Phytoestrogens
Add phytoestrogens to your diet. Phytoestrogens (see page 20) are found in foods such as soya, chickpeas, lentils and garlic. These foods can have an overall balancing effect on your hormones, and they stimulate the production of sex hormone binding globulin (SHBG; see page 27).[3] SHBG is a protein produced by the liver that binds sex hormones such as oestrogen and progesterone in order to control how much is circulating in the blood at any one time. This can be very useful in preventing functional cysts.

Antioxidants
Include plenty of foods that contain antioxidants (see page 17). Good choices include carrots, leafy green vegetables, nuts, seeds, cauliflower and oily fish. Antioxidants help to mop up free radicals (see page 17) that can cause abnormal cell growth, which can lead to cell mutation and cancer.

Garlic

Garlic has a protective effect on cells. The American Institute for Cancer Research recommends that we eat two to five cloves of garlic a week or take garlic supplements. The positive effect is there whether the garlic is raw or cooked, so include it in your diet when you can.

Supplements

The supplements below will enhance the dietary changes you are making, working to balance hormones, improve immunity, enhance liver function and protect against abnormal cell growth. Some of these supplements are recommended simply because they will encourage optimum health, which will allow your body to function normally.

Vitamin C

This is an important nutrient for boosting immune activity. If the immune system is working efficiently, it can destroy abnormal cells, and this is important to prevent abnormal cysts.

Zinc

Zinc is also crucial for the immune system, but it plays an additional role in the reproductive system. Zinc is needed for normal egg development as it helps cells reproduce, and it can also protect your body against free radical damage. Free radicals (see page 17) can cause cell and damage (to the DNA), so it is important that they are kept under control.

B vitamins

The B-complex vitamins are needed by your liver to convert excess oestrogen into weaker and less dangerous forms. B vitamins are, therefore, essential, when you are working to balance your hormone levels.

Antioxidants

Add a good antioxidant formula to supplement your diet. This should include vitamins A and E and the mineral selenium. Antioxidants help to protect your cells against damage and any abnormal cell changes.

Herbs

The herbs are used to help balance the hormones, which will encourage the ovaries to function normally. This can help to prevent functional cysts.

False unicorn root (*Chaemaelirium luteum*)

This is the herb of choice for functional cysts because it improves the functioning of the ovaries and helps to normalise the hormones that the ovary produces (oestrogen and progesterone).

Peony (*Paeonia lactiflora*)

Peony is a Chinese herb that helps to prevent the recurrence of ovarian cysts and normalise ovulation.

Echinacea (*Echinacea purpurea* or *E. angustifolia*)

Echinacea is useful for boosting immune system function as it can increase white blood cell count and activity. These increased levels can help the body to engulf abnormal cells.[4]

Echinacea appears to be more effective when taken on a slightly infrequent basis. Take it for ten days, with a three-day break, and then repeat for another ten days.

Milk thistle (*Silymarin marianum*)

This is an important herb for the liver, acting as a tonic. It can encourage the detoxification process, which means that abnormal cells will be destroyed and excess hormones excreted.

The Integrated Treatment Plan

If you suffer from chronic functional cysts, it is worth following the natural approach. Taking the Pill is not the answer in the long term (see page 225). If you need to have a cyst aspirated, begin the natural approach straightaway and follow it for six months in order to try to prevent another one forming.

If you have an abnormal cyst, it is better to have it surgically removed and then work on reaching optimum health. Follow the suggestions below for at least six months in order to prevent a recurrence. Find a good gynaecologist who will operate as conservatively as possible (taking steps to preserve your ovary). At the same time, it is essential that you take steps towards optimum health. You will often have a period of time before the surgery in which to adopt a good healthy diet (see page 16), and this will help to ensure that you recover quickly following the operation. During this period, you should also adopt the supplement plan outlined below, and take these before and after the surgery. Stop taking the supplements when you go to hospital.

Homeopathic remedies can be extremely useful for encouraging a speedy recovery from surgery. Arnica, for example, is often used alongside other remedies to promote healing. See a qualified homeopath for appropriate treatment before you go into hospital.

Your Supplement Plan

- A good multivitamin and mineral supplement, e.g. The Healthy Woman by the Natural Health Practice

- Vitamin C (1,000mg per day)

- Vitamin B complex (providing 50mg of most of the B vitamins per day, including levels found in your multivitamin supplement)

- A good antioxidant formula (including vitamins A, E and selenium)

- Zinc (15mg per day)

- Linseed oil (1,000mg per day)

> ### Note
>
> Each nutrient represents the total intake for one day, so if your multivitamin and mineral already contain 5mg of zinc, for example, you only need to add in a separate zinc supplement containing 10mg per day.

Herbs

If you are prone to functional cysts, take a tincture containing equal parts of false unicorn root tincture and peony 1 teaspoon three times a day for six months. Take milk thistle in the same way.

If you have had an abnormal cyst, take milk thistle as above, and add 1 teaspoon of echinacea tincture, three times a day. Take echinacea for ten days on, three days off, and ten days on, for a period of three months.

In Summary

- If you suffer from any of the symptoms of cysts, either functional or abnormal, see your doctor for a diagnosis.

- If you have suffered from cysts in the past, you will need to focus on preventing a recurrence.

- Follow the hormone balancing diet from Chapter 1.

- For both types of cysts, eliminate sugar, coffee, cigarettes and alcohol.

- Take steps to encourage the health of your liver (see page 37).

- Drink plenty of water in order to flush the toxins from your system.

- Ensure that you are not constipated by including plenty of wholegrains, and fresh fruit and vegetables in your diet.

- Eat foods that are rich in phytoestrogens.

- Eat foods that contain antioxidants, and take a good antioxidant supplement to ensure healthy cells.

- Add garlic to your diet.

- Take steps to boost your overall immunity (see page 179), which can prevent abnormal cell development.

- Take supplements (see page 230) and herbs (see above).

POLYCYSTIC OVARY SYNDROME

Polycystic ovary syndrome is something quite different to suffering from ovarian cysts, which are discussed in detail on pages 220–231. Polycystic ovaries are ovaries that are actually covered with very small follicles in which the egg develops.

What is Polycystic Ovary Syndrome?

In each menstrual cycle, follicles grow on the ovaries. Within those follicles eggs develop, one of which will reach maturity faster than the others and be released into the Fallopian tubes. This is known as ovulation. The remaining follicles (sometimes hundreds) will degenerate. In the case of polycystic ovaries, however, the ovaries are much larger than normal, and there are a number of undeveloped follicles that appear in clumps, rather like a bunch of grapes. Polycystic ovaries are not particularly troublesome and in many cases they will not even affect your fertility. Where the problem starts, however, is when the cysts cause a hormonal imbalance, leading to a series of other symptoms. These symptoms are the difference between suffering from PCOS and from polycystic ovaries.

So a woman can have polycystic ovaries without having PCOS, but all women with PCOS will have polycystic ovaries.

What Symptoms Could You Experience?

With the most extreme form of PCOS, you would tend to be overweight, have no or very few periods, be prone to acne, grow unusually heavy body hair, often on the face, breasts and insides of the legs, and be susceptible to mood swings. And with this can come problems with fertility and often recurrent miscarriages. Women with PCOS may be seven times more likely to develop diabetes because of problems with blood sugar balance.

Blood tests would also reveal a hormone imbalance, which can include:

- high levels of LH (luteinizing hormone)
- higher than normal male hormones (such as testosterone)
- low progesterone

Luteinizing hormone (LH), which is released by the pituitary gland, controls the development and release of the egg from the ovary. The other hormones, testosterone and progesterone, are produced in the ovaries themselves.

How Do You Know If You Have PCOS?

Your doctor will normally diagnose PCOS by ultrasound together with hormone blood tests. The hormones measured should include FSH, LH, the androgens (male hormones), prolactin (see page 135) and thyroid function, and the sample should be taken early in the menstrual cycle. The hormone tests help to determine the severity of the problem and to rule out any other endocrine (hormone) abnormalities.

What Causes Polycystic Ovary Syndrome?

No definite cause has been established, but it has been suggested that the problem stems from the ovaries, which are unable to produce the hormones in the correct proportions. This in turn gives the message to the pituitary gland that the ovaries are not working properly and this gland then releases high levels of LH. But PCOS also seems to affect a number of other different kinds of hormonal pathways in the body. Problems with the thyroid and adrenal glands may make some women more susceptible to PCOS. Problems with insulin (insulin resistance) have also been implicated, and PCOS does seem to run in families.[5]

And it may even be more complicated than that. Sometimes it is not just the *amount* of hormones produced by the body that can cause an imbalance. Scientists have found that some women are simply unable to deal effectively with the hormones, which can be the root of the problem. Sex hormone-binding globulin (SHBG) is a protein produced by the liver that binds sex hormones, such as oestrogen and testosterone, in order to control how much of them are circulating in the blood at any one time.

It appears that overweight women have much lower levels of SHBG in their blood, which results in more circulating testosterone and increasingly bad PCOS symptoms, such as an excess of hair, which can be one of the most distressing symptoms.[6]

So, it appears that PCOS is a bit of a 'chicken and egg' situation. Do the high levels of androgens (male hormones) create the weight gain or does the weight gain cause the hormone imbalance? It is also known that women with PCOS are more likely to have problems balancing blood sugar, and they can be insulin-resistant. Insulin-resistance happens when insulin levels are high (hyperinsulinaemia), but that insulin cannot transport glucose into the cells. This, in turn, leads to high levels of blood glucose (sugar). And again, back to the chicken and egg, does the weight gain cause the insulin resistance or does the problem with insulin cause the weight gain?

Excess insulin leads to an increased appetite, which can cause over-weight. The more circulating insulin, the more the ovaries produce testosterone and so the cycle continues. It's extremely difficult to know which problem is the cause and which is the effect.

What Treatment Can You Be Offered By Your Doctor?

The choice of treatment will depend upon whether or not you want to become pregnant. If you don't, the Pill is normally offered in order to provide a regular 'cycle'.

Drugs

The contraceptive pill

A low dose oral contraceptive pill is usually offered when you do not want to become pregnant. This will produce a regular (although arti-ficial) cycle and a withdrawal bleed every month. The Pill will work to regulate 'periods' for as long as you take it, but as soon as you stop, the symptoms will recur. When you come off the Pill, you will be back at square one again. Remember: the Pill does nothing to address the underlying problem. Some of the listed side-effects of the Pill are nausea, vomiting, headache, thrombosis, changes in weight, changes in sex drive, depression and breast tenderness.

Clomiphene

If you are trying to conceive, you have to start to ovulate. One of the most common drugs used is clomiphene citrate. Clomiphene is an anti-oestrogen drug that tricks the brain into thinking that there is no oestrogen in the blood. Because the oestrogen is blocked, the pituitary gland gets the message to increase the supply of follicle-stimulating hormone (FSH). The FSH reaches the ovaries and egg production is stimulated. If the clomiphene is suddenly stopped, the brain recognises that there is a massive amount of oestrogen and this results in a LH surge that releases the egg from the ovary.

Clomiphene is an effective drug for artificially inducing ovulation but, ironically, it may also increase the chances of a miscarriage by somewhere in the region of 20 to 30 per cent.[7] It is thought that the clomiphene interferes with the womb lining, preventing the fertilised egg from implanting.

It is suggested that clomiphene is only used for a maximum of six months and normally other types of medication, such as gonado-trophins, might be tried if the clomiphene is unsuccessful.

Metformin

Metformin is a drug that has traditionally been used to treat non-insulin dependent diabetes (NIDD), also know as type II diabetes. Because there is a link between PCOS and abnormal secretion and the action of insulin, metformin is now being used in the treatment of PCOS. Side-effects can include nausea and an upset stomach.

Surgical techniques

Wedge resection

In the past this was a popular treatment, which involved removing a wedge of the ovary. This often helped to restore ovulation, but it had the unfortunate side-effect of creating scar tissue on the ovaries which would, of course, prevent conception.

Laparoscopic ovarian diathermy

This is now used instead of the wedge resection and in this technique part of the ovary is burned away in order to correct the hormonal imbalance. Alternatively, the follicles can be drilled, which seems to allow the ovaries to become sensitive to the production of FSH, causing ovulation to occur. Using either of these techniques on only one ovary can help. This treatment is normally viewed as a last resort as the benefits may only last for about six months.

THE DRAWBACKS OF MEDICAL TREATMENT

There are a wide variety of symptoms that can accompany PCOS, including acne, excess hair and mood swings. There are, beyond all doubt, many drugs and other methods that can be used to treat these symptoms, including taking the Pill to regulate your cycle, antibiotics for the acne and electrolysis for the hair removal. However, while the symptoms can be controlled using these methods, the underlying problem will continue unchanged. Stop the treatment and what happens? The symptoms flood back and you return to square one.

What Natural Treatments Could Be Effective?

The aim of the natural approach is to address the imbalances that we know are associated with PCOS. Symptoms disappear because the underlying cause has been addressed.

There are six stages involved in this treatment programme:

1. Improve your diet, based on the recommendations outlined in Chapter 1.

2. Balance your blood sugar levels.

3. Use nutritional supplements that are known scientifically to help with PCOS.

4. Ensure that your body can excrete excess hormones efficiently by working on liver function.

5. Improve certain lifestyle factors, such as stress and exercise.

6. Use specific herbs in the long term to help correct any hormone imbalances.

7. Use other herbs to help improve liver function.

Dietary changes

Over the last few years, research into the nutritional approach to PCOS has revolutionised the treatment of this problem.

As women with PCOS lose weight, hormone levels start to return to normal. Testosterone levels fall, serum insulin levels go down, SHBG levels go up and the symptoms of PCOS diminish, with significant improvements in the growth of excess hair as the women lose weight.[8]

Along with the weight loss comes a remarkable change in ovarian function. In one study, 82 per cent of the women who were not previously ovulating showed improvements, with a number of successful pregnancies during the study, even though many of these women had a long-standing history of infertility.[9]

So dramatic have been some of the results, it has now been suggested that changing a woman's diet should be the first move if she is overweight and failing to conceive. One study found that 11 out of 12 women who had been overweight and not ovulating conceived naturally after reducing their weight.[10]

It has also been discovered that normal-weight and overweight women with PCOS have similar levels of testosterone (the 'male' hormone), but overweight women have lower levels of SHBG (see page 27).[11] Because SHBG binds testosterone in the blood, it means that if there is less SHBG, then there are going to be much higher levels of free testosterone and consequently more 'male' symptoms, such as hair growth and acne.

In general, women with high levels of luteinizing hormone (LH) in the first half of their menstrual cycle seem to have a greater risk of miscarriage. So miscarriages are more likely to occur in women with PCOS because of the high levels of LH. But, in a study of women with PCOS who were asked to change their diets, the rate of miscarriages dropped from 75 per cent to 18 per cent once they had lost weight.[12]

A BMI (body mass index) (see page 446) of over 25 is considered overweight. The good news is that losing only a small amount of weight (say 10 per cent) can be enough to improve hormone profiles, make your periods more regular, stimulate ovulation and increase your chances of becoming pregnant.[13]

Following the hormone-balancing diet from Chapter 1 which will not only help you to lose weight without dieting, but will help to get your hormones back in balance. (If you need extra help to lose the weight, then see my book *Natural Alternatives to Dieting*.)

Phytoestrogens

It is important to include foods that are phytoestrogens (natural oestrogens), such as soya, chickpeas, lentils etc. These phytoestrogens have an effect on SHBG (see page 27). Phytoestrogens help to stimulate the production of SHBG.[14] That is, if the level of SHBG goes up, more of the excess circulating hormones, such as testosterone and LH will be controlled. The result? Your symptoms should abate.

THE IMPORTANCE OF TIMING

When you eat is just as important as what you eat when controlling the symptoms of and treating PCOS. Because PCOS is so tied up with the way your body balances blood sugar, it is important that you make some adjustments to your diet, to help your body work effectively and control blood sugar imbalances.

Chapter 13 (see page 459) describes the concept of the glycaemic index (GI), which tells you how quickly or slowly certain foods will raise insulin levels. What you need to focus on are the 'slow-releasing' foods, which will ensure that your blood sugar levels do not rollercoaster during the day. That same section explains about the effects of sugar on the body, and makes it clear why sugar is one of the main 'no-nos' for PCOS sufferers.

So, not only do you have to watch *what* you are eating, but you must learn *when* to eat.

Many women suffer from the misconception that the best way to lose weight is to cut out meals. It seems logical that if you miss a meal you will take in fewer calories, thereby losing weight. I'm afraid, however, that this is one case where your body will outwit you. Bodies are designed to protect us from harm. If your body twigs that there is not enough food about, it assumes that you are entering a period of famine and slows your metabolism accordingly. It also hangs on to fat, in the event that another meal may not appear for some time. What this means in the short term is that when you do eat your next meal, even if it is just a few hours later, you will be eating it on a much slower metabolism. It's fairly obvious that missing meals is counter-productive.

But if you suffer from PCOS, there is another reason why *timing* of meals is crucial.

After you eat there is a naturally high level of glucose in the blood. (The glucose level is even higher if you had sugary foods.) Your body takes what it immediately needs for energy and then produces insulin from the pancreas in an attempt to lower the level of excess glucose. Any glucose that is not used immediately for energy is changed into glycogen and stored in the liver and muscles to be used later. The glucose level in the blood then reduces to normal.

If you miss meals your blood sugar level can drop and you can experience any of the following symptoms:

- irritability
- palpitations
- crying spells
- anxiety
- forgetfulness
- fatigue
- headaches
- aggressive outbursts
- lack of sex drive
- dizziness
- confusion
- inability to concentrate
- insomnia
- muscle cramps

When your glucose level drops, the hormone adrenaline is released from the adrenal glands and 'glucagon' is produced from the pancreas. Glucagon works in the opposite way to insulin and increases blood glucose by encouraging the liver to turn some of its glycogen stores into glucose in order to give you some quick energy.

At the low point, you will probably feel that you need a 'quick fix', such as a bar of chocolate, to give you a lift. That may seem like the obvious solution, but its effect is short-lived. The glucose enters the bloodstream too fast, which means that more insulin has to be released.

Any food or drink that has a stimulant effect (such as tea, coffee, chocolate and all sugars) will keep you on this roller-coaster of blood-sugar ups and downs. We often go for chocolate because it combines caffeine and sugar together, offering two 'quick fixes' in the one food! Anything refined, such as white flour, will also hit the bloodstream fairly fast.

And there's more! The adrenal glands obviously secrete adrenaline, but what you may not know is that they produce androgens (male hormones) as well. If they are overstimulated, they can secrete too much of the male hormones. Excess androgens will stop ovulation, and when ovulation ceases, the ovaries begin to secrete even more testosterone. It's a bit of a double whammy!

It's fairly clear from this description that all of the systems in your body are interconnected. That is why the natural approach, especially with PCOS, works so well. Because this condition involves so many different systems in the body, it's essential you choose an approach that looks at you as a whole person, not just a collection of different organs and systems.

This never-ending cycle has to be broken and one way to start is to make sure that your blood sugar doesn't drop too low, which would cause adrenaline to kick in. The key to doing this is to eat little and often. You really shouldn't go more than three hours without food. What you eat every three hours also makes a difference, because sugary or refined foods will just exacerbate the problem, sending your blood sugar rocketing up and then slumping straight back down again. You need to eat breakfast, lunch and dinner and, in between, have a small amount of complex carbohydrates to keep your blood sugar 'topped up'. Complex carbohydrates include those starchy foods described in Chapter 1 (see page 17). Always stick to wholegrain foods, or unrefined carbohydrates, which are 'slow-releasing'. It's fine, for example, to have a slice of wholemeal toast, but white bread or toast will start the roller-coaster off again. You should also include some good quality protein such as fish, eggs or beans, as the combination of both protein and good quality carbohydrate can have a more beneficial effect on insulin than just the complex carbohydrate on its own.

Supplements

The use of certain vitamins and minerals can be extremely useful in helping to correct PCOS, when taken while you are working on your diet. If you have been using the Pill to regulate your periods, you may have an even greater imbalance between a number of key vitamins and minerals (see pages 121–2). Correcting this imbalance will go a long way towards treating the root cause of the problem.

Chromium

Chromium is an extremely important mineral if you have PCOS. It helps to encourage the formation of glucose tolerance factor (GTF), which is a substance released by the liver and required to make insulin more efficient. A deficiency of chromium can lead to insulin resistance, which is a key problem in the case of PCOS; too much insulin can be circulating but it is unable to control your blood sugar (glucose) levels.

Chromium is the most widely researched mineral used in the treatment of overweight. It helps to control cravings and reduces hunger. Chromium also helps to control fat and cholesterol in the blood. One study showed that people who took chromium picolinate over a ten-week period lost an average of 1.9kg (4.2lb) of fat while those on a placebo (sugar tablet) lost only 0.2kg (0.4lb).[15]

Warning
If you are diabetic and on medication, you should speak to your doctor before taking chromium

---

Clare

Clare was 29 when she came to see me. She'd been diagnosed with PCOS five years earlier. Her periods had started when she was 14, but they had been irregular right from the beginning. By the time she was 19, they had stopped completely and she had started to grow excess hair on her face and the insides of her legs, and she felt generally 'hairier'.

Clare was put on the Pill and started to go for electrolysis. Over this period, she had also gained weight and was now 13.5 stone (at 5ft 10in). She had had breaks from the Pill but had not had any proper periods (in other words, periods that were not induced by the Pill) for ten years. When I first saw Clare she had been on Dianette, which is an anti-androgenic (anti-male hormone) contraceptive pill, but had stopped two months previously. She felt that over the ten years she had been in treatment, nothing had actually addressed the fundamental problem. Every time she came off the Pill, she was back to square one. Her doctor's advice had been to stay on the Pill until she was ready to have a baby, at which time she could come back for fertility treatment.

I discussed the impact of blood sugar imbalance on PCOS, and she agreed that there were parts of the day when she would start to shake and feel faint. On my advice, she started to eat little and often, and I gave her a supplement programme that included chromium, zinc, essential fatty acids and herbs to improve her liver function. She also took a herbal mix to help with the PCOS. Four months later her periods started, and she is now having regular periods. In her words, she 'feels wonderful', and has no need for the herbs at all now.

B vitamins

The B vitamins are very important in helping to correct the symptoms of PCOS. Vitamins B2, B3, B5 and B6 are particularly useful for controlling weight, and here's why: Vitamin B2 helps to turn fat, sugar and protein into energy; B3 is a component of the glucose tolerance factor (GTF), which is released every time blood sugar rises; and vitamin B3 helps to keep the levels in balance. Vitamin B5 has been shown to help with weight loss because it helps to control fat metabolism. B6 is also important for maintaining hormone balance and, together with B2 and B3, is necessary for normal thyroid hormone production. Any deficiencies in these vitamins can affect thyroid function and consequently affect the metabolism.

The B vitamins are also essential for the liver to convert your 'old' hormones into harmless substances that can then be excreted from the body.

Zinc

Zinc is one of the key minerals that we need in our daily diets and it has a wide range of functions. Unfortunately, because our soil has been depleted by overfarming there is very little natural zinc found in our food. Furthermore, processing and refining strip out what little might be remaining. So no matter how good your diet, you may not be getting anywhere near the levels of zinc you need. There are two approaches to this: you can eat whole organic food, which has much more rigorous controls on farming methods, or you can add a zinc supplement to your diet. But why is zinc so important?

Zinc is an important mineral for appetite control and a deficiency can cause a loss of taste and smell, creating a need for stronger-tasting foods, including those that are saltier, more sugary and/or spicier (and often more fattening!). Zinc is also necessary for the correct action of many hormones, including insulin, so it is extremely important in balancing blood sugar. It also functions together with vitamins A and E in the manufacture of thyroid hormone.

Magnesium

Magnesium levels have been found to be low in people with diabetes, and there is a strong link between magnesium deficiency and insulin resistance.[16] It is, therefore, an important mineral to include if you are suffering from PCOS.

Co-Enzyme Q10 (Co-Q10)

This is a vitamin-like substance that is contained in nearly every cell of your body. It is important for energy production and normal carbohydrate metabolism (the way our bodies break down the carbohydrates we eat in order to turn them into energy). One study showed that people on a low-fat diet doubled their weight loss when they supplemented with Co-Q10 as compared to those who did not take it.[17] Co-Q10 has also been proven useful in controlling blood sugar levels.[18]

Garcinia cambogia

If you are really struggling with sugar cravings, or you find it difficult to resist bingeing on just about anything, this is the supplement for you. Garcinia cambogia is a small tropical fruit called the 'Malabar tamarind'. It comes from central Asia, where the rind is used in Thai and Indian cooking. The garcinia contains HCA (hydroxy-citric acid), which enables carbohydrates to be turned into usable energy instead of being deposited as fat. The HCA in this fruit seems to curb appetite, reduce food intake, and inhibit the formation of fat and cholesterol. It seems to be particularly helpful when teamed with chromium (see page 240). I use one which combines the HCA and chromium in the same capsule, which saves you taking two different supplements (to obtain a combined capsule, get in touch with me, see page 507).

Herbs

Herbs are extremely useful in the treatment of PCOS. Making changes and adding supplements to your diet will help to control weight and balance blood sugar, while herbs go a step further, targeting any problems involving hormone balance.

Herbs can also be very beneficial in encouraging the function of your liver, in order to make sure that it is metabolising the hormones efficiently and then eliminating them.

Agnus castus (vitex/chastetree berry)

This is one of the most important herbs for PCOS because it helps to stimulate and normalise the function of the pituitary gland, which controls the release of LH (luteinizing hormone).

Black cohosh (*Cimicifuga racemosa*)

Black cohosh helps to suppress LH levels, which are usually high in PCOS, so this is a useful herb for this condition.

False unicorn root (*Chaemaelirium luteum*)

This herb helps to normalise the balance of hormones and to encourage healthy development of follicles.

White peony (*Paeonia lactiflora*)

The white peony is an excellent herb for helping with PCOS as it works in a similar way to false unicorn root by encouraging the healthy development of the follicles and trying to rectify any hormone imbalance especially with the male hormones (androgens).

Saw palmetto (*Serenoa repens*)

Saw palmetto is a herb that is traditionally considered in light of its success in treating prostate problems caused by an imbalance of hormones (including excess testosterone). It is a small palm tree found in North America and the berries of the tree are used. With these changes in the hormones it helps to regulate the cycle.

Research has shown that saw palmetto works as an anti-androgen, which can be very helpful given the high levels of testosterone in PCOS.[19]

Add saw palmetto to your treatment plan if you have excess hair growth, or have been told you have high levels of androgens.

Milk thistle (*Silybum marianum*)

This is one of the key herbs for the liver, which acts as your waste disposal unit, and it is therefore essential for the treatment of PCOS. It helps to protect your liver cells against damage and to promote the healing of damaged cells, so improving the general functioning of the liver and all its detoxifying properties.

Dandelion (*Taraxacum officinale*)

Dandelion is another liver cleanser, and it helps to get rid of accumulated 'old' hormones.

Because all these herbs are valuable for helping with the symptoms and imbalances of PCOS, the easiest way to take them is to combine them in one tincture. Take 1 teaspoon, three times a day. But take the milk thistle and dandelion as a separate tincture.

Stress

When we are under stress, adrenaline is released as part of our 'fight or flight' mechanism (see page 44). It's fairly clear what effect adrenaline can have on PCOS (see page 232), so it is important to do whatever you can do to manage or reduce stress in your life. The best way to do this is to prioritise so that you aren't taking on too much. The next best thing is actively to find ways to relax.

Exercise

We all know that exercise is good for us, but it is particularly important if you have PCOS. In conjunction with a healthy diet, exercise helps to control weight. On page 323, I explained that your 'shape' can affect your risk of breast cancer and heart disease. Again, it seems that being apple-shaped (with weight around your abdomen) rather than pear-shaped (with weight around your hips) can hold more health risks. It has also been found that having high levels of abdominal fat (apple-shaped) increases your chances of developing insulin resistance. Therefore, if you use exercise (and diet) to reduce abdominal fat, you will have a better chance of keeping your blood sugar levels in balance and reducing the symptoms of PCOS. Try to exercise at least three times a week. The ideal is five times a week for 30 minutes.

The Integrated Treatment Plan

The aim of this plan is to encourage optimum health, where your body will be able to balance itself. This can be undertaken by changing your diet, and using vitamins, minerals and herbs, which are known to have a balancing effect on hormone levels.

I have made some suggestions below depending on your age and whether or not you want to become pregnant. If you are already taking medication and want to try the natural approach, you will need to speak to your doctor about stopping the drugs. You can't combine drugs and a natural treatment plan in the case of PCOS. Perhaps you have opted for surgery? In this case you should definitely use all of the natural recommendations in order to optimise the effects of the surgery.

If you do not want to get pregnant

Allow six months to get yourself really healthy by following the nutritional recommendations, and including the supplements and herbs. Put the conventional medical approach (drugs or surgery) aside for that time and see what difference the natural approach can make. While your body is re-balancing, you will probably still need to address any excess hair, using electrolysis or another means. As your body approaches optimum health, your hair growth should slow down.

If you are under 35 and want to get pregnant

Because you have time on your side, I would suggest that you follow the natural approach for six months, without medication, to see if you conceive naturally. You can take the herbs for three months (while trying *not* to conceive), then stop taking them while you try to conceive over the next three to six months.

If you are over 35 and want to get pregnant

Ideally you should give yourself at least three months to correct any vitamin and mineral deficiencies and to achieve optimum health before you conceive (for extra help see my book *Natural Solutions to Infertility*, Piatkus, 2000), which will also minimise your chances of experiencing a miscarriage. If you already trying to conceive, then make sure your multivitamin and mineral is designed for pregnancy so that the folic acid content is at a good level (400mcg) and that you get no more than 2,500iu of vitamin A per day (see page 375). There is a supplement called Fertility Plus for Women which would give you the correct balance (see Staying in Touch, page 510, if you can't get it locally).

All of the suggested supplements are known to be safe while you are trying to conceive, apart from Co-enzyme Q10 or Garcinia cambogia. After three months on the herbal programme, stop taking the herbs before you begin trying to conceive.

If time is of the essence in terms of trying to get pregnant, then you may need medical help. However, it important that you make sure you have been properly investigated to find out exactly what is going on. The difficulty is that sometimes women are given drugs like clomiphene citrate when they are not getting pregnant, without any tests being done. Clomiphene citrate, for example, should *only* be given if you are *not* ovulating, so it is important to know whether you actually need it. You want the correct treatment for your particular situation, not just a blanket approach.

It's possible to take clomiphene and to follow the natural approach simultaneously; however, omit the herbs from the programme, sticking only to the dietary recommendations and the supplements.

Your Supplement Plan

- A good multivitamin and mineral supplement, e.g. The Healthy Woman by the Natural Health Practice

- Chromium (200mcg in total each day; take into consideration the amount in your multivitamin and mineral)

- Zinc citrate (30mg in total each day)

- Magnesium (300mg in total each day)

- Co-enzyme Q10 (30mg three times a day)

- Vitamin B-complex (providing 50mg of most of the B vitamins per day)

> ### Note
> Each nutrient represents the total intake for one day, so if your multivitamin and mineral already contains 15mg of zinc, for example, you only need to add in a separate zinc supplement containing 15mg per day.

Herbs

Take a blend of *Agnus castus*, black cohosh, false unicorn root, peony and saw palmetto (if you have 'male' symptoms). Tincture form is best – take 1 teaspoon, three times a day throughout your cycle *except* when you have your period. Resume taking the herbs when your period stops.

Take a separate tincture blend of milk thistle and dandelion root (1 teaspoon, three times daily).

Both herbs can be taken over six months, unless I have suggested otherwise in the treatment plan above.

In Summary

- It is essential that you have a doctor's diagnosis to rule out any other cause of your symptoms. For example, make sure you are not suffering from diabetes.

- Follow the hormone balancing diet in Chapter 1 (see page 16).

- Take steps to reach your natural weight.

- Eat three good meals a day, focusing on slow-releasing foods (see page 17) which ensure that your blood-sugar levels do not roller-coaster. Wholefoods (complex carbohydrates) should replace all refined foods in your diet. Make sure you go no longer than three hours without a meal or a snack. And include some good quality protein such as fish, eggs and beans.

- Increase the phytoestrogens in your diet (see page 20).

- Take steps to reduce stress, which can lower adrenaline levels.

- Exercise at least three times a week.

- Ensure that you are getting enough of the key nutrients, including B vitamins, magnesium, zinc, co-enzyme Q10 and chromium.

- Take supplements (see page 240) for six months.

- Take herbs (see page 243) for six months.

CHAPTER 8

Infections and Other Problems

Infections or problems 'down there' are all too familiar to many women. Two types of infections are particularly widespread: thrush and urinary tract infections (UTIs). There are, however, other conditions that can affect the vagina and cervix, and these infections are becoming increasingly common.

VAGINAL INFECTIONS

When the birth control pill took over as the main form of contraception for women, it replaced a variety of other methods, all of which acted as a barrier to sperm reaching an egg for fertilisation. But these barrier methods did more than prevent sperm getting through, they also prevented diseases from entering the reproductive organs. Today, many women have had more than one sexual partner and there has been a dramatic increase in sexually transmitted disease (STDs). Some of the classic STDs, such as syphilis, are in decline (the result of early detection and improved methods of treatment), but they have been replaced by another group of infectious agents, which can cause discomfort and more serious problems.

What are Vaginal Infections?

The two main infections are caused by either a bacteria (bacterial vaginosis) or by a tiny parasite, known as trichomonas vaginalis.

Bacterial vaginosis

This is the most common cause of abnormal vaginal discharge among women (see below).

Trichomonas vaginalis

This is caused by a tiny parasite called a 'trichomonad', which lives in the vagina. It is spread by having sexual intercourse with someone who has the infection.

Are there any Symptoms?

Bacterial vaginosis

There are a number of potential symptoms, including:

• itching, soreness and redness around the vagina, vulva or anus

• grey or yellow vaginal discharge with a fishy smell, especially after sex

• a burning sensation when passing urine

• pain during intercourse

You may suffer from some or all of these symptoms.

Trichomonas vaginalis

Unfortunately, there are fewer symptoms for this type of infection, and you may not even have any, which can make diagnosis a bit more difficult. You may, however, experience:

• yellow or green vaginal discharge which is frothy and smells fishy

• soreness and itching around the vagina.

What Can Cause Vaginal Infections?

Bacterial vaginosis

This inflammation of the vagina develops when normal vaginal lacto-bacilli ('healthy' bacteria) are replaced by an overgrowth of gardnerella vaginalis (unhealthy bacteria), anaerobic lactobacillus (unhealthy bacteria) and mycoplasmas (small organisms that infect your vagina or urinary tract).

In other words, there is a sudden imbalance in the natural bacteria of the body. Scientists are not sure what causes this imbalance, but when this infection is present the normal – slightly acidic – quality of the vagina changes to become more alkaline. The acid/alkaline balance in the body is known as a 'pH balance'. It is suggested that a sudden shift in balance from acid to alkaline allows other bacteria to take hold.

Trichomonas vaginalis

This condition is sexually transmitted and is, therefore, only present if you have been in contact with someone carrying the parasite.

Getting a Diagnosis

If you are suffering any irritation around the vagina, or if you have an unusual discharge, it is very important that you see your doctor.

A swab will be taken and sent to the laboratory to work out which infection, if any, is present. You may find that you are suffering from a simple, and easily treatable yeast infection (thrush; see page 263), but you could be suffering from one of the infections listed above, which can be more problematic. If you find you carry one of these infections, your partner will also need to be screened.

THE IMPORTANCE OF TREATING BACTERIAL VAGINOSIS

It is extremely important that you are screened for this infection before you become pregnant, because it can cause a miscarriage or bring on premature labour (see page 383).

What Treatment Can You Be Offered By Your Doctor?

Treatment normally involves drugs, which are chosen depending on the type of infection that shows up during screening.

Bacterial vaginosis

The recommended treatment usually takes the form of drugs, such as metronidazole, doxycycline or clindamycin. These are taken orally (by mouth), but it is possible to use them in gel or cream form, which can be applied directly into the vagina. Both doxycycline and clindamycin are antibiotics, so they will, unfortunately, eliminate the healthy bacteria as well as the unhealthy bacteria, leaving you open to an attack of thrush. Metronidazole is an anti-microbial that efficiently eliminates anaerobic bacteria. Side-effects can include nausea, vomiting and other gastrointestinal disturbances.

Trichomonas vaginalis

This condition is also treated with metronidazole, which is normally taken orally. Metronidazole is the drug of choice for eliminating parasites, such as those causing trichomonas.

Over-the-counter medications

There are now a variety of different medications available over the counter from your local chemist. A word of warning: don't ever attempt to self-treat. What you assume is simple thrush may in fact be something more serious. Before using any drugs, no matter how gentle they are, or sure you are of the cause of your discharge, you must get a diagnosis from your doctor. Treating an infection with the wrong drug can not only lead to further imbalance, but it can be dangerous. Left untreated, many infections can lead to PID (pelvic inflammatory disease; see below), which presents a serious risk to your health.

PELVIC INFLAMMATORY DISEASE (PID)

PID is an umbrella term for any inflammation of the organs in the pelvis, and it is normally caused by an infection in any of the repro-ductive organs, including the womb, ovaries, Fallopian tubes, cervix, womb lining and/or vagina. PID is sexually transmitted and the symp-toms can be very extreme. They include:

- foul smelling vaginal discharge

- fever

- pain in the lower abdomen

- breakthrough bleeding between periods

- back pain

- pain on intercourse

- a need to pass urine more frequently

- pain when urinating.

It is believed that the infection spreads from the area around the cervix and migrates upwards. The two most common organisms that are implicated in PID are Chlamydia trachomatis and Neisseria gonor-rhoeae.

If you suffer from *any* of the symptoms listed above, you should see your doctor immediately. It is essential that a proper diagnosis is made

---

and that any other reason for the symptoms, such as ectopic pregnancy or appendicitis, are ruled out.

All too often you may be unaware that you are suffering from an infection until it is too late. Chlamydia in particular is known as a 'silent illness' because only a small number of women experience symptoms such as a discharge in the early stages of the disease. On the other hand, men will often experience a burning sensation on passing urine. So if your partner is experiencing symptoms, and you have regular intercourse, it's a good idea to see a doctor to check that you are not suffering from anything yourself.

A number of countries, such as Sweden, routinely screen for chlamydia and the fall in the number of chlamydia cases in these countries has been dramatic. At present there is no routine scanning in the UK.

The chlamydia bacteria can lie dormant in your body for many months before passing through the cervix. It can travel virtually unnoticed from the cervix to the womb and up the Fallopian tubes. If untreated, it can damage the tubes, resulting in blockages or scarring that can lead to infertility or an increased risk of ectopic pregnancy (where the fertilised egg implants into the Fallopian tube instead of in the womb). Women can be screened for chlamydia with a cervical swab and/or a urine test. If the condition is caught early enough, it can be treated successfully with antibiotics before it turns into PID.

HOW DOES THE BACTERIA TRAVEL UPWARDS?

Scientists have found that sperm, menstruation and trichomonads (the parasites that cause trichomonas vaginalis) can all play a part in the movement of the bacteria from the cervix upwards into the other reproductive organs.

Sperm are designed to travel upwards to the Fallopian tubes in order to fertilise an egg. It seems that certain organisms can 'hitch a ride' on the sperm to make their way further into the body.[1]

For most of the month, women have a protective mucus that acts as a barrier to most organisms. However, around ovulation, this mucus changes in consistency to become stretchier and more alkaline to help the passage of the sperm. Unfortunately, it also leaves the 'gate' open for other organisms, particularly those in hitchhiking mode. Furthermore, menstrual blood offers a favourable environment to a type of infection known as Neisseria gonorrhoea, which is one of the causes of PID. So you may be particularly vulnerable around the time of your period.

Parasites (trichomonads) can also move from the vagina to the Fallopian tubes and carry other unwanted organisms with them (literally 'hitching' a ride).

WHAT TREATMENT CAN YOU BE OFFERED BY YOUR DOCTOR?
Treatment for PID involves taking oral antibiotics. If your PID is severe, you may need to be hospitalised for intravenous antibiotic treatment. PID can be life-threatening, so if you suffer from any of the symptoms, it is essential that you see your doctor immediately for treatment.

What Natural Treatments Could Be Effective?

It is important that you have proper medical treatment because of the potential severity of PID. It is also essential that the cause of the infection is determined so that the appropriate medication can be given. Some antibiotics are sensitive to one type of infection such as chlamydia, but resistant to others, such as gonococci.

In the case of both bacterial vaginosis and trichomonas vaginalis, I feel it is crucial that you go for conventional medical treatment and then work on prevention. Use the natural approach in addition to the conventional treatment to enhance healing and to speed up recovery time.

Prevention is important not only for vaginosis and trichomonas, but also for PID. The aim is to improve your immune system so that it can fight off infections more effectively, and also to make sure that the bacteria inside the vagina is at a beneficial level. In other words, you want to establish the correct pH balance in the vagina so that other bacteria do not grow. Any woman who has suffered from PID will be at risk of a recurrence, so preventative measures are absolutely essential.

Because most of these infections are sexually transmitted, precautions need to be taken. By this I mean using a barrier (such as a condom) during intercourse.

The natural approach is based upon prevention and there are a number of steps:

• Get medical treatment in order to eliminate the infection.

- Improve your diet, based on the recommendations outlined in Chapter 1, in order to ensure that medical treatment is effective. Continuing to eat well will help to prevent a recurrence.

- Use nutritional supplements that are known scientifically to support the medical treatment.

- Use nutritional supplements to help prevent a recurrence by boosting your immune system function.

- Use herbs that are known to boost your immune system, helping it to fight off any future infections.

Dietary changes

It is important that your diet is as healthy as possible to encourage resistance to any colonisation of bacteria. Follow the dietary suggestions outlined in Chapter 1 (see page 16).

Yoghurt

As well as taking acidophilus supplements, it is worth well adding live, organic, plain yoghurt to your diet. Researchers have also been looking at the possible use of yoghurt inserted into the vagina in order to prevent bacterial vaginosis because none of the medical treatments can actually prevent another infection.[2] The conclusion is that yoghurt could be extremely useful preventatively. The yoghurt helps to provide beneficial bacteria in the vagina in order to keep negative bacteria under control. Inserting yoghurt into the vagina can be rather messy (it is usually smeared around a tampon and inserted that way) and a vaginal cream containing acidophilus that comes with an applicator can often be more convenient.

Alcohol

Avoid alcohol while you have an infection. For one thing, alcohol can lower immunity, which is essential for successful recovery and, indeed, prevention. Furthermore, alcohol is a source of sugar, which can 'feed' infection, change the pH balance of the vagina and, again, lower immunity. Taking this one step further, eliminate sugar and all refined carbohydrates (such as white bread). A healthy diet can help to strengthen your immune system, and to keep the pH of your vagina balanced in order to fight off any infections and to cope with any infection you may be suffering.

Supplements

Supplements are recommended to boost your immune system so that it can more effectively fight off infections. They can also help to encourage the success of your medical treatment. Ultimately, however, your supplement plan is designed to prevent future attacks, using nutrients that are known to be helpful in the prevention of vaginal infections.

Vitamin C

This vitamin is essential for the proper functioning of the immune system. It also helps with the formation of collagen, which is very important if you are suffering from a vaginal infection or PID. Collagen is a protein that is found in abundant supply in the body. It maintains the integrity of skin, ligaments, tendons and bone. If the collagen matrix (which is the main component of connective tissue) is intact, infection is less likely to spread, and your organs are less likely to become scarred by the infection. The bacteria can spread through the connective tissue, so having extra vitamin C at this time will help to strengthen the connective tissue, make it more resistant, and decrease the time it takes for your body to repair damaged tissue.

Beta-carotene

Beta-carotene is a type of vitamin A that is known to help your body produce collagen, and it also helps to keep your cartilage strong. It is important that you have adequate levels in your body to help stop the spread of infection. Beta-carotene is also a powerful antioxidant (see page 17) and is found in high concentrations in the ovaries. However, if there isn't enough in the body, levels in the ovaries will be inadequate, and the ovaries will be less likely to be able to fight off attacking infectious agents. Studies show that adequate levels of beta-carotene can help to prevent excess cell damage. Beta-carotene is also vital for immune function and for the normal growth of the type of tissue found in the vagina.[3]

Vitamin E

We now know that vitamin E encourages an increased resistance to chlamydial infections.[4] As well as taking a vitamin E orally, you can open up a capsule and apply the oil to the inflamed area – or insert a yeast-free capsule into the vagina to help soothe the tissues and encourage healing.

B Vitamins

These water-soluble vitamins are often deficient in women with vaginal infections. They are needed for healthy cell replication, which is particularly important when cells (such as those in the vagina) are bombarded with infection.

Zinc

Zinc is an important mineral for the immune system and needs to be taken when an infection is present. Not only does it help to boost immunity, which can encourage faster healing, but it can help to prevent a recurrence.

Garlic

Often called 'nature's antibiotic', garlic is very important while you are trying to fight off an infection because it has strong antibacterial properties. So not only can it help to deal with the present infection, but it can also help to prevent a recurrence by making the body an inhospitable place for invaders.[5]

Acidophilus

Lactobacillus acidophilus, a 'healthy' bacteria known as flora, normally inhabits the vagina in good numbers. Infections such as bacterial vaginosis tend to 'get hold' when the balance between healthy and unhealthy bacteria in the body changes. Therefore, it makes sense that if the bacteria in your body is largely healthy, it is less likely that opportunistic bacteria can take over. What's more, lactobacillus is toxic to Gardnerella vaginalis, which is the main cause of bacterial vaginosis.[6] Acidophilus needs to be taken orally, but I would also suggest that you use it internally by either inserting an acidophilus capsule directly into the vagina[7] or a vaginal cream that contains acidophilus or live organic yoghurt.

Herbs

Herbs are taken to help increase the effectiveness of your immune system. They can be useful while you are taking medication, but they are also extremely effective when used following an attack in order to prevent a recurrence. Some herbs work on the infection directly.

Barberry root bark (*Berberis vulgaris*)

This is an excellent herb to help combat a vaginal infection and to prevent a recurrence. It contains a substance called 'berberine', which acts both to boost the immune system and to attack bacteria.[8]

Myrrh resin (*Commiphora molmol*)

Myrrh is effective against bacteria and a useful herb for vaginal infections together with barberry. It helps stimulate the production of white blood corpuscles, so will help your immune system fight the battle and will also help to directly eliminate the bacteria.

Calendula (*Calendula officinalis*)

This herb is more commonly known as marigold and is especially beneficial for vaginal infections because it has anti-microbial effects and healing qualities.

Tea tree oil (*Melaleuca alternifolia*)

Tea tree oil has been the subject of recent research into its beneficial effect on vaginal infection. It appears to have anti-microbial properties and was especially successful in treating trichomonas.[9] This essential oil is not taken by mouth but used vaginally to combat trichomonas and bacterial vaginosis. It is possible to buy tea tree oil pessaries, which you insert into the vagina, from a healthfood shop.

Another trick is to add a few drops of the essential oil of tea tree to your bath, together with three cups of pure apple cider vinegar, which can be very helpful when you have a vaginal infection.

Echinacea

This is the herb of choice for boosting the immune system and strengthening its ability to fight off infection. Studies show that echinacea is more effective if taken with short breaks (the immune system benefits are less effective if it is taken continuously). I would suggest ten days on and ten days off, ten days on etc. for maximum benefit.

Self-help

- Wipe from front to back after a bowel movement to ensure that nothing is transmitted from the bowels to the vagina.

- Use barrier methods of birth control or ensure that you are both tested and free from infections.

- Change tampons frequently when you menstruate or, preferably, use sanitary towels.

- Using an IUD (coil) can increase the risk of getting PID, so it's worth choosing another form of birth control, particularly if you have suffered from PID in the past.

- Wear cotton underwear and looser-fitting clothes so that you are not providing a warm, moist breeding ground for bacteria.

- Stop smoking. This may seem like an unusual suggestion, but it is now known that smoking can increase the risk of PID if you are suffering from a vaginal infection.

- Women with multiple partners have a four times higher risk of contracting PID than women in monogamous relationships, which makes it all the more important that barrier methods are used, or that you and your partners are screened regularly.[10]

The Treatment Plan

In this situation you need to make sure that the symptoms are investigated and to use the natural approach to get yourself into optimum health.

The Integrated Approach

I would recommend medical treatment for the vaginal infection. At the same time, change your diet, and take the recommended supplements and herbs. This integrated approach can help the drugs to be more effective, while at the same time encouraging your body to become stronger for the future. Once you have eliminated the infection, the aim is to stop it recurring.

Your Supplement Plan

- A good multivitamin and mineral supplement, e.g. The Healthy Woman by the Natural Health Practice

- Beta-carotene (50,000iu per day)

- Vitamin B-complex (providing 50mg of most of the B vitamins per day)

- Zinc (30mg per day)

- Vitamin E (300iu, open the capsule to use as an oil to rub into sore tissue)

- Linseed oil (1,000mg per day)

- Garlic capsules (4,000mcg of allicin per day)

- Vitamin C (1,000mg, twice daily)

- Acidophilus (containing 4 billion beneficial bacteria)

Note

Each nutrient represents the total intake for one day, so if your multivitamin and mineral already contains 15mg of zinc, for example, you only need to add in a separate zinc supplement containing 15mg per day.

Herbs

Take a tincture of barberry root bark, myrrh resin and calendula, 1 teaspoon three times a day for three months. Take a tincture of echinacea (1 teaspoon three times a day) for ten days, stop for three days and repeat for ten days etc. Continue to repeat in this manner for three months. Use tea tree oil (as described on page 259) while there is an infection, and to prevent a recurrence.

In Summary

- Always get a diagnosis from your doctor before beginning any treatment plan. If you suffer from any of the symptoms listed above, a laboratory test is essential to establish the type of infection you have.

- Don't attempt to use over-the-counter drugs without a full diagnosis and the approval of your doctor.

- Follow the dietary recommendations in Chapter 1 (see page 16) to give your body the best fighting chance against the infection.

- Avoid eating sugar, which can 'feed' the infection, and lower immunity.

- Use a barrier method of birth control if you have a new partner or if either one of you is suffering from an infection.

- If you have any of the symptoms of PID, see your doctor immediately.

- Avoid alcohol while you have an infection, which can encourage its growth and lower immunity.

- Take steps to boost your immune system, using supplements and herbs.

- Use the natural approach while you are suffering an attack, to speed up healing, and following recovery to prevent a recurrence.

- Take supplements for three months.

- Take herbs as described on page 261.

THRUSH (VAGINAL)

Vaginal thrush affects millions of women during their lifetime and many women will have several bouts of thrush every year. Some women suffer from thrush on a monthly basis, which can be enormously uncomfortable, inconvenient and even embarrassing.

What is Vaginal Thrush?

Thrush is an infection caused by a yeast (fungus) called *Candida albicans*, which occurs naturally in the gut, in the skin and in the vagina. Under normal circumstances, it is kept under control by other 'friendly' bacteria in the body, but occasionally it overgrows, which is when problems start.

What Symptoms Could You Experience?

With vaginal thrush you usually get a thick, white, sticky discharge, accompanied by soreness and irritation. The discharge can often look like cottage cheese and can have an unpleasant smell. If you are suffering from thrush, you may experience pain during sex and when passing urine. The outside of the vagina may also feel sore and swollen.

The most irritating symptom is an intense itching around the outside of the vagina, which is definitely worse in some cases than in others.

Men are also susceptible to thrush, which appears as a discharge from the penis, with soreness and/or reddened skin.

What is the Cause?

Because the yeast *Candida albicans* occurs naturally in the vagina and other parts of your body, something has to happen in order for it to grow out of control.

There are a number of factors that can cause this:

• taking antibiotics

- natural hormonal changes (for example, during pregnancy, around your period or during menopause)

- taking hormones such as the Pill or HRT

- becoming run down (by overwork, for example)

- suffering from continual stress

- a compromised immune system (you may feel that you are always 'coming down with something')

- undiagnosed or poorly controlled diabetes

- sex with someone who has thrush

- long-term steroid use.

Your body is literally teeming with millions of bacteria, and under ideal circumstances they are kept in a healthy balance. In other words, the healthy bacteria keep the unhealthy bacteria in check. When your immune system is compromised, say because of illness or a poor diet, the proportion of the different bacteria can alter, allowing candida to grow out of control.

When antibiotics are given for infection, they do not discriminate between the 'good' bacteria and the 'bad' bacteria in the body. They wipe out everything, which means that there is not enough of the 'good' bacteria to keep yeasts (and other 'invaders') such as thrush at bay. What's the result? Candida is no longer controlled and it begins to overgrow.

Taking the Pill alters the levels of natural hormones in the body (including those in the vagina), so you can become more susceptible to thrush. Hormonal changes during pregnancy and before a period can also make you more susceptible to a yeast overgrowth because the environment in the vagina changes, allowing the yeast to grow.

When diabetes is not properly controlled, you will have high levels of sugar in your blood and urine. There are three problems here: first of all, sugar compromises the function of the immune system, which means that it is unable to fight off invaders. Secondly, yeast 'feeds' on sugar, which means that it is more likely to overgrow. Finally, because there is extra strain on your body, it is less likely to be able to cope with 'normal' levels of yeast. If you have persistent yeast infections, it's worth checking to see that you are not suffering from diabetes. Regular yeast infections can be an indication of undiagnosed diabetes.

How Do You Know You Have Definitely Got Vaginal Thrush?

Because a discharge can be caused by other infections (such as gardnerella; see page 251), it is important to know what type of infection or overgrowth you have. This will, of course, determine the most appropriate treatment.

Candida Test

This is a test for yeast (candida) overgrowth. You can have yeast overgrowth in the vagina, which is more commonly known as thrush, but it is also possible to have yeast overgrowth in other parts of the body. Candida can also form in the intestines (see page 274).

Persistent vaginal thrush can be one of the symptoms of candidiasis, but other symptoms can include food cravings, especially for sugar and bread, fatigue, a bloated stomach with excess flatulence, a 'spaced out' feeling, and becoming tipsy on a very small amount of alcohol. Both men and women can suffer from candidiasis.

Diagnosis is made by your doctor who will take a sample of vaginal discharge on a swab which is then sent to the lab for testing.

What Treatment Can You Be Offered By Your Doctor?

Thrush is usually treated with anti-fungal drugs, which are available in different forms. These are now available over the counter in pharmacies, but you should not attempt to self-treat unless you are certain that you are suffering from thrush and not another sort of infection, or perhaps an underlying problem, such as diabetes.

Creams and pessaries

Anti-fungal creams are rubbed into the vulva or into the vagina and pessaries are inserted directly into the vagina. Both can be rather messy. They can be effective if the full course of treatment is taken, although the success of the treatment varies between brands. If you do not finish the course, there can be a recurrence. You are particularly likely to experience a repeat infection if you do not address the cause (see page 263).

Oral treatments

These are anti-fungal medications taken by mouth. Drugs containing fluconazole require only a single dose for a bout of thrush. These types of drugs do, however, have numerous side-effects, which can include mild nausea, abdominal pain, diarrhoea, flatulence or rashes.

Your partner can have thrush with or without symptoms, so if you suffer from recurrent bouts of thrush, it's important that he is treated as well. Otherwise, the yeast is simply passed back and forth and drugs will, in the long run, become ineffective.

Oral treatments for thrush should not be used when you are pregnant, so if you plan to treat the condition medically, see your doctor instead of using over-the-counter products.

What Natural Treatments Could Be Effective?

The aim of the natural treatment is to ensure that your body has all the nutrients it needs to function optimally, thereby boosting your immune system. The programme focuses on certain foods and supplements in order to do this. You'll also encourage the friendly bacteria in your system, to create a normal balance that keeps the yeast under control.

Dietary changes

As well as following the hormone balancing diet, outlined in Chapter 1, you can help to eliminate the thrush by focusing on a few dietary changes. You will definitely need to avoid sugar, and any foods containing sugar, as they will promote the growth of yeast. You also need to cut out foods that contain yeast, and any products that are fermented, such as bread and wine.

Yoghurt
Live yoghurt containing the culture acidophilus or bifidus, which are found naturally in your gut, is the most beneficial type of yoghurt. These cultures represent some of the 'healthy' bacteria, which can help

to prevent an overgrowth of yeast in the body. When yoghurts are heat-treated they lose their original bacterial culture, so they will not help to control symptoms or treat the problem. Buy natural yoghurt that is 'live' and organic. These can be marketed in different ways, so read the labels carefully. 'Bio' usually means 'live' and 'bio' yoghurts will contain a culture like lactobacillus, which will do the job. I mention organic because non-organic produce can contain antibiotics and chemicals, that form part of the animal's diet (cows, sheep or goats; whatever type of milk product you choose). Fruit yoghurts should be avoided because they have a very high sugar content, which will 'feed' the yeast.

When researchers gave women one *Lactobacillus acidophilus*-containing yoghurt a day over six months, there was a threefold decrease in bouts of thrush.[11]

Essential Fatty Acids (EFAs)

Make sure that you are getting enough of these essential fatty acids (see page 27), which have anti-fungal properties. EFAs are contained in nuts, seeds and oily fish, and can be taken in supplement form (see below).

Garlic

I have suggested below that you take supplementary garlic while you are trying to get rid of thrush, but if you (and your friends!) can bear it, it will help to chew a clove of raw garlic every day. Alternatively, add raw garlic to salads or salad dressings. Garlic loses some of its anti-fungal properties when it is heated, so try to eat it raw if you can.

Supplements

I have recommended a general multivitamin and mineral supplement to ensure that you are not nutritionally deficient. Other supplements known scientifically to help with thrush and to boost the immune system are also suggested.

Beta-carotene

Levels of beta-carotene (a type of vitamin A) have been found to be low in the vaginal cells of women who have thrush. It is suggested that this may affect the immune response of the cells in the vagina, which encourages (or at least allows) the yeast to overgrow.[12]

Zinc

Zinc deficiency has been connected with women who have recurrent thrush.[13] Adequate levels of zinc are critical for the optimum functioning of your immune system. People who are deficient in zinc will be susceptible to recurrent infections or infestations of any kind (that's why you may seem to suffer from one cold or tummy bug after another when you are run down). If you are zinc deficient, your immune system can be compromised and your body will not be able to control yeast overgrowth.

Essential fatty acids (EFAs)

The essential fatty acids that are contained in oily fish and in nuts and seeds have anti-fungal, anti-bacterial and anti-viral actions,[14] so it is important to take supplementary EFAs while you are combating an attack of thrush. If you have a tendency to recurrent thrush, it's worth taking a capsule of linseed oil every day over a period of six months. Try also to ensure that you are getting enough of these essential fats in your food.

Garlic

Garlic is well known for its effect on the immune system, and it has both anti-bacterial and anti-fungal properties. Take garlic as a supplement when you are trying to eliminate an attack of thrush, and as prevention if you are prone to attacks. In clinical studies, garlic extracts have been to found to prevent the growth of candida.[15] One of the active ingredients in garlic is called 'allicin', and it appears that this is the ingredient with the ability to prevent an overgrowth of yeast. When buying supplements, choose one with a high level of allicin.

Probiotics

A probiotic is the opposite of an antibiotic, which means that it encourages rather than destroys bacteria in the body. That's not as alarming as it sounds! What probiotics do is increase the growth of 'healthy' bacteria in the body, which is known as flora. By taking probiotics, you are aiming to increase the amount of beneficial bacteria in your system, which in turn helps to control the amount of yeast overgrowth. As well as eating live plain organic yoghurt (see page 266), it is important to take supplements of *Lactobacillus acidophilus,* one of the best-known and effective probiotics. Yoghurt has shown to be helpful in *preventing* attacks of yeast, but a probiotic supplement goes one step further to actually *treat* a yeast infection. The difference is that lactobacillus levels in yoghurt are high enough to work on a preventive basis, but they will not be concentrated enough to deal with an infection. Make sure the one you buy has to be kept in the refrigerator, because these are viable cells that need to be kept at a low temperature.

Some companies make a vaginal cream containing the beneficial bacteria, which can be inserted directly into the vagina with an applicator. There are also acidophilus capsules that can be inserted into the vagina. Alternatively, you can use live yoghurt in the same way. Some women slather a tampon with yoghurt, and insert it into their vaginas, removing the tampon after 30 minutes or so, which should be enough time for the yoghurt with all its beneficial bacteria to be absorbed by the body. This method can be effective but like anything that is used internally, messy! Furthermore, if you already have a yeast infection, there can be no doubt that levels of beneficial bacteria are not high enough. Even if you choose one of these external methods, it's sensible to take a good probiotic alongside.

If you are currently suffering from thrush, add in fructooligosaccharides (FOS), which are the naturally occurring, water-soluble fibre in fruits and vegetables. These act as a food source for the growth of friendly bacteria.

Angela

Angela was 42 when she came to see me because she was feeling tired all the time. On most days she felt that she was dragging herself out of bed, but she normally felt better by the end of the day. Two years before her visit, she had been made redundant and her father had died. Her bowels were regular but she was experiencing quite a bit of bloating. She'd been on progestogen-only contraception for 10 years, 12 years earlier. I organised a stool sample for Angela and it showed a high level of *Candida albicans*, plus a bacteria called *Citrobacter freundii* and a parasite called *Blastocytis hominis*. We talked about whether she wanted to approach this with natural remedies, which work effectively but are slower, but Angela had been feeling so unwell for so long that she felt she needed something faster. I wrote to Angela's doctor and she was given the appropriate medication. On the follow-up visit, Angela said that she was 'fundamentally and profoundly changed'. She was now working full-time, whereas before she was managing only one hour a day. The bloating was gone.

Herbs

Herbal treatment is aimed at treating an active attack of thrush and also working to prevent future attacks.

Golden seal (*Hydrastis canadensis*)

This is the herb of choice for vaginal thrush, because it contains a substance called berberine, which acts both to stimulate the immune system and to combat yeasts and bacteria.[16] It has become an endangered herb because of overuse, so if you can't obtain it then use barberry root bark (*Berberis vulgaris*) instead.

Calendula (*Calendula officinalis*)

This herb is also known as marigold and works as an anti-fungal, which is very beneficial when treating yeast. It is also anti-microbial, so can be helpful when fighting any kind of infection.

Pau d'arco (*Tabebuia impetiginosa*)

This is a brilliant herb for candida because it has both immune-enhancing and anti-fungal properties. In order for it to be effective you need a product from the whole bark of the tree *Tabebuia impetiginosa*. Some products contain only the active ingredient 'lapachol'. If these are taken in high doses, they can cause nausea and vomiting. This is another example (see page 56), of the need to use the plant as nature provided. In other words, using the active ingredient alone can result in side-effects. When you take pau d'arco as a tincture made from the whole bark, there are no side-effects.

Tea tree oil (*Melaleuca alternifolia*)

Research has been undertaken into the effects of tea tree on candida and other vaginal infections,[17] and it has been shown to be an excellent anti-fungal and anti-bacterial agent herb.

This essential oil (the same type of oil that is used in aromatherapy) is not taken by mouth, but used vaginally to combat the thrush. It is possible to buy tea tree oil pessaries from a healthfood shop. Try adding a few drops of tea tree essential oil to your bath when you have thrush. If you are prone to thrush, it can be used on a preventative basis.

Echinacea

Because your immunity will be compromised if you suffer from recurrent thrush, one of the aims of herbal treatment will be to boost your immune system.

Echinacea is one of the best herbs for increasing immune system function. One study showed that women suffering from recurrent thrush, who were given echinacea, had a 43 per cent reduction in the number of attacks.[18]

For optimum benefit to the immune system, it seems that echinacea is more effective if taken with short breaks. I would suggest ten days on and three days off.

Salt baths

To help soothe the irritation and itching, either wash yourself in a salt solution (1 teaspoon of salt to 1 pint of water) or add a handful of sea salt to your bath.

PREVENTING VAGINAL THRUSH

Once you have successfully treated a bout of vaginal thrush, you will need to focus on preventing a recurrence. Apart from taking the supplements noted above, and changing your diet accordingly, the following tips will help:

- Wear cotton underwear and looser-fitting clothes because yeast grows in a warm, moist environment. If you need to wear tights for work, or simply prefer them, choose a brand with a cotton or open gusset – or wear stockings or hold-ups. You are three times more likely to get thrush if you wear nylon underwear or tights.[19]

- Have a break from using tampons and use sanitary towels to allow the blood to flow naturally (see page 46).

- Avoid perfumed soaps and bubble baths, as these can alter the natural balance of your vagina.

- Use drops of tea tree oil in the bath, which can act as an anti-fungal.

- Take a good probiotic (see page 268), to encourage the growth of fungus-fighting 'healthy' bacteria.

- After opening your bowels, wipe yourself from front to back as yeast can be present in the digestive system (see below), and you could be passing the yeast from your bowel to your vagina.

The Integrated Treatment Plan

The aim is to improve the function of your immune system so that your body is balanced enough to fight off future attacks. Natural remedies are also used to treat a bout of thrush.

There are four steps involved in treatment:

1. Follow the dietary recommendations from Chapter 1 in order to reach a state of optimum health. Eliminate foods and drinks known to encourage thrush.

2. Take nutritional supplements known to be effective in the treatment and prevention of thrush.

3. Take short-term herbs to combat an active attack of thrush.

4. Take long-term herbs to prevent a recurrence.

If you decide to take drugs to treat thrush, it is important to follow the dietary recommendations, and to take the recommended supplements. Continue to take the supplements and to eat well when you have finished your medication, and then add the long-term herbs to the programme. Continue for three months to boost your immune system to prevent another attack.

Your Supplement Plan

- A good multivitamin and mineral supplement e.g. The Healthy Woman

- Beta-carotene (25,000iu per day)

- Zinc (30mg per day)

- Garlic capsules (containing up to 5,000mcg of allicin, taken once a day)

- *Lactobacillus acidophilus* (with approximately 4 billion bacteria)

- FOS (10g per day, sprinkled on food)

- Linseed (flaxseed) oil (1000mg per day)

Note

Each nutrient represents the total intake for one day, so if your multivitamin and mineral already contains 15mg of zinc, for example, you only need to add in a separate zinc supplement containing 15mg per day.

Herbs

In the short term, take separate tinctures of golden seal or barberry (if golden seal is unavailable) and calendula. Also take a separate tincture of pau d'arco while you have thrush (1 teaspoon of each, three times a day), and use tea tree in the bath and in pessary form. Take echinacea during an attack (1 teaspoon three times a day),

For the long term, take echinacea in tincture form: 1 teaspoon a day for the next three months – four weeks on and one week off – to boost your immune system.

To make this programme simpler, I have formulated the Natural Yeast-opack made by the Natural Health Practice, which contains the above nutrients and herbs. If you can't get this locally then call 01892 750511 and it can be posted to you.

In Summary

- Always investigate the cause of any vaginal irritation, itching or discharge before treating as thrush.

- If you have chronic thrush, consider whether or not you may be suffering from diabetes.

- Begin the hormone balancing diet (see page 16).

- Include live yoghurt, garlic and essential fatty acids in your diet, all of which help to reduce a yeast overgrowth.

- Avoid foods that contain yeast, or that are fermented.

- Take steps to boost your immune system, using the herbs and supplements outlined on pages 272 to 273.

- Make sure your partner is also treated, if you suffer from thrush. Otherwise you will pass it back and forth.

- Try to reduce any stress in your life.

- Be sure to include an acidophilus supplement in your diet on a daily basis, particularly if you have been taking antibiotics, or suffer from chronic thrush.

- Follow the self-help tips on page 271.

- Take supplements (see page 272) for three months.

- Take short-term herbs during an attack, and long-term herbs for three months.

Warning

Apart from following the dietary recommendations, do not treat yourself during pregnancy. See a qualified practitioner before you take any herbs or supplements, or use anything internally.

CANDIDA IN THE DIGESTIVE SYSTEM

Candida can exist in parts of the body other than the vagina. For example, oral thrush is common in babies, and appears as white patches on the inside of the mouth. Candida can also form in the intestines.

In the intestines, the yeast form of candida can become 'mycelial' (that is, it forms root-like growths). These roots can penetrate the intestine walls, and cause the gut to 'leak'. Small pieces of undigested food then escape into the bloodstream. This condition is known as 'leaky gut syndrome', and can be the result of an overwhelming infestation of candida in the body, known as 'candidiasis'.

Persistent vaginal thrush can be one of the symptoms of candidiasis, but other symptoms can include food cravings, especially for sugar and bread, fatigue, a bloated stomach with excess flatulence, a 'spaced out' feeling, and becoming tipsy on a very small amount of alcohol. Both men and women can suffer from candidiasis.

If you suffer from these symptoms, you will need to take the candidiasis in hand and often food allergies (see page 72) need to be checked as well. To do this, you'll need expert advice. Please either contact me (see page 507), or see a nutritional therapist (see page 506) for an individual assessment and treatment plan.

A stool test, which can be organised by post, can be used to detect an overgrowth of yeast in the digestive system. The test also shows the levels of beneficial bacteria in your body. But don't assume that because you have these symptoms, there is candida at the root. Many of my patients have believed they were suffering from candidiasis – even going to the extent of following an anti-candida diet for some time – before a stool test showed that a parasitic infestation rather than candida was at the root. The symptoms of both conditions are remarkably similar, so it is essential that you have the appropriate tests to get the correct treatment.

CYSTITIS

Nearly half of all women will experience a painful attack of cystitis at some point in their lives.

What is Cystitis?

Cystitis is an inflammation of the bladder, and it can be the result of infection, irritation or bruising, or even a combination of these three factors. Women are more prone to cystitis than men because the tube (urethra) that runs from the bladder to the outside of the body is much shorter (about 5cm/2in) in women than it is in men (about 18cm/7in). This means that bacteria can more easily travel to a woman's bladder than it can to a man's. What's more, the opening to the urethra is close to both the anus and the vagina in women (in men, it's quite a distance away), which provides even easier access for bacteria to enter the urethra and to make its way up to the bladder.

What Symptoms Can You Experience?

The symptoms of cystitis make the diagnosis crystal clear, and if you have ever suffered from cystitis in the past, you'll recognise them immediately. The two most common symptoms of cystitis are:

- an overwhelming urge to urinate every few minutes, normally with little urine to pass

- burning pain during urination

Other symptoms may include:

- dragging pains in the lower abdomen and back

- nausea and vomiting

- a painful burning sensation at the outer end of the urethra

- dark, often foul-smelling urine, which may also contain some traces of blood

- fever, if there is an infection present.

What Can Cause Cystitis?

There are two main types of cystitis: bacterial (infectious) and non-bacterial.

Bacterial

Bacterial cystitis is responsible for about 50 per cent of all cases of cystitis. Bacteria (normally the E. coli bacteria; see below) enters the urethra in one of a variety of different ways. Once in, it can stick to the walls of the bladder and occasionally travels to the kidneys. The urinary tract itself is normally kept clean by the rush of urine when we eliminate waste products, but infection can develop in the urethra if the bacteria sticks to the walls and multiplies. It then travels up the urethra to the bladder, causing inflammation and infection.

Women who use tampons are more susceptible to bacterial cystitis than women who use towels. The chemicals from tampons can irritate the delicate lining of the vagina, encouraging inflammation and bacterial infection, which then travels to the urethra. Furthermore, the string on a tampon can act like the fuse on a stick of dynamite: providing bacteria with easy access to the body.

Non-bacterial

Non-bacterial or non-infective cystitis is normally caused by bruising or irritation. This type of cystitis is often nicknamed 'honeymoon cystitis' because sex can irritate or bruise the entrance to the urethra, causing inflammation. This inflammation can also make infection more likely. Sex can also cause infectious cystitis; when body fluids are mixed, bacteria can more easily be transferred to the urinary tract.

Other causes of non-bacterial cystitis include chemical irritants, including soaps and bubble baths. Even swimming pool chlorine can irritate the delicate lining of the urethra. Vibrations, such as riding a motorcycle, can also cause bruising, which leads to symptoms of cystitis. Drinking too little can make the urine over concentrated, causing irritation of the urethra and the bladder, which is never properly emptied. Some foods can also irritate the bladder and the urethra, including spicy foods, alcohol, strong coffee and any foods to which you may be allergic. Fresh fruit juice is also highly acidic, and this can cause irritation in some people.

Some women experience cystitis during pregnancy because the urethra is relaxed by the extra progesterone produced by the body. In later pregnancy, urine can remain trapped in the bladder due to the size of the expanding foetus, also causing inflammation.

Cystitis is also common around the menopause because, as oestrogen levels fall, the walls of the vagina become thinner and the walls of the urethra shrink, encouraging bacterial infection and making women more susceptible to irritants.

Are The Symptoms Different If You Have An Infection?

Whether your cystitis is caused by an infection, or simply irritation or bruising, your symptoms will be much the same. Any of these agents will cause inflammation, which in turn causes a tingling sensation that sends a signal to the bladder to empty itself. When this occurs, urine flows down the urethra and passes over the inflamed tissue, causing pain and the characteristic burning sensation. When infection and inflammation spread up the urinary tract to the bladder, it reacts by increasing the urge to pass urine.

As the bladder becomes full, stretch-sensitive receptors in its walls are stimulated and you become aware of the fullness. The frequency and urgency are common because the inflamed bladder wall is being irritated by the urine.

As a result, the kidneys are forced to produce more urine for the bladder to excrete. In most situations, there is inadequate water in the body to produce the necessary quantities, and the urine tends to be more concentrated and higher in uric acid. Under normal circumstances, urine is mildly acidic, but when uric acid levels are high, this increased acidity causes the burning sensation that you experience when urinating. Many over-the-counter cystitis remedies work by lowering the acidity of the urine.

INTERSTITIAL CYSTITIS

This is a chronic, persistent form of cystitis that is not caused by an infection. Interstitial cystitis is an inflammation of the space between the bladder lining and bladder muscles (the interstitium). Ulcers and tiny haemorrhages appear on the bladder wall, and you will experience an increased need to urinate. No bacteria is normally found in the urine, but sufferers experience frequent muscle pain and spasms. This type of cystitis is believed to be aggravated by food allergies.[20]

How Do You Know For Sure You Have Cystitis?

Your doctor will test a midstream urine sample for bacteria. E. coli (Escherichia coli) is the most common bacteria causing cystitis. E. coli is naturally present in the bowels where it is normally harmless. Problems begin when it enters the urethra and bladder. It's important to note, however, that this naturally occurring E. coli is different from the E. coli (0157) that causes food poisoning (in contaminated meat, for example).

When infectious cystitis is untreated, infection can spread from the urinary tract to the bladder and on to the kidneys, causing more dangerous complications, such as a kidney infection. Always see your doctor if you experience symptoms such as:

- fever

- lower back pain

- blood in your urine

- shivery or achy feelings.

What Treatment Can You Be Offered By Your Doctor?

Non-infective cystitis can be easily treated with over-the-counter medications that work to make the urine less acidic.

Bacterial cystitis is treated with antibiotics. Although antibiotics will undoubtedly eliminate the infection, they also wipe out the friendly bacteria in the gut, which can lead to recurrent infection and thrush (candida, see Chapter 8). Similarly, it is believed that an overgrowth of candida can trigger cystitis, so regular antibiotics may become necessary.

If you have used antibiotics to address cystitis in the past, it is important to put into action the recommendations below in order to prevent a recurrence. If you don't, chances are that you will experience another bout of cystitis. It has been found that many women who were given antibiotics for a respiratory infection ended up with a urinary tract infection.[21] It is believed that antibiotics used to kill off the bacteria causing the respiratory infection allowed another bacteria to overgrow in the urinary tract.

What Natural Treatments Could Be Effective?

The natural approach to cystitis involves treating the underlying cause of cystitis while encouraging your body to heal itself. The fundamental aim is to help you restore your health so that you are less susceptible to future attacks of cystitis.

There are several stages involved in this treatment programme:

1. Improve your diet, based on the recommendations outlined in Chapter 1.

2. Use nutritional supplements that are known to reduce infection, build immunity and prevent recurrences.

3. Use herbal remedies to encourage the body to fight infection and prevent recurrences.

4. Undertake practical measures to prevent cystitis from recurring in future.

Dietary changes

• Follow the hormone balancing diet outlined in Chapter 1 (see page 16). Although cystitis is not caused by a hormone imbalance, this healthy diet will encourage your immune system to function more effectively in order to fight off infection.

- Some women find that acidic food and drinks can cause cystitis to flare up. For this reason, it is important to avoid caffeine in tea and coffee, alcohol, meat, spicy foods and fruit juices. Drink plenty of water every day to help dilute the acidic urine.

- It is important that you avoid all sugars, including those hidden in foods such as tomato sauce. Read all labels. Refined carbohydrates, such as the white flour found in pastries, cakes and pies, should also be avoided.

- Certain other foods can aggravate cystitis and these include strawberries, potatoes, tomatoes, spinach and rhubarb.

- As a food allergy can also be a culprit this may be worth investigating (see page 72).

- Eating live organic yoghurt on a regular basis can help with the balance of friendly bacteria in the vagina.

Cranberry juice

It has been known for some time that cranberry juice does help cystitis and that it significantly reduces the bacteria associated with urinary tract infections.[22] It was originally believed that cranberry juice reduced the symptoms of cystitis by making the urine more acidic – but this is obviously not a desirable effect, as it is the acidic urine that causes the burning sensation.

We now know that cranberry works in a completely different way. It seems that certain substances called condensed tannins in cranberries can stop bacteria such as E. coli from sticking to the walls of the urinary tract.[23] For bacteria to infect your urinary tract, they must first stick to the mucosal (mucous membrane lining) walls of the tract. If they are unable to do so, they cannot multiply and are flushed from the body when you urinate. If you have had chronic cystitis in the past, it is worth using cranberries as a preventative measure.

It is interesting that other members of the same botanical family (Ericaceae), such as blueberries, also have the same effect on bacteria in the urethra. Other fruits and vegetables do not.

Don't, under any circumstances, buy cranberry juice with sugar (or artificial sweeteners) thinking it will help your cystitis. Sugar has a terrible effect on your immune system[24] and will compromise the ability of your own body to fight any infections. It has been found that sugar reduces the process called 'phagocytosis', where white blood cells engulf and consume bacteria and foreign substances. Sugar also encourages candida (see Chapter 8), which can in turn lead to cystitis.

Cranberries and blueberries do not need to be taken in liquid form. Supplements (normally dried berries) are acceptable.

Garlic

Garlic has often been called 'nature's antibiotic' and it has been found to control many bacteria that have been implicated in cystitis such as E. coli, proteus, klebsiella and staphylococcus.[25] In order to get the full benefits of the garlic you will need to eat it raw. That may sound daunting, but it can easily be added to salad dressings or crushed and used as a garnish on Italian meals. Take a garlic supplement if you (or anyone around you!) can't stand the smell or taste.

Supplements

The aim is to use supplements that have been found to have a beneficial effect in the treatment of cystitis – partly because they promote a good acid/alkaline balance and also because they try to prevent bacteria from sticking to the urinary system and the bladder. The supplements are also designed to help restore your health, which will naturally encourage your immune system to eliminate any unhealthy bacteria.

Suggested dosages will follow in the treatment plan (see page 286).

Vitamin C

Vitamin C is an important vitamin in all cases of infection, and it also helps to boost immune activity. Many studies have shown that vitamin C helps to increase immune function.[26] In the case of cystitis, vitamin C has been shown particularly to inhibit the growth of E. coli.[27] Buy the vitamin C in an ascorbate form (the label will read magnesium or calcium ascorbate). If the label says 'ascorbic acid', it will be too acidic for cystitis sufferers.

Beta-carotene

Vitamin A and beta-carotene (the precursor to vitamin A, found in brightly coloured fruits and vegetables) help to maintain healthy cells. By keeping cells healthy, you are more likely to prevent an invasion by bacteria. Vitamin A is also important for a healthy immune system.

Bromelain

This is a digestive enzyme that comes from pineapples. Bromelain is known for its anti-inflammatory properties, and it has been shown to have a beneficial effect on urinary tract infections, including cystitis.[28]

Zinc

Zinc is an important mineral for the immune system, and it needs to be taken both when an infection is present and to prevent a recurrence. It is recognised for its anti-infectious properties (in other words, it can help to prevent an infection from taking hold).[29]

Lactobacillus acidophilus

This probiotic (see page 268) helps to restore the 'good' or 'healthy' bacteria (known as flora) in your body. When you have an attack of cystitis it may be beneficial to use a vaginal cream that contains acidophilus, as well as taking it orally. *Lactobacillus acidophilus* is available in a variety of different forms, including supplements and live organic yoghurts. For best effect, you should try to incorporate all of these forms into your diet when you are suffering from an attack.[30]

Herbs

Specific herbs are chosen to help reduce the amount of bacteria present, soothe the inflamed tissue and to boost your immune system to fight off this bacteria. The best approach is to use herbs that do both of these things at the same time.

Corn silk (*Zea mays*)

This herb is used to soothe bladder irritation and to ease pain in the urinary tract. It helps to protect the inflamed tissue.

Yarrow (*Achillea millefolium*)

This herb has anti-inflammatory properties, so it helps to soothe the sore tissues in the bladder. It seems to target particularly the urinary system, where it can heal irritation and help to fight the infection.

Horsetail (*Equisetum arvense*)

This herb also has anti-inflammatory actions, so can help your inflamed bladder, but also helps to control the levels of bacteria that can be causing the inflammation.

Blend equal parts of corn silk, yarrow and horsetail (in tincture form) and take 1 teaspoon three times a day while the infection is present.

Uva ursi (*Arctostaphylos uva-ursi*)

This herb contains a substance called 'arbutin', which is transformed in the urinary tract into hydroquinone. Hydroquinone is an antiseptic that is effective again E. coli bacteria. This herb should only be taken for two weeks.

Golden seal (*Hydrastis canadensis*)

Golden seal is effective against E. coli and many of the other bacteria that can cause cystitis. It is particularly useful in cases where there is bleeding.[31] Because golden seal is endangered due to overharvesting, it is better to minimise its use and just take for a short time with the uva ursi. Golden seal should not be used during pregnancy. If you have a history of heart disease, glaucoma or diabetes, consult your doctor or practitioner before using this herb.

Uva ursi and golden seal can be very effective in the short term in order to try and prevent the need to take antibiotics. The best approach is to have a mix of the two herbs, but only take for a maximum of two weeks.

Echinacea

In order to fight off infections without the need for antibiotics, and to prevent further infections causing cystitis, you will need to strengthen your immune system. Echinacea is the herb of choice here, as it has been shown to increase the white blood cell count and activity in order to effectively engulf bacteria and viruses.[32]

Echinacea appears to be more effective when taken on and off. I suggest taking it for ten days, then taking a break of three days, before repeating for another ten days.

TREATING INTERSTITIAL CYSTITIS

The herb gotu kola (*Centella asiaticas*) has been shown to be helpful in interstitial cystitis because it helps to improve the integrity of the connective tissues that make up the intersititium (see page 279).[33]

Furthermore, the amino acid L-arginine has been found to reduce significantly the symptoms of interstitial cystitis.[34] It is believed that L-arginine helps the manufacture of a vasodilator (opens blood vessels) called nitric oxide, which opens up and relaxes blood vessels, thereby reducing muscle pain and spasms. Take approximately 1,500mg per day for six months.

> **Note**
> If you suffer from herpes attacks (as either cold sores or genital herpes) you should not supplement with arginine because it stimulates the virus.

Self-help

Bicarbonate of soda can help to make your urine more alkaline, and will relieve the burning sensation. Dissolve 1 teaspoonful of bicarbonate of soda (also called baking soda) in about ½ a litre of warm water and drink twice daily, or sip throughout the day. This treatment is not appropriate for anyone suffering from epilepsy.

Add a blend of tea tree, juniper, cypress and eucalyptus essential oils to your bath every night (1–2 drops of each). Alternatively, a few drops of these oils can be added to a large jug of warm water and poured over the affected area while sitting on the toilet.

The preventive recommendations below are also useful during an attack of cystitis.

Barley water

Barley water helps as it acts as an anti-inflammatory agent for the urinary system. Buy whole barley, put 1.5oz (40g) in 2 pints (1200ml) water and bring to the boil. Simmer for 30 minutes. For the last ten minutes you can either add a slice of lemon or the juice of one lemon. The barley water can be sipped during the day. This not only gives you extra fluid, but has other beneficial anti-inflammatory properties as well.

Homeopathy

Homeopathy can also be extremely beneficial for cystitis. The most common remedies used are Cantharis and Sarsaparilla, but as the remedy is matched to the specific symptoms it is worth while seeing a qualified homeopath. This is particularly important if you suffer from chronic cystitis.

Prevention

Once you manage to get rid of a bout of cystitis, it's important to prevent a recurrence. Cystitis can be notoriously difficult to treat when it becomes persistent. Follow the recommendations below to prevent another attack.

- urinate regularly, and don't hold it when you have to go

- if you suffer from repeated attacks, take showers instead of baths

- avoid perfumed bath products, soaps, shampoos, toiletries and douches

- wipe yourself from front to back after urinating or defecating

- wash the area from front to back with a little cool water to ensure that you remove all traces of infectious agents

- always pat the area dry rather than rubbing

- make sure that you are aroused enough when having sex, or use a lubricant

The Integrated Approach

You should start the natural approach as soon as the symptoms begin. If the symptoms are getting worse after 48 hours, if you develop a fever or if there is blood in the urine, you need to see your doctor. Antibiotics may be necessary. Go on to prevent another attack by following the self-help measures described above.

If you do need antibiotics, follow the dietary and supplement recommendations. When you have finished the antibiotics, take a course of probiotics (acidophilus) for three months to help replenish the beneficial bacteria.

Your Supplement Plan

During an attack and to prevent cystitis in the future, take the following supplements:

- A good multivitamin and mineral supplement, e.g. The Healthy Woman by the Natural Health Practice

- Vitamin C at 500mg four times per day when the cystitis is present (use the calcium or magnesium ascorbate form of vitamin C, not ascorbic acid)

- Beta-carotene (25,000iu per day)

- Zinc (30mg per day)

- Bromelain (500mg, three times a day between meals)

- Cranberry supplements

- Acidophilus (containing approximately 4 million bacteria)

Note
Each nutrient represents the total intake for one day, so if your multivitamin and mineral already contains 15mg of zinc, for example, you only need to add in a separate zinc supplement containing 15mg per day.

Herbs

Take herbs in tincture form (see page 57).

Short term

- Take a tincture, which contains a mix of equal parts uva ursi and golden seal for two weeks, 1 teaspoon three times a day

- During that same two weeks, use a tincture of echinacea 1 teaspoon three times a day for the first ten days, then stop for three days. Repeat

Long term

As well as the short-term herbs, take a blend of corn silk, yarrow and horsetail in equal parts. Take 1 teaspoon three times a day for at least a month.

To make this programme simpler, I have formulated the Natural Cystopack made by the Natural Health Practice, which contains the above nutrients and herbs. If you can't get this locally, then call 01892 750511 and it can be posted to you.

CERVICAL ABNORMALITIES AND SMEAR TESTS

What Causes Cervical Dysplasia?

Dysplasia – also known as CIN, or cervical intraepithelial neoplasia – describes the irregularities and abnormalities that can occur in the cells of the cervix.

It is now known that the human papillomavirus (HPV), which is also the cause of genital warts, is the major cause of cervical dysplasia. It is an infection that is linked to 99.7 per cent of all cervical cancers.[35]

The current thinking is that women with mild and/or borderline smear results should have HPV testing, which could prevent them being unnecessarily overtreated.[36]

Smear Tests and Cervical Abnormalities

What is a smear test?

A cervical smear test is a simple test designed to detect abnormalities in the cells of the cervix. It is also called a Pap (Papanicolaou) smear after the doctor who invented it. A small instrument called a speculum is inserted into the vagina and a spatula is put inside this in order to reach the neck of the womb (the cervix). Cells are gently scraped from the surface of the cervix, smeared on to a glass slide and then sent to a laboratory for examination.

The cells are graded according to the degree of change that is seen under a microscope. If changes are found in cells from the cervix then a colposcopy is often suggested (see below).

If you have had a hysterectomy and your cervix was removed then you do not need to have any more smears.

RELIABILITY OF THE SMEAR TEST

The major problem with the cervical smear test is that these changes are often read incorrectly. There are a number of 'false positives', where

---

you can be given a diagnosis of cervical cancer when, in fact, the changes are benign (harmless). There are also 'false negatives', where you can be told that everything is fine when there is evidence of cancer of the cervix. If you have been told the smear is positive (even though it is not – a 'false positive'), you would at least be sent for a colposcopy (see below) and the diagnosis can be confirmed. The worse scenario is getting a false negative, because there could be a risk of undiagnosed cancer, and no further tests would be arranged.

These mistakes have led to a number of deaths from cervical cancer, which should have been picked up earlier, and also to many emergency hysterectomies. But in the case of false diagnoses of cancer, women have gone through needless emotional suffering and anxiety. Sometimes, too few cells are taken, which means that you have to repeat the smear. This can obviously be a source of great anxiety for many women.

The problem is that technicians have to analyse the smears under a microscope. They have to try to pick out abnormal cells from a total of maybe 400,000 cells. This means that there is always going to be a big risk of human error because the process is repetitive and tiring.

To help prevent the possibility of human error, other ways of analysing cervical smears are in the pipeline. One way involves the use of a computer to scan the 400,000 or so cells in the smear and then grade them on a sliding scale of abnormality. Cells that the computer considers to be abnormal are then displayed on a computer screen, and these are then checked by a technician. The system still relies on people reading the screen and making judgements, but it greatly reduces the possibility of missing abnormalities.

Another system 'lights up' the abnormal cells with a fluorescent dye, which makes them easier to see.

There is pressure on us to have regular smears not just because it should pick up abnormal cervical cell changes, but because your doctor benefits financially. It has been said that, in the UK, doctors get bonus pay if more than 50 per cent of the women on their lists receive the test and triple the bonus pay if 80 per cent have smears.[37]

Classification of Cell Changes (CIN)

Any changes in the cervical cells are graded according to a standard system. There are three categories of dysplasia (cell changes) known as Cervical Intraepithelial Neoplasia (CIN) and classified as CIN 1, 2 and 3, according to whether the changes are mild, moderate or severe. Severe dysplasia (CIN 3) is also called 'carcinoma in situ', which means that there is cancer confined to one particular place, such as the cervix. A further stage of the cancer would be invasive, and tests would show that it had spread to other areas such as the pelvic organs.

THE 'WAIT AND SEE' APPROACH

Many women will develop CIN but it disappears and the cervix returns to normal. So, when the results show only mild cervical changes, the best approach seems to be to wait six months and then repeat the smear.[38] Also, many more women develop CIN than ever develop cancer, and the CIN can persist without causing any problems or developing into cancer.

What to Do

Research is showing that a plan of action should be followed, depending on the results of the smear:

If smear results are inconclusive   Then you should have the smear repeated

If smear is mild and/or borderline   Then you should be tested for HPV. If the HPV test is negative, then repeat the smear in six months' time together with another HPV test. If the second HPV is negative, and the cervical abnormality has not progressed, then it is recommended that no treatment is offered.

If HPV test is positive   You should go for a colposcopy, as the HPV tests cannot distinguish between the three stages of CIN (1 to 3).

It is, however, possible to have HPV, but never experience any abnormal cell changes (dysplasia). HPV infections can come and go, and most young women will shake them off with no ill-effects. However, if HPV infection is persistent after the age of 30, there is a greater risk of developing cervical cancer.

If you test negatively for HPV, you will have little or no risk of developing cervical cancer. As a quote from the *Journal of Pathology* says, 'the extreme rarity of HPV-negative cancers reinforces the rationale for HPV testing in addition to, or even instead of, cervical cytology *smears* (my italics) in routine cervical screening'.

RELIABILITY OF THE HPV TEST

The reliability of the HPV test is very different to that of the regular smear test. The HPV test has a 95 per cent or greater detection rate,[39] compared to 76 per cent by the conventional smear method, and it is not subject to human error.

The sample is taken from the same area of the cervix as the smear test, but high-risk HPV (see below) is not visible on the smear. Only special DNA testing can detect this. Unlike the smear test, the answer is either positive or negative. You either have HPV or you don't, which is very different from a normal smear test where the cells are graded.

What is HPV (Human Papillomavirus)?

There are as many as a hundred different types of HPV. Some types cause warts or verrucas, but do not cause genital warts. The types of HPV that cause genital warts are highly contagious, but usually benign. Using condoms helps to prevent transmission, but they are not completely effective because the warts can be very small, and both inside and outside the body. There can, as a result, still be direct skin contact. But there are a number of HPV types that are classed as 'high risk', and it is these types that are linked to cervical cancer. HPV testing can determine which type you have.

Cervical Dysplasia – Risk Factors

The following factors increase your risk of developing cervical dysplasia and cervical cancer:

• multiple sexual partners

- smoking

- being sexually active at a young age

- the Pill.

Smoking doubles and even can triple your chances of developing abnormal cervical cell changes.[40] Nicotine becomes concentrated in the glands of the cervix and can act as a carcinogen (cancer-triggering compound). It is also thought that smoking may alter your immune system's response, making it harder for it to stop the cells from changing abnormally.

It is unclear why women are more at risk with the Pill. Obviously because the Pill is not a barrier method of birth control, there will be more chance of infection. However, some experts believe that the hormones in the Pill may be to blame.

See your doctor if you experience any of the following symptoms:

- bleeding between periods
- bleeding after intercourse
- continuous vaginal discharge.

Other Reasons For Unusual Bleeding Between Periods

If you suffer from any of the above symptoms, it is important to see your doctor so that cervical dysplasia can be ruled out. There can, however, be other reasons why you have been bleeding between periods, and these include the following:

Cervical erosion – This occurs when the cervix appears inflamed, with a red spot or an ulcer, and can occur after childbirth or when taking the Pill. If the erosion is causing persistent bleeding then it can be treated. If there is no bleeding, it can be left alone. A smear should be performed to check that the cervix is healthy. Cervical erosions are not cancerous and do not develop into cancer.

Cervical polyp – This is a wart-like growth that is attached to the cervix. A polyp can cause bleeding, but it is not usually painful. Again a smear is usually performed to double-check that the cervix is healthy. The polyp can then be 'snipped' off.

What Treatment Can You Be Offered By Your Doctor?

The treatment suggested will depend on the degree of cell changes seen, but they can include drugs or surgery.

Colposcopy

The colposcope is literally a pair of binoculars on a stand. It enables the doctor to see an enlarged, three-dimensional view of the cervix, while a speculum is used gently to separate the walls of the vagina.

The results of the smear test may have shown cell changes, but the colposcopy shows where the CIN is and its extent. To help to make the CIN more visible, the cervix is often painted with dilute acetic acid (vinegar), and sometimes with an iodine solution. Acetic acid makes the CIN whiter than a healthy cell and iodine stains it brown.

When the abnormal area on the cervix is identified, a sample (biopsy) is taken, which is then sent to the laboratory for testing.

Treatment will depend on what is found under the microscope and these options are listed below. Remember that a smear test is only a screening tool and cannot be used for diagnosis. The colposcopy, together with the biopsy gives you the diagnosis.

Drugs

Imiquimod

Women who are found to be HPV-positive, but with a normal or borderline smear test, can be offered a cream called Imiquimod. This drug is classed as an 'immune response modifier', which means that it is aimed at improving the immune system response so that the body fights off the infection itself. This is exactly the same aim as the natural approach to HPV (see page 296).

HPV Vaccine

At the moment a vaccine is under trial, and it should be available in the next five years. It is suggested that the vaccine would be used for older women and eventually to vaccinate children before they become sexually active.

The Surgical Approach

The choice of surgical treatment is dependent on what is seen during a colposcopy.

Diathermy

If, during the colposcopy, the cells examined from the biopsy show abnormalities and the abnormal area is on the outer surface of the cervix, the cells can be destroyed using diathermy (heat). This is performed under a local anaesthetic and it takes only about 15 minutes to destroy the cells. Because the tissue has been burned by the heat, you could experience bleeding for up to three weeks after the treatment. The diathermy effectively eliminates the abnormal cells and there is a low rate of recurrence afterwards, although you would be asked to have regular yearly smears just to be on the safe side.

Laser therapy

Instead of using diathermy, the abnormal cells are destroyed by laser. There would also be some bleeding after this treatment for a number of weeks. Laser therapy seems to be used less frequently than in the past.

Cryosurgery

Here the abnormal cells are frozen by using a small probe. There can be mild, period-like pains during the treatment and some discharge for a few weeks afterwards.

Cone biopsy

If the whole of the abnormal area cannot be seen because it involves the inner part of the cervix, it may be necessary to cut away the abnormal tissue rather than destroying it. A heated loop is used to take out a cone-shaped piece of tissue, which is sent to the lab for analysis. So a cone biopsy is diagnosis and treatment at the same time. Cone biopsy may involve a general anaesthetic but can also be performed under a local. There will usually be bleeding for up to three weeks after the treatment while the tissue heals. After a cone biopsy, you would be asked to have six-monthly smears for a while and then to have them yearly. The recurrence rate is very low. There can be two problems following a cone biopsy, but both are very rare. If the amount of abnormal tissue that had to be removed was extensive, an incompetent cervix may be the result. This would make it difficult to stay pregnant. There may also be a reduction in the amount of mucus produced from the cervix, which can affect fertility.

Natural Approaches to Cervical Dysplasia (Abnormal Cell Changes)

The natural approach is twofold: aiming both to prevent (in other words, reduce the likelihood of getting this problem in the first place); and to treat (encouraging any abnormal cell changes to revert back to normal) the problem.

It is important to remember that cervical dysplasia is a sexually transmitted disease. It is extremely rare for virgins to have abnormal cell changes on the cervix. Therefore, basic methods of prevention include:

- using condoms during intercourse, unless you are always with the same partner

- reducing your exposure to men who have genital warts

- trying to limit the number of sexual partners

There are a number of stages involved in preventing abnormal cervical cell changes:

1. Improve your diet, based on the recommendations outlined in Chapter 1.

2. Use nutritional supplements that are known to be deficient in women with cervical cancer.

3. Use certain nutrients to boost the functioning of your immune system in order to be able to fight any viruses.

4. Use herbs to boost the immune system.

5. Use certain herbs that are known to be effective against viruses and warts.

- It is now thought to be unlikely that HPV can be transmitted between women.

- Spontaneous regression of cervical dysplasia is possible as long as your immune system is working efficiently. It is estimated that up to 70 per cent of women can have been infected with HPV over our lifetimes, but only 10 women per 100,000 get cervical cancer.

Dietary changes

Research has found that women with abnormal cervical cells and cervical cancer are deficient in many of the powerful antioxidants (see page 17). It makes sense that alongside the dietary recommendations from Chapter 1, you should pay particular attention to increasing your intake of the foods that contain these antioxidants. Antioxidants can protect your cells from DNA damage, which can cause cell mutation and cancer. Furthermore, the *Obstetrics and Gynaecology News* suggested in May 1999 that cruciferous vegetables, such as broccoli, cabbage and Brussels sprouts, can help to encourage abnormal cervical changes to regress back to normal.

Supplements

What most doctors don't know is that 67 per cent of women with cervical cancer are deficient in one or more nutrients, despite the fact that this information has been published in one of the leading medical journals for gynaecologists, *The American Journal of Obstetrics and Gynae-cology*, as far back as 1985.[41] These deficiencies can include folic acid, beta-carotene (vitamin A), vitamin C, vitamin B6, vitamin E, zinc and selenium.

You will notice that nearly all of the supplements mentioned below are noted for their antioxidant properties and their effects on the immune system. The idea is that if you have optimum levels of these nutrients, you can prevent abnormal cell changes and even cell mutations. In many cases, it is even possible to reverse abnormal cell changes back to normal.

Vitamin A and beta-carotene

It has been found that women with cervical cancer only have one-half the level of vitamin A in their blood, compared to women with normal cervical cells[42] and that women with either cervical dysplasia (cell changes) or cancer had low levels of beta-carotene.[43]

Although beta-carotene is fairly well known, and many women get lots from carrots, which are an excellent source, there are other carotenes that are equally important. Lycopene, for example, is found primarily in tomatoes, and is more readily absorbed by your body when the tomatoes are cooked than when they are raw. It is also present in red fruits and red peppers. Some scientists think that lycopene may be more effective in reversing dysplasia than beta-carotene.[44] In one study, simply adding lycopene to cancer cell cultures inhibited their growth.[45]

Because of the benefits of the other carotenes, it is best to take a supplement that contains a mix of the different carotenes.

Vitamin E

Vitamin E has been found to be low in women with cervical abnormalities. One study looked at 168 women with normal smears who did not have an HPV infection and compared them to 228 women with CIN and an HPV infection. For both groups the researchers measured the blood levels of vitamin E and found that those women with the abnormal smear tests had significantly lower levels of vitamin E.[46]

Vitamin C

Vitamin C, which is a powerful antioxidant and immune-system booster, is significantly lower in women who have cervical dysplasia and 'carcinoma in situ' (see pages 290–1).[47] Also, those women whose daily intake of vitamin C was less than 88mg had a four times higher risk of developing cervical cancer than women with higher intakes.[48]

It is interesting to note that smoking, which is one of the most important co-factors in relation to the development of cervical dysplasia, alters the levels of vitamin C. Vitamin C levels in the cells of the cervix and vagina of smokers is significantly lower than in non-smokers.[49]

Vitamin B6

Up to one-third of women with cervical cancer can have a vitamin B6 deficiency. A lack of vitamin B6 could be compromising the immune system.[50]

Folic acid

One of the early signs of a folic acid deficiency is actually abnormal changes in the cells of the cervix.[51] And it has been found that women who test positive for the high-risk type HPV are five times more likely to have cervical dysplasia if they are deficient in folic acid.[52]

It has been known for some time that using the Pill can cause a folic acid deficiency, which then leads to negative cell changes in the cervix.[53] Ironically, it is possible that when a woman's blood levels of folic acid are tested, they can seem normal or even high. However, the deficiency shows up in the actual tissues of the cervix. It is believed that the Pill blocks the uptake of folic acid by the cells.

To confirm this, women have been given folic acid even when there weren't obvious deficiencies, but when they were taking the Pill. Abnormal cell changes in the cervix were completely reversed when the folic acid was added.[54]

Remember that if you take folic acid you should always make sure you are taking vitamin B12 as well, or a multivitamin and mineral that contains B12, so that you do not mask a vitamin B12 deficiency (pernicious anaemia).

Selenium

This mineral is a powerful antioxidant and is deficient in women with abnormal cells in the cervix.[55] Selenium can help prevent abnormal cell changes, so is an essential nutrient in the treatment and prevention of cervical dysplasia.

Zinc

Zinc is an important mineral to take for abnormal cell changes. It is an essential component of genetic material and a zinc deficiency can cause chromosome changes. It plays a vital role in cell division and is extremely important for the optimum functioning of your immune system.

Herbs

The choice of herbs to be used for cervical dysplasia relate to their ability to help boost your immune system. Anti-viral properties are also important, in order to try to control the HPV.

Echinacea (*Echinacea purpurea* and *E. angustifolia*)

This is the herb of choice for cervical dysplasia and HPV because it has both a positive effect on your immune system function and it is also anti-viral. Echinacea has been shown to increase the white blood cell count and activity in order to effectively engulf bacteria and viruses.[56] This is ultimately important when the aim is to control the human papillomavirus (HPV).

It seems that echinacea is more effective if taken with short breaks. A good regime is ten days on, three days off, ten days on, and so on.

Cat's claw (*Uncaria tomentosa*)

This herb is also excellent for the immune system as certain components isolated from cat's claw (a herb, not the real thing!) are able to increase the ability of the white blood cells to engulf viruses.[57]

Astralagus (*Astralagus membranaceus*)

This herb is also both an immune stimulant and anti-viral. Research has found it to be effective against a number of different viruses.[58]

Thuja *(Thuja occidentalis)*

This is an important herb for the treatment of genital warts and HPV. Like echinacea it stimulates phagocytosis (the ability of the white blood cells to engulf viruses and bacteria). But thuja is able to do this at an earlier stage of phagocytosis than echinacea and it also has anti-viral properties.[59]

Golden seal (*Hydrastis canadensis*)

Golden seal is an excellent herb for cervical dysplasia (abnormal cell changes), but unfortunately it has become endangered because it has been overharvested. This herb helps to tone and heal the mucous membranes in the cervix and can help to fight infection by boosting immune system function. Because it is endangered and is now being produced commercially, I have suggested below that you add it in a small amount to the overall tincture of herbs as it is so valuable with this problem.

The Integrated Treatment Plan

If you have been told to follow a 'wait and see approach', begin the dietary suggestions (see page 297), and take the supplements and herbs to try to reverse any abnormal cell changes before the follow-up smear in approximately six months' time. If the follow-up smear is normal, continue to eat well and take the supplements, but stop taking the herbs. If the follow-up smear is still abnormal, you need to follow the medical advice given to you for treatment. See a qualified nutritional therapist for more individual nutritional advice.

If you have been told you need a colposcopy and possibly treatment, with or without a positive HPV test, then follow all the recommendations for six months following treatment. The aim is to prevent a recurrence. If the next check is normal, continue to eat healthily and take the supplements. Stop taking the herbs. If the follow-up shows a problem, take medical advice and see a qualified nutritional therapist for more personal nutritional advice.

Your Supplement Plan

- A good multivitamin and mineral supplement, e.g. The Healthy Woman by the Natural Health Practice
- Mixed natural carotenes (50,000iu per day)
- Vitamin B-complex (containing 50mg of most of the B vitamins per day)
- Folic acid (800mcg per day)
- Vitamin C (1,000mg per day)
- Vitamin E (300iu per day)
- Selenium (200mcg per day)
- Zinc citrate (50mg per day)
- Linseed oil (1,000mg per day, for general health)

> **Note**
> Each nutrient represents the total intake for one day, so if your multivitamin and mineral already contain 25mg of zinc, for example, you only need to 'top up' that nutrient with an extra supplement to the recommended amount.

Herbs

- Echinacea: use ten days on, three days off, ten days off etc, 1 teaspoon three times per day over six months.

- Blend equal parts of the herbs cat's claw, astralagus and thuja together and add a small amount of golden seal. So if the equal parts are 10ml, for example, which makes 30ml of cat's claw, astralagus and thuja in total, then add in 5ml of golden seal. Take 1 teaspoon three times a day for three months.

CHAPTER 9

Breasts

Both in a physical and metaphorical sense, breasts are of major importance in a woman's life. The female breast primarily exists as a source of nourishment for babies, but it is also part of her sexual armoury – a means of sexual pleasure for both herself and her partner. Breasts are affected by hormones – cyclically, in association with a woman's periods, and during pregnancy – and can be affected by a number of problems, among them breast cancer, a basic fear for many women. Although advice on the latter is beyond the scope for this book, there are practical ways in which the risk factors for this disease can be lessened.

CYCLICAL BREAST PROBLEMS

Up to 70 per cent of women in the West experience breast changes that fluctuate with their menstrual cycles. Their breasts can feel so tender, swollen and/or lumpy that the discomfort is hard to cope with. Some women complain that they can't bear to be hugged, and find sleeping very difficult because they can't get comfortable.

The symptoms are grouped under a variety of different umbrella terms, including cyclical breast pain, cyclical mastalgia (which literally means breast pain), cyclical mastitis or fibrocystic breast disease. Despite their severity and the disruption they can cause, most breast problems are benign, not cancer. However, don't be tempted to ignore them. Any unusual changes in your breasts should be reported to your doctor.

What Can Cause Fibrocystic Breasts?

Because the symptoms are linked to the menstrual cycle then it could be easy to say that the breast tenderness and lumpiness are 'caused' by the hormone changes in the cycle. But it is interesting to note that women who live in Asian countries like Japan don't experience the same degree of breast changes, although they have the same hormones circulating each month.[1] What's the main difference between Eastern and Western women? Apart from geography, it's largely diet. Later in this section you'll see how to eliminate breast discomfort simply by changing your diet.

YOUR HORMONES AND BREAST CHANGES

The two main female hormones circulating during your menstrual cycle are oestrogen and progesterone. Oestrogen acts as a 'builder' in the body, as it helps to build up the lining of the womb ready to receive a fertilised egg. Progesterone is released after ovulation (in the second half of your cycle), and this is the hormone that helps to maintain a pregnancy once you have conceived. Progesterone also increases the blood supply to the breasts and 'readies' the cells in the breasts to secrete milk if you become pregnant. Some experts think that breast discomfort is increased in women whose ratio of oestrogen

---

to progesterone is out of balance – in other words, when oestrogen is too high in relation to progesterone – or when cycles are anovulatory (no ovulation), which causes 'oestrogen dominance'. It is, however, interesting that when women become pregnant, the first indication of their condition is often the fact that their breasts feel larger and more tender.

When you become pregnant the hormone progesterone continues to rise, so it's possible that excess progesterone may be at the root of the problem. Prolactin is a hormone secreted by the pituitary gland and it reaches a high level in women who are breastfeeding. It is thought that some women may be sensitive to even normal levels of prolactin.

Finding Out If There Is a Reason For Your Breast Discomfort

The medical profession seems to be unsure about what really causes breast discomfort, but if your discomfort definitely varies with your cycle, improving when your period begins, or fairly soon afterwards, then there is unlikely to be anything sinister at the root. However, it always pays to be vigilant about examining your breasts, so even if you can dismiss your pain as being cyclical, you should continue to check your breasts regularly.

KNOW YOUR BREASTS

You need to become familiar with your breasts in order to spot anything unusual. This involves examining them regularly, as follows:

1. Stand in front of a mirror, raise your arms above your head and move from side to side to get a good look at your breasts. Get to know how they feel, and look at the shape and outline. Become aware of the position and shape of the nipples.

2. Lie on your back with your head on a pillow. Examine one breast at a time. Raise your right arm and put it behind your head. Using

the tips of your left fingers, feel around the right breast in small, circular movements. Check both breasts and armpits in the same way.

What to look for:

- any small lump in the breast or armpit

- a dimple or dent in the skin when lifting your arm

- any reddish, ulcerated or scaly area of skin on the breast or nipple

- any bleeding or discharge from the nipple or moist, reddish areas that don't heal easily

- any change in nipple position (for example, pulled inwards or pointing in a different direction).

The best time to check your breasts is just following your period. If you discover anything that concerns you, make an appointment to see your doctor at the same point in your cycle the following month. If you go for an examination just before your period, it is more difficult to assess which changes are harmless, and related to hormonal fluctuations, and those that should be taken more seriously.

The majority of women find lumps themselves when they are showering. Often partners are the first to notice a change. If you are concerned about anything at all, see your doctor.

If your doctor finds anything suspicious during a physical breast check, then you will probably be referred for a mammogram. For more information on whether a mammogram is a good idea and what other choices you have, see below.

What Treatment Can You Be Offered By Your Doctor?

Because the pain and tenderness are related to your hormone cycle, the conventional approach is to manipulate the female hormones to try to eliminate the problem. While this can control the problem in the short term, the root cause will not have been addressed. When medication is ceased, the symptoms will return again. Furthermore, all drugs have potential side-effects, and you will have to assess the benefits versus the risks of any prescribed medication programme.

Because the natural approach to this problem is so effective, it is definitely worth trying it first.

Drugs

Bromocriptine

This drug works by lowering the level of prolactin (the hormone that is high in breastfeeding women). Unfortunately, prolactin is not always high in women with cyclical breast discomfort. The side-effects of bromocriptine can be very extreme and can include nausea, vomiting, dizziness, hallucinations, leg cramps and a dry mouth.

Prolactin levels can be increased when under stress, but if prolactin is high, as shown by a blood test, then you should be referred to a specialist to rule out any problems with the pituitary gland, which produces the prolactin.

The contraceptive pill

The Pill is the drug of choice because it offers a synthetic dose of hormones, which creates a 'false' cycle. In reality, your hormone levels will be artificially altered, and the 'period' that you experience at the end of your cycle is, in fact, simply a withdrawal bleed. In some women, the Pill makes breast discomfort worse.

Some of the listed side-effects of the Pill are nausea, vomiting, headache, thrombosis, changes in sex drive, depression, changes in body weight and, ironically, breast tenderness.

Danazol

This synthetic, weak male hormone stops ovulation, which suppresses the cycle. The logic is that if you are not having a cycle, you will not have the hormone fluctuations, thereby eliminating the breast tenderness. The side-effects can include severe mood swings, nausea, dizziness, rashes and headaches. Because danazol is a male hormone, side-effects can also include facial hair, acne, increased sex drive and weight gain.

Gonadotrophin releasing hormone (GnRH) analogues

These are synthetic hormones that put your body into a state of temporary menopause. They are normally offered in the form of an injection or as a nasal spray. Not surprisingly, hot flushes are a common side-effect, but others include headaches, mood swings, vaginal dryness and insomnia. You might also want to ask yourself how long it is safe to take a drug like this, and what the possible effects on your bone density might be.

Tamoxifen

This is an anti-oestrogen drug that is primarily used to prevent the recurrence of breast cancer. It has been successfully used for cyclical breast pain, but it is often accompanied by uncomfortable menopausal symptoms such as hot flushes. The other concern is that young women taking this drug could be putting themselves at risk of osteoporosis, and there is also an increased risk of womb cancer.

'Natural' progesterone

I have deliberately put this in the drug section, to make it clear that progesterone is a hormone and, when taken into the body, it should be classed as a drug. Progesterone is different from progestogen, which is the synthetic hormone used in the Pill and HRT. The 'natural' in front of the word progesterone just means that it is chemically identical to the progesterone that you produce from your ovaries. This is discussed in more detail in the chapter on PMS (see page 88), but it is important to make the point here that when you use a progesterone cream, you are using a drug, not a natural remedy.

A number of books suggest that if cyclical breast discomfort is caused by an imbalance of oestrogen to progesterone, then increasing progesterone in the body would be the answer to the problem. It has also been suggested that the cream is applied to the breasts in the second half of the cycle, to prevent cyclical breast pain.

I have concerns about this recommendation. In our breasts and womb we have separate oestrogen and progesterone receptors that 'pick up' the relevant hormone for that particular receptor. In the womb there are both oestrogen and progesterone receptors. There is a kind of 'lock and key' effect: the hormones are the keys, and they fit into the receptors (the locks). Each key has a different lock. In the womb, progesterone has a protective effect on the endometrium (womb lining) and it encourages the shedding that occurs every month when you are not pregnant. In the breasts, however, progesterone has a stimulatory effect because it prepares the cells in the breasts to produce milk in anticipation of a pregnancy. It also increases the blood supply to the breast.

So we can have a situation where the same hormone can behave one way in one part of the body and seemingly the opposite way in another part of the body. For example, Tamoxifen is the drug used to prevent breast cancer by blocking the oestrogen receptors in the breast. But when picked up by the receptors in the womb, the Tamoxifen can actually increase the risk of womb cancer because it has a stimulatory effect on the receptors in the womb lining.

In the *British National Formulary* (a guide to all drugs for pharmacists), one of the side-effects listed for progesterone (which is listed separately from progestogen) is breast discomfort. A number of women have reported to me that when they used the progesterone cream, their breasts had actually seemed larger. Furthermore, some studies have shown that progesterone may in fact be a risk factor for breast cancer.[2]

Surgical techniques

In Chapter 5, I mentioned the gynaecologist who suggested that the best approach to PMS was to remove the ovaries and womb. This 'treatment' was also suggested for cyclical breast discomfort. Obviously, you can't suffer pre-menstrual symptoms – breast or otherwise – if you are not having a cycle. But it seems to me that we are losing sight of our priorities here. Removing your reproductive organs because of breast pain is both extreme and unnecessary. Following a hysterectomy (one where the ovaries are removed as well, see page 474), you are plunged into an immediate surgical menopause, regardless of your age or health. You may then be given HRT to overcome the symptoms of the menopause, which has its own dangers and side-effects, one of which can be breast discomfort and enlargement.

Not only is this surgical approach needless, but it would be hard to justify the use of any of the above drugs for cyclical breast discomfort as an effective long-term solution. In my opinion, the risks and side-effects are simply not acceptable. The natural alternatives are simple and effective, requiring just a few changes to your lifestyle and diet.

What Natural Treatments Could Be Effective?

The natural approach is to look at breast discomfort in a number of ways at the same time. Breast tenderness is not really a medical illness, so why treat it medically with strong drugs, given all the risks involved? The natural approach involves giving your body the tools it needs to heal itself and using good food, supplements and herbs to correct any imbalances with female hormones. The second stage is to ensure that your liver is functioning optimally to eliminate excess oestrogen. It also entails making sure that your digestive system is working efficiently, and that your bowels are operating regularly to excrete toxins and hormones. Finally, this approach involves removing any foods or drinks that are known to aggravate breast tissue discomfort.

You will need to undertake the following steps:

1. Follow the hormone balancing diet in Chapter 1.

2. Control levels of excess oestrogen and progesterone that your body may be producing, or taking in from your environment.

3. Improve the function of your liver. Your liver is responsible for ridding your body of excess and 'old' oestrogen.

4. Use herbs and supplements to balance hormones and to relieve the pain.

Diet

What you eat and drink will make the most difference to the breast problems you experience during your cycle. I have seen some women eliminate all symptoms in just one cycle by making a few changes. Follow the hormone balancing diet (see page 16) and also pay particular attention to the following recommendations.

Methylxanthines

Any food or drinks that contain substances known as methylxanthines should be avoided as they have been shown to increase breast discomfort.[3] What are they? Methylxanthines are a family of substances that include caffeine, theophylline and theobromine. These methylxanthines are found in coffee, black tea, green tea, chocolate, cola and decaffeinated coffee, as well as in medications that contain caffeine, such as headache remedies.

Unfortunately, these substances really do need to be permanently removed from your diet to have effect. Avoiding them in the second half of your cycle will not work. Furthermore, cutting down doesn't seem to be effective. If you are sensitive to methylxanthines, you need to ensure that they don't feature in your daily diet at all. Some women can, for example, drink five cups of coffee every day without experiencing any noticeable breast changes throughout their cycle. Other women may be far more sensitive, responding to a single cup of coffee. I know of countless women who have experienced a dramatic reversal of symptoms simply by cutting out that one cup of coffee.

Fiona

Fiona was 38 when she came to see me, complaining of excruciating breast tenderness in the second half of her cycle. She found it difficult to sleep because she couldn't get comfortable and didn't want her partner to touch her as it was so painful. She was a small, petite woman, and she felt that her breasts got so large pre-menstrually that they were out of all proportion to her size and she felt 'top heavy'. Fiona even had to wear a larger bra size in the second half of her cycle.

Fiona's health was good and she had no real problems other than this extreme breast tenderness and enlargement. We discussed her lifestyle and diet, and then she mentioned that she could drink up to ten cups of coffee a day. I talked about the relationship between coffee and breast discomfort, and initially she found it hard to believe that just one thing could be making all the difference. I suggested that she eliminate the coffee very gradually, otherwise she could get terrible withdrawal symptoms such as headaches, and shaking. She substituted half of her regular cups with decaffeinated coffee over the next week and gradually weaned herself from coffee over the next month. Eventually even the decaffeinated coffee has to go. Although the caffeine is not present, it still contains the methylxanthines (see page 310), which are implicated in breast problems. It was, however, a good way to make the transition from ten cups of coffee a day to none.

She gradually substituted the coffee for grain coffees and herb teas, and over the next three months the problem cleared up completely.

Fats

A diet high in saturated fats is known to stimulate oestrogen over-production and it has been shown that a low fat diet is beneficial for breast pain.[4] But don't fall into the trap of thinking that a 'no fat' diet would be even better. As I explained in Chapter 1, there are 'good' and 'bad' fats. In the case of cyclical breast discomfort, these 'good' fats are crucial. Only the saturated fats (found mainly in animal products, apart from fish) need to be reduced. It's important that you increase your intake of oily fish (such as mackerel, sardines, salmon etc.), nuts, seeds and vegetable oils to help reduce the symptoms. These essential fatty acids help to control substances called prostaglandins. One of these prostaglandins, PGE2, can cause heat and inflammation in the breasts.

Fibre

A link between fibrocystic breast disease and constipation has now been established. One study showed that women who had fewer than three bowel movements per week had a four-and-a-half times greater chance of having breast problems than women who had a bowel movement every day.[5] It is important that you have an adequate intake of fibre in the form of wholegrains, vegetables and fruits to ensure regularity. Adding wheatbran is not the ideal solution as it can irritate the bowel in sensitive people, and can prevent the uptake of essential nutrients in the digestive tract.

Phytoestrogens

These weak, naturally occurring oestrogens (see page 20) can help to keep any excesses of oestrogen in check and may explain why the majority of Asian women do not experience breast discomfort as we do. Phytoestrogens are effectively 'plant' oestrogens, and they are found in foods such as soya, chickpeas and lentils. Include them all in your diet as often as you can.

Supplements

Certain supplements have been recommended to support the changes you are making with your diet. Once the breast discomfort has been alleviated, you can continue to take only the multivitamin and minerals mentioned in the treatment plan, as long as you are still eating well.

Vitamin E

Vitamin E has been shown to help reduce breast pain and tenderness in a number of studies, and is worth supplementing over a couple of months to see if it helps ease your symptoms.[6] Vitamin E is found in foods such as almonds, leafy green vegetables, oats, soya, sunflower seeds and oil, wheatgerm and wholegrains, but you should also take a good supplement.

B vitamins

If there is a deficiency of the B vitamins in your body, your liver will be unable to inactivate 'old' oestrogens, which can be playing havoc with your cycle (see pages 37–8) and creating an excess of oestrogen because 'old' hormones are not being eliminated properly. Taking a B-complex supplement can help to reduce breast symptoms for this reason.

Lactobacillus acidophilus

Cyclical breast changes may be due to an excess of oestrogen over progesterone. *Lactobacillus acidophilus* helps to lower the level of enzymes that work to reabsorb the 'old' oestrogens in your body. These pro-biotics (beneficial bacteria) also help to improve the transit time of a bowel movement. The longer waste material stays in your system the more 'old' hormones and toxins can be reabsorbed back into your body.

Essential fatty acids (EFAs)

Essential fatty acids are not only an important part of a healthy diet, but they can also make a big difference to problems associated with hormones (see pages 27–30). Aim to get plenty in your daily diet (in the form of nuts, seeds, oily fish, walnuts, and oils such as corn and sunflower). Apart from this, however, it's a good idea to take a daily supplement. Research has shown that supplementing with evening prim-rose oil which contains GLA (gamma linolenic acid, see pages 154–6) can have a significantly positive effect on breast discomfort.[7] The GLA helps to control the production of a 'bad' prostaglandin called PGE2, which can cause heat and inflammation in the breasts if levels are too high. GLA also increases the level of another 'good' prostaglandin, PGE1, which can help to balance the effect of prolactin on the breasts.

It is now possible to get evening primrose oil on prescription in the UK. The GLA content is normally 40mg per capsule and you may need to take up to eight capsules a day to achieve the desired effect (the suggested dosage is between 240 and 320mg per day). The GLA content in each capsule varies tremendously between supple-ment producers, so it's worth scouting around for a brand containing higher levels of GLA.

Evening primrose oil is only one of the important oils studied for its effect on breast discomfort. Other oils, such as starflower oil, blackcurrant seed oil and borage oil may be just as effective.

> **Warning**
> Check with your doctor before taking any capsules containing GLA if you have a history of epilepsy.

WHICH EFA SHOULD YOU TAKE AS A SUPPLEMENT?

You may be surprised to find that the treatment plan does not include evening primrose oil but GLA and also EPA. The reason for this can be simply explained. Evening primrose oil contains mainly linoleic acid (LA) and a small amount of GLA. In order to experience the benefits, your body has to convert the LA into GLA. If your body doesn't make this conversion (and this can happen if you are deficient in certain nutrients, such as vitamin B6, zinc and magnesium, you are under stress or you have too much alcohol or sugar in your system) your body won't get the benefit.

Our bodies are constantly trying to achieve balance – in other words, finding the status quo. No one wants an overactive or an underactive thyroid, for example. The same goes with the hormones. Too much oestrogen is just as much a problem as too much progesterone. Balance is the key. The tendency has been for women to go overboard taking supplements of evening primrose oil. In fact you need both GLA (Omega 6) and EPA (Omega 3) oils (see pages 154–6).

The Omega 3 fatty acids are especially important for healthy breasts because they have been shown to inhibit tumour growth,. Many studies have shown that the Omega 3 fatty acids have a protective role to play against breast cancer.[8]

Herbs

The aim of the herbal remedies is to help balance your hormones and to ensure that your liver processes oestrogen efficiently so that any excess is excreted properly. The herbs also help support the changes you are making with your diet in order to speed up the process.

Agnus castus (vitex/chastetree berry)

This herb can be enormously useful in the treatment of breast tenderness because of its ability to balance the female hormones.[9]

Cleavers (*Galium aparine*)

This herb is particularly useful for breast tenderness as it helps to eliminate waste and toxins. It also stops fluid retention and general congestion in the breasts. It enhances the functioning of the lymphatic system, which forms part of your body's defence system to filter out unwanted material before it gets into your bloodstream.

Ginkgo biloba

A trial conducted by a hospital in France has shown that women who took ginkgo had significantly less pre-menstrual breast pain than those who took a placebo.[10] Ginkgo helps to increase circulation and can also reduce swelling.

HERBS FOR THE LIVER

The liver, which is the major organ of detoxification, helps to eliminate accumulated 'old' oestrogen so it is important that it is functioning efficiently. Both milk thistle and dandelion are excellent herbs for optimising liver function. If your body does not excrete oestrogen then you can end up with an accumulation which then further upsets the balance of oestrogen to progesterone.

Your Bra

Research, carried out by Professor Robert Mansel at the University Hospital of Wales and Simon Cawthorn from Frenchay Hospital in Bristol, is suggesting that wearing bras could be causing breast pain. They asked a hundred pre-menopausal women to go without a bra for three months, and then go back to wearing one for three months and keep a diary recording the differences. They found that the number of totally pain-free days went up by 7 per cent when the women stopped wearing a bra. A book called *Dressed to Kill*[11] had previously suggested that bras might be increasing our risk of breast cancer by suppressing the lymphatic system – a vital part of the immune system and the body's first line of defence against the spread of cancer. It is our lymphatic system that filters toxins and accumulated waste from our blood. Anything that stops the flow of lymph such as tight clothing, like a bra, can cause an accumulation of these toxins.

The connection between clothing and disease has been noticed before. The kind of tight corsets worn by women in the late 19th and early 20th centuries which really constricted the waist were associated with high rates of heart, liver and kidney problems. More recently, male infertility and possibly testicular cancer has been linked to men wearing tight underpants.

As yet there is no substantial connection between wearing a bra and increasing breast pain or cancer. However, it makes sense to err on the side of caution. Do not sleep in your bra and wear loose-fitting cotton nightwear that does not constrict your breasts. Choose bras made of natural fibres like cotton so that at least your breasts can breathe through the natural fibre rather being trapped inside nylon. On days when you are just 'pottering' around the house, go without a bra, unless you are pregnant or breast-feeding, in which case you need to wear one, except in bed.

Exercise

As mentioned in Chapter 1, exercise is important for keeping oestrogen in balance. Make sure that you wear a good supportive bra for exercising, especially during the pre-menstrual period.

Other treatments

Acupuncture and homeopathy can be excellent alongside the other recommendations to enhance the functioning of the liver and to encourage hormone balance.

The Treatment Plan

If you are experiencing pain, tenderness, lumpiness or swelling in your breasts, it is crucial that you see your doctor for a diagnosis before going any further. You will need to rule out the possibility of more serious problems, although these are rare.

If you are given a diagnosis of cyclical breast changes, and told that you have nothing to worry about, then go ahead and put into place the natural advice offered here. You may be offered medication to help with these harmless but uncomfortable breast changes, but I would suggest that you try the natural suggestions over the next three months before you take the medication.

Over many years of practice, I don't think I have ever had anyone come back to say that the nutritional approach for breast discomfort hasn't worked. There is no question that it is effective, and can make a dramatic difference to your symptoms and, indeed, your overall health.

Your Supplement Plan

- A good multivitamin and mineral supplement, e.g. The Healthy Woman by the Natural Health Practice

- Vitamin E (400–800iu per day as d-alpha tocopherol)

- GLA (300mg per day)

- EPA (300mg per day)

- Vitamin B-complex (providing 50mg of most of the B vitamins per day)

- Acidophilus (containing approximately 4 million bacteria)

- Ginkgo biloba (300mg per day) – this is a herb but take in supplement form

---

Note
Each nutrient represents the total intake of one day, so if your multivitamin and mineral already contains 25mg of vitamin B6, for example, you only need to add in a separate B complex containing 25mg per day.

Herbs

Herbs are taken over a period of six months and the best way to do this is to take an equal mixture of *Agnus castus*, cleavers and milk thistle in tincture form. Take 1 teaspoon three times a day. If your breast discomfort disappears fairly quickly, reduce the dose to 1 teaspoon twice a day for the next two weeks. Work down to 1 teaspoon once a day, and then stop.

In Summary

- Always have the cause of breast pain, lumps or tenderness investigated before taking any drugs, or beginning a natural treatment programme.

- Begin a self-examination programme of your breasts at home and make sure that you practise it on a regular basis.

- If tests show that there is nothing medically wrong, begin the natural treatment programme before trying any drugs or considering surgery.

- Begin the hormone balancing diet (see page 16).

- Make sure that your diet does not contain any methylxanthines (caffeine; see page 35).

- Avoid saturated fats, increase your fibre intake and make sure that you are getting plenty of foods containing phytoestrogens.

- Add acidophilus to your diet, and take regularly throughout your cycle. EFAs (essential fatty acids) should also form a good part of your diet.

- Take steps to find your natural weight and stay there. Exercise is important both to reduce stress levels before your period, to keep your weight down and to keep a normal level of oestrogen.

- Take supplements, as suggested (see page 319), throughout your entire cycle.

- Take herbs as required (see page 314).

PREVENTION OF BREAST CANCER

According to the Breast Cancer Awareness Campaign, 1 in 12 British women will develop breast cancer, and there are 29,000 new cases diagnosed each year in the UK. This year 14,800 women will die of breast cancer in Britain, which has the highest mortality rate for breast cancer in the world. The figures are only slightly better in the US, where one in nine women develop the disease each year. However, in 2000, 182,800 new cases of female invasive breast cancer will be diagnosed in the US, and 40,800 women will die from the disease.

When caught early enough, many cases of breast cancer are treatable and there are many women who have gone on to lead full, healthy lives. This is why it's particularly important to be vigilant about self-examining your breasts on a regular basis. There are many natural treatments available to complement the conventional treatment for breast cancer, but in this section we will focus on the ways in which breast cancer could be prevented. The research coming out from the scientific and medical literature over the last few years suggests that this is possible.

WILL I BE MORE SUSCEPTIBLE TO BREAST CANCER IF I HAVE BREAST PROBLEMS DURING MY CYCLE?

First and foremost, it's important to establish that being prone to breast problems throughout your cycle does not mean that you are at a higher risk of developing breast cancer. What breast pain, tenderness and lumps do tell you, however, is that your hormones are not functioning correctly. By achieving optimum health, through diet, and by addressing any vitamin and mineral deficiencies, your body will be given the opportunity and the tools it needs to correct any imbalances you may be suffering. The key word in natural medicine is 'prevention'. It's a great deal easier to prevent a problem than it is to try to correct once it has appeared.

Furthermore, by adopting a healthier lifestyle you will be more likely to *prevent* breast cancer (see below).

What Is Cancer?

Cancer is a group of diseases caused by cells growing unrestrainedly in any of your body's organs or tissues. Cancer differs from other abnormal growths (such as benign, or harmless, tumours) in two ways. As it grows, it spreads and infiltrates the tissues around it and may block passageways, destroy nerves and eat away at bone. Cells from cancer may spread through the blood vessels and lymphatic system to other parts of the body, where new growths occur.

Certain things need to happen for cancer to be triggered in the body. First of all, DNA in the cells must become damaged, and then something is required to make those damaged cells grow and develop.

Free Radicals and Cancer

In Chapter 1, there is an explanation of how free radicals can attack DNA in the nucleus of a cell, causing cell mutation and cancer. Nature provides us with the protection against these free radicals in the foods that we can eat every day in our diets. The foods we need to eat are those that contain antioxidants, and you can choose to include them in your diet, to help prevent damage to the DNA in your cells. You may also decide that it is worth taking an antioxidant supplement, as good research has shown that antioxidants can have a beneficial effect in preventing cancers in general.[12] In fact, some research has showed partial remission of breast cancer in women taking antioxidants.[13]

An Eastern Diet

A few years back scientists started looking at women around the world, and they realised that different cultures have different rates of breast cancer. Japanese women only have one-sixth the rate of breast cancer we have and yet when Japanese women move to the West and adopt a Western diet their breast cancer rate rises to Western levels.[14] For some time experts have suspected that the biggest factor in breast cancer is diet. They have also found that as the diet in Japan, for instance, becomes more Westernised, the breast cancer rate is going up. Japanese women not only eat more fish, which gives them

Omega 3 fatty acids known to inhibit tumour growth, but also soya, which is a phytoestrogen that can reduce the risk of breast cancer. They also eat very little dairy produce.

The Oestrogen Link

Breast cancer is most often 'oestrogen dependent': in other words, tumours often grow and develop in the presence of oestrogen. The oestrogen receptors in the breasts lock on to circulating oestrogen and excess oestrogen will stimulate the breast tissue.

Oestrogen is not all bad news; in fact, it is a very beneficial hormone that we need to protect our bones and hearts, and it is responsible for giving us our female characteristics. However, as with most things in life, too much can be as much of a problem as too little. Once again, balance is the keyword.

This all-important balance is dependent on a number of factors:

1. How much oestrogen you are exposed to from the environment; in other words, the xenoestrogens ('bad' oestrogen; see page 40).

2. How much oestrogen your body is producing – from your ovaries or fat cells (if you are overweight) – or if there is an oestrogen dominance because your hormones are out of balance.

3. Whether your body can efficiently eliminate excess oestrogen coming from the environment and/or produced by your own body. Your liver needs to be able to convert the carcinogenic oestrogens into harmless substances and to excrete them out of your system.

This entire concept is explained in detail in Chapter 1, and in order to work towards preventing breast cancer, you will need to follow the hormone balancing diet on page 16.

Phytoestrogens

It is also extremely important that you include phytoestrogens (naturally occurring oestrogens found in plants that appear to have an oestrogen-balancing effect on female health) in your diet (see page 20). Not only do they have the ability to help reduce levels of carcinogenic oestrogen, but they also stimulate the production of a protein called SHBG (sex hormone-binding globulin) that is produced by the liver. SHBG binds sex hormones such as oestrogen and testosterone in order to control how much of them are circulating in the blood at any one time.[15] The fewer hormones there are circulating, the fewer are available to stimulate breast tissue and possibly cause cancer. This means that the phytoestrogens are able to lower the risk of hormone-related cancers such as breast cancer because they control the amount of free and active oestradiol, which is the more carcinogenic kind.

What's the Cause?

No one knows for certain what causes breast cancer. Overweight, excess consumption of saturated fats, alcohol, emotional stress, family history, exposure to pesticides and radiation, the hormonal changes of the menopause have all been linked to this condition but no conclusive cause has emerged. However, research does indicate that some women seem to be more at risk than others. These women may have a mother or sister who has had breast cancer. Obese women, those who never had children, and women who gave birth for the first time after the age of 35 seem to have a higher risk, as do women who started the Pill at a very young age and stayed on it for more than four years. Breastfeeding also seems to have a preventative effect, as women who did not breastfeed their babies appear to be slightly more at risk.

Let's look at some of these cases in detail:

Genetic factors

The risk of developing breast cancer is higher if you have close female family members (mother or sister) who also have had breast cancer. Two faulty genes have been linked to an increased risk of breast cancer: BRCA-1 and BRCA-2. You may require monitoring because of this possible inherited tendency and it makes sense to adopt as many of the preventative recommendations as you possibly can, to reduce the possibility of breast cancer developing.

Hormone replacement therapy (HRT)

It is now well established that HRT increases the risk of breast cancer, although scientists have not always agreed on the degree of risk. Two studies published in 2000 have shown a 24 and 40 per cent risk higher risk of developing breast cancer.[16] These were not small or insignificant studies. The study showing the 40 per cent risk looked at the data for 46,355 women. So, if you have a family history of breast cancer or are concerned about whether or not you are at risk, then you should think seriously about whether or not to take HRT. Remember that the menopause is not an illness but a natural event in most women's lives and the symptoms of the menopause can be managed naturally without the use of HRT (see my books *Natural Alternatives to HRT* and *Natural Alternatives to HRT Cookbook* for more details). You may decide that the risks associated with HRT are simply not worth it.

Weight

Overweight is a problem when it comes to excess oestrogen, which makes it another risk factor for breast cancer. But *where* we pile on those pounds matters almost as much as *how many*. Researchers have found that women who put on weight around their middle (apple-shaped women) are more likely to develop breast cancer than women who are pear-shaped (with weight around their hips). Research has also shown that apple-shaped women are also more likely to suffer heart disease, so it seems that carrying weight around the middle is generally not good for our health.

Doctors at the Harvard School of Public Medicine in the US studying 47,000 nurses over a ten-year-period found that those who had plump stomachs were 34 per cent more likely to suffer from breast cancer than women with pear-shaped figures.[17] When the researchers narrowed down the study to only post-menopausal women who had never taken HRT, the apple-shaped women were 88 per cent more likely to get breast cancer.

If your waist–hip ratio is more than 0.8, you will need to take action! Here's how to calculate it:

1. Measure your waist, at the point where it is narrowest.

2. Measure your hips at their widest point.

3. Divide your hip measurement by your waist measurement to calculate the ratio.

For example:

86cm (34in) waist divided by 94cm (37in) hip = 0.9

This measurement would be considered marginally high, possibly putting you at a higher risk of breast cancer.

Fats

Scientists have found that the higher a country's intake of dietary fat (the total fat in the diet, not just dairy), the higher the risk of breast cancer.[18] Furthermore, the more 'damaged' the fat (fats that are altered to become unhealthy by deep-frying or processing, for example), the greater the risk of breast cancer.[19] This ties in with current thinking about free radicals. We now know that free radicals (see page 17) can be produced from 'damaged' fats, and we also know that they can have a damaging effect on DNA, thereby making them carcinogenic. It makes sense, then, that these damaged fats could trigger the onset of cancer.

On page 314 we discussed the Omega 3 oils, which help inhibit tumour growth. There is another oil that was not considered, and this is olive oil, which is an omega-9 fatty acid. Studies show that it can lower the risk of breast cancer[20] so it can be used successfully as a preventative measure.

The best advice is to alter the balance of the oils you consume so that you are eating more Omega 3 (fish and linseed) and Omega 9 oils (olive oils), and fewer Omega 6 oils (evening primrose oil and margarines).

Stress

There's no question that your general health can be affected by stress, but you may not realise that a hectic lifestyle and high stress levels can also increase your risk of breast cancer. Research has shown that the risk of developing breast cancer can be increased by three to four times when a woman has suffered severe stress in the previous five years.[21] Stress affects the way our bodies produce hormones and also the efficiency of our immune system, so it is important that you keep both at optimum levels of health.

Cosmetics and deodorants

If cancer is triggered by damage to DNA, it is important to look at the toxins or pollutants to which we may be exposing ourselves. Many of these have the potential to damage cells. Obviously life in the 21st century precludes avoiding chemicals of every kind, but there are certain things that we can control.

The most important way to avoid toxins is to change your diet (see Chapter 1). Other than that, consider the fact that scientists are investigating the link between the use of deodorants/anti-perspirants and breast cancer. Deodorants and anti-perspirants are obviously applied under the armpit and Dr Philippa Darbre from Reading University in the UK is investigating whether chemicals known as 'parabens', which are used as a preservative in many deodorants, can explain why more cancers develop in a certain area of the upper breast. I avoid anti-perspirants altogether, and would choose a chemical-free deodorant.

So, think about what you are putting on your body, and that means considering the face creams, suntan lotions, body lotions, hair-removing agents and anything else that you may use. Read the ingredient list. Ask yourself whether you could choose a more natural alternative to the brand you are using, particularly if you are using it around the breast area.

It was once suggested that we should only put on our skins substances that we would be happy to eat. It is definitely a thought, but not always easy to put into practice. But do what you can – using vitamin E oil on your skin, for example, is a much better option than chemical-laden moisturising cream.

Pesticides

The problems associated with pesticides, plastics and xenoestrogens (foreign oestrogens) has been explained in detail in Chapter 1 (see page 40). It is, however, worth reconsidering them in light of their effect on the breasts and breast cancer in particular. Because breast cancer can be 'oestrogen driven', there are obvious concerns about the impact of xenoestrogens on the condition. As a result, scientists examined the breast tissue of women with breast cancer to see if they contained more organochlorines (pesticides) than women with benign breast problems. In fact, significant residues of organochlorines were found in women with breast cancer as compared to those without.[22] The best advice is to eat as much organically grown food as possible and to avoid exposure to pesticides by avoiding their use in the garden.

You should also take steps to include phytoestrogens (see page 20) in your diet, because although we are bombarded with these xenoestrogens, we can do something about it. Studies have shown that genistein, the isoflavone (a type of phytoestrogen) in soya, can inhibit the growth and development of breast cancer cells induced by pesticides.[23]

WHAT ABOUT MAMMOGRAMS?

Mammograms have been put forward as an ideal way to detect breast cancer. However, the logic behind using this test may be flawed. A mammogram involves using an X-ray to detect small changes in the breast before you can feel or see them. However, X-rays have been linked to breast cancer so you may end up triggering the very same condition that you are trying to detect.

There have been concerns about mammograms since the 1980s. A study in Canada looked at 89,000 women over an eight-year period. Half of the women in the group received mammograms every year and the other half did not. The scientists found that those women who had had the mammograms had a 52 per cent increase in deaths from breast cancer compared to the women who had not been screened in this way.[24]

And then in 1999 came the results of a massive ten-year study on 600,000 women. This study, which was conducted in Sweden, showed no reduction in deaths from mammogram breast screening. Doubts were thrown on this study, possibly because some researchers were concerned about the outcome, so the data was independently reanalysed together with research from other previous trials. The conclusion, which was published in the *Lancet* medical journal, was that 'screening for breast cancer with mammography is unjustified'.[25] At the moment around £34 million is spent in the UK on breast screening and some experts suggest that this money would be better spent on treatment and research rather than on unjustified screening.

The researchers of the original study also warned about the negative effects of the X-rays and the possibility of being wrongly diagnosed, then subjected to unnecessary tests and surgery. They had found from their study that 100,000 women had been given a false positive (told they had cancer when they didn't): that's an alarming rate of one in six. Out of these women, 16,000 had undergone a biopsy (where a needle is inserted into the breast and tissue is extracted and sent to a lab for analysis) and more than 400 women had surgery, including mastectomies.

Screening for breast cancer

Apart from mammograms (see panel) there are a variety of other ways to screen for breast cancer.

Ultrasound

It is also possible to scan the breasts using ultrasound. Ultrasound has been proved particularly useful for women who have dense breasts. Women who have not entered the menopause, and women on HRT are more likely to have dense breasts (where the tissue is thicker). After the menopause (and providing HRT is not taken) breast tissue becomes less dense, so it is fairly easy to spot subtle changes using a mammogram. If your mammogram shows anything unusual, you will be referred for an ultrasound scan. It seems sensible, therefore, to skip the mammogram stage altogether. The problem is that ultrasound costs a great deal more than mammogram screening, because it is much more labour intensive, and each breast has to be scanned separately.

Obviously it is better to avoid X-raying your breasts if possible, or keeping it down to a minimum. If you have a strong family tendency towards breast cancer then the best protocol may be to have three-yearly mammograms and intersperse these with ultrasound scans every year in between. Otherwise, I would suggest that you use the recommendations on page 303 for checking yourself as most lumps are detected by the women themselves. But if you are concerned or feel a lump then you could opt for an ultrasound.

Most women can check their breasts at home, safely and effectively (see page 303), and the majority of lumps are detected by self-examination. If you are concerned, or you feel a lump, opt for the ultrasound if you have a choice.

Other screening methods

Other screening tools are being used to detect breast cancer, but many are not yet available in the UK. Here's what's on offer elsewhere in the world.

Hair tests

Professor Veronica James of the Australian National University has developed a test that aims to detect breast cancer from a single strand of hair. She has found that hair taken from a woman who has or is likely to develop breast cancer (in other words, she carries the inherited breast cancer gene BRCA-1) has a different molecular structure (when viewed by X-ray) than hair taken from women who don't have breast cancer and don't carry the genes likely to cause the disease.[26]

Electrical Scanner

This hand-held machine has been approved by the US Food and Drug Administration on the grounds that it may reduce the number of unnecessary biopsies performed each year. The scanner distinguishes between benign and cancerous lumps by measuring electrical changes on the skin's surface. It has been known for many years that cancerous cells cause electrical disturbances and the scanner can pick up these disturbances on the surface of the skin. Cancerous tumours can be 40 times more conductive than benign tissue and the scanner can measure this.[27]

CHAPTER 10

Infertility

Over the past 20 years, fertility problems have increased dramatically. At least 25 per cent of couples planning a baby in the UK will have trouble conceiving, and more and more couples are turning to fertility treatments to help them have a family. On average, young couples can expect to wait an average of three years before conceiving, and, as a result, very few doctors will consider a diagnosis of infertility until after at least a year has passed. For a growing number of older women waiting until their careers are established before they try to conceive, conception can be more difficult.

FERTILITY PROBLEMS

From a medical point of view, infertility is believed to be caused by the following factors, and in these proportions.

Problem	Percentage of cases
Ovulatory failure (including polycystic ovary syndrome)	20
Tubal damage	15
Endometriosis	5
Male problems	26
Unexplained	30

If the mathematics don't add up, it's because many couples experience more than one problem when trying to conceive: for example, you may suffer from endometriosis, but your partner may also have a low sperm count.

Interestingly, the most common cause of infertility is 'unexplained', which means that following thorough investigations, doctors can find no specific or identifiable medical problem at the root. But this is where a natural approach can come into play. If a couple fails to become pregnant, there is obviously something causing the problem. It's no good labelling infertility 'unexplained'. The answer is to look deeper – at lifestyle factors, nutritional deficiencies and even emotional elements. As the old saying goes, you can't find something that you aren't looking for.

Fertility is multi-factorial – in other words, there are many things that can affect your ability to conceive, and they are not all medical! To find the cause of fertility problems, it is important to look at every aspect of your health, your emotions and your lifestyle. I discuss this in some detail on pages 331 to 339, but if you want to investigate the subject further, please see my book *Natural Solutions to Infertility* (Piatkus, 2000).

Are You Infertile?

Infertility generally means an inability to conceive, but there are many reasons why you are not able to become pregnant, and many of these may be temporary. A diagnosis of infertility does not necessarily mean that you will always be infertile. It simply means there is a problem that needs to be addressed. In the case of unexplained infertility, the more correct phrase should be 'subfertility', because if given the right advice to boost your fertility, chances are you can become pregnant.

If you are quite young (between 20 and 30 years), with no known problems, you can expect to wait about 12 months to become pregnant. If nothing happens after that time, approach your doctor for tests.

However, if you are over 35 and 6 months of trying has not produced the desired result, see your doctor. Biologically (see page 350) it is harder for women over 35 to conceive, and you may need intervention earlier than someone who is younger.

What Can Cause My Infertility?

Your doctor will arrange a series of tests to establish what – if any – problems exist. Remember, unless you have been trying to become pregnant for at least a year, your doctor will not consider you to have fertility problems.

Although this book focuses on women's health issues, there can be no doubt that it takes two to make a baby. For that reason, factors affecting male fertility and their subsequent treatment are addressed in this chapter. Some 40 per cent of fertility problems are associated with men, yet the focus, particularly in the early stages of investigation, tends to be on the female partner. Testing for problems should always be undertaken on both partners at the same time. If you are not conceiving, it is extremely important that both you and your partner are examined, and that you put into place the recommendations suggested on pages 343 to 353 of this chapter.

Tests For Women

Blood tests

A blood test is normally the first step in assessing female fertility problems, and it is undertaken to see whether or not you are ovulating. Tests normally take place on day 21 of your cycle, and they will measure your progesterone level. If the test shows that you are ovulating normally, your doctor will probably suggest that you carry on trying to conceive for another few months. If you are not ovulating, you will probably be referred to a gynaecologist, who will take things further.

INFECTIONS AND FERTILITY

Many people are unaware of the fact that some infections can prevent conception. For this reason, it's essential that both you and your partner are screened for infection. Your tests should screen for cytomegalovirus (CMV), mycoplasmas/ureaplasmas, chlamydia, anaerobic bacteria, group B haemolytic streptococci, gardnerella vaginalis, klebsiella, toxoplasmosis and candida. You will also need to ensure that you are immune to rubella (German measles), which can affect the health of your baby once you do become pregnant. For more on these infections, see pages 250–88.

In some cases, your GP will organise screening, although you may need to visit a GUM (genitourinary medicine) clinic at your local hospital. If you have a positive result for any infection, you will need to ensure that it is treated properly and that you are retested and given the all-clear before attempting to conceive again.

Further tests

If a blood test shows that you are ovulating normally, but you fail to conceive, further tests will be necessary, and you will be referred to a gynaecologist, who will check to see that your Fallopian tubes aren't blocked, and anything else that may be preventing conception, including endometriosis (see Chapter 8) or fibroids (see Chapter 10).

Some of the most common tests you might be offered are listed below.

Laparoscopy

This diagnostic procedure involves inserting a laparoscope (a narrow instrument with a telescopic lens) through a small incision below the navel and into the abdomen. It allows your specialist to examine your uterus, Fallopian tubes, ovaries and other abdominal organs to ascertain any problems that may be preventing conception.

Hysterosalpingogram (HSG)

This is an X-ray procedure in which a special opaque dye is injected through the cervix to see the inside of the uterus and to assess whether or not the Fallopian tubes are 'patent', or open, and to what degree. The test is always undertaken in the first half of your menstrual cycle, when you know you cannot be pregnant.

Hysterosalpingosonogram (HSS)

This examination is similar to the HSG, but ultrasound instead of X-rays are used to assess your Fallopian tubes. It is also a valuable tool for examining the uterine cavity for fibroids or other problems.

Hysteroscopy

In this procedure, a hysteroscope (a lighted scope) is inserted through the cervix in order to view the inside of the womb to pick up any abnormalities.

The monitored cycle

In most countries, fertility testing offered by health services involves a series of tests undertaken across several months. In other words, each test is often done during a different cycle. You may have a blood test one month, a laparoscopy in the second month and further tests later on. Though widely used, this approach does not provide you with information about how your body actually works over one complete cycle.

Bearing this in mind, the North London clinic in which I work has pioneered an investigation process called a 'monitored cycle', which is designed to provide more complete information by closely monitoring a single menstrual cycle. A monitored cycle looks at both hormonal balance and reproductive function, and the way they work together.

Monitored cycle using ultrasound and blood tests

Between days one and three at the beginning of the cycle, a blood test is taken to measure oestradiol, which is produced by the ovary, and luteinizing hormone (LH) and follicle-stimulating hormone (FSH), which are produced by the pituitary gland. Your egg reserve will also be checked. This blood test also checks hormone output from the thyroid gland, and prolactin levels, both of which are essential for normal reproductive function.

Then, three scans are performed during the cycle to show the thickness of the womb lining, as well as the size and growth of, and the blood flow to, the developing follicle (egg) in the ovary. One scan is undertaken following ovulation to assess the functioning of the corpus luteum, which pumps out the hormone progesterone, that is required to maintain a pregnancy. This scan will also determine whether the womb lining is thick enough for a fertilised embryo to be implanted and sustained.

This type of monitored cycle is also now available as an investigation by some health services, so do ask about it.

Monitored cycle using saliva

A total of 11 saliva samples are collected at home at specific times across one cycle, and sent to the lab for analysis. This simple test will chart the level of the hormones oestrogen and progesterone across the month, to work out a pattern that may reveal:

• early ovulation

• anovulation (no ovulation)

• problems with the phasing of the cycles, such as a short luteal phase (second half of the cycle)

• problems with maintaining progesterone levels.

This test can be done even if you have irregular cycles. The graph opposite shows a cycle charted from one of my patients. This 34-year-old woman was having trouble conceiving and was also having breakthrough bleeding for a few days before each period started.

Her cycle was 26 days but the tests showed that she was ovulating around day 17, which meant that there were just 9 days between ovulation and her period. It was immediately clear that she was suffering from a luteal phase defect, which means that the second half of her cycle is less than 12 days.

The graph also shows that her progesterone output was almost finished by day 21 of her cycle, which meant that it was only high for 4 days after ovulation. The breakthrough bleeding was explained by this early drop in progesterone. This woman's progesterone output meant that she would find it very difficult to maintain a pregnancy. In fact, chances are she had become pregnant in the past but was unaware of it.

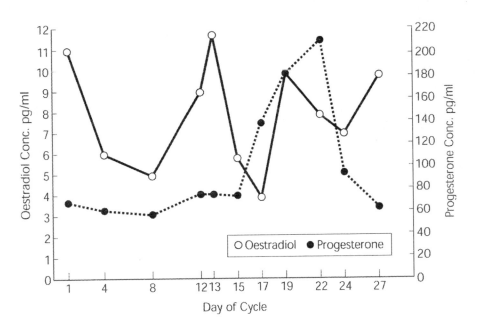

Example of a Female Hormone Test using saliva

Rosalind

Twenty-nine-year-old Rosalind was concerned because she had just started using a home testing kit for ovulation and realised that over the last three months she had not been ovulating at all. She wanted to start a family and obviously this was of concern. Her hair mineral analysis showed that she was low in zinc. Her diet was pretty good, but she had an overwhelming weakness for chocolate. I also suggested some herbs (including *Agnus castus*) to help balance her hormones. Over the next two cycles she ovulated each time. She then reduced the dose of the herbs over the next cycle, making sure she was still ovulating.

Which monitored cycle?

The monitored cycle using ultrasound and blood tests gives extra information, in that the development and thickness of the womb lining can be assessed at the same time as looking at hormone balance. It gives your doctor an idea whether or not your womb lining is actually thick enough for an egg to implant.

However, the saliva-monitored cycle is very convenient as a first step because you don't need to go into a clinic during the cycle. Samples can be taken at home (see page 334) and then sent to a laboratory for analysis.

Tests For Men

Semen analysis

Semen analysis is the most basic male fertility test and it can be easily undertaken at home, or in a clinic setting. Your partner will be asked to provide a semen sample by masturbating directly into a sterile container. He will be asked to abstain from sex for a minimum of 48 hours before giving a sample, but no longer than 7 days. Some clinics prefer that the sample is taken on-site, while others will allow your partner to produce the sample at home and to bring it directly to the lab (usually within an hour of it having been taken).

The semen sample will be examined and the following things will be measured:

• the number of sperm per millimetre (the sperm count)

• the percentage of sperm moving (the number of motile sperm)

- the quality of that movement (progression, which is graded from 1 to 4; 1 is the highest score and 4 is the lowest)

- the percentage of abnormal sperm

- the volume of semen.

According to the World Health Organisation, which sets recommendations for semen analysis, there should be more than 20 million sperm, of which at least 30 per cent should be normal and at least 50 per cent should be actively moving.

If there is a problem with your partner's sperm, then he should be referred to a urologist who can assess the reason. The normal course of action involves testing for infection (see page 332), as well as checking hormone levels. A physical examination will pick up any obvious blockages. For example, he may have a varicocele (an enlarged vein around the testes) that could be inhibiting sperm production and perhaps motility. There is some evidence that a varicocele can overheat the testes, causing problems with fertility; however, many men have completely harmless varicoceles that have not affected their fertility. Unfortunately doctors cannot predict which men with varicoceles will benefit from having them treated, and if you are having trouble conceiving, it is probably wise to have them treated. This normally involves tying off the affected veins.

A urologist may organise hormone tests for your partner, and these could include FSH, LH, prolactin, testosterone and thyroid hormones. If FSH levels are high, it may indicate that there is a problem with sperm production in the testes. Some medications, such as clomiphene citrate and tamoxifen, have been used to treat male infertility, but they are controversial and it is not known how beneficial they are.

Anti-sperm antibody test

Some men produce antibodies that cause their sperm to clump together (agglutinate), lose motility (mobility) or prevent fertilisation. Antibodies are often produced in response to an infection causing a man's immune system to recognise his own sperm as a foreign body that needs to be destroyed.

The most common test for antibodies is the MAR (mixed antiglobulin reaction) test, which usually comprises part of a normal semen analysis. If antibodies are present, the sperm will appear in clumps instead of moving freely.

Treatment for anti-sperm antibodies may include steroids, which can have many side-effects, including weight gain, stomach bleeding and depression. IVF (see below) treatment may still be possible if the sperm is capable of penetrating the egg. If not, ICSI (intracytoplasmic sperm injection) may be appropriate (see page 341).

What Treatment Can You Be Offered By Your Doctor?

Your doctor may suggest one of a variety of different treatments, but the first course of action is likely to be drug-based.

Drugs

If tests show that you are not ovulating, but your Fallopian tubes and your partner's sperm are normal, drugs for inducing ovulation will normally be the first line of treatment. There are many drugs now available, and they are aimed at stimulating ovulation, correcting hormonal imbalance and ensuring that an egg is released each cycle. These drugs do not make you more fertile in the long term; they simply work during the month in which they are taken.

Clomiphene citrate

This drug stimulates ovulation if you are not ovulating and it is also used if you have infrequent periods and long cycles. It is taken for five days early on in the cycle. It should not be used for more than six cycles, as there is an increased risk of ovarian cancer when it is taken for more than 12 cycles.[1] Side-effects can include bowel upsets, bloating, headaches, dizziness, breast discomfort, blurred vision, hot flushes and depression.

Other Drugs

Other drugs can be used, such as human chorionic gonadotrophin (HCG), which helps the dominant follicle to release its egg. Human menopausal gonadotrophin (HMG), which is a combination of FSH and LH, is given by injection and is used when clomiphene has not been very successful. The side-effects from these are similar and can include mood swings, depression and breast tenderness.

Progesterone

If tests show that your progesterone levels are not being maintained in the second half of the cycle, then it is possible to conceive and then have a period without knowing you are pregnant, because the progesterone levels were not high enough to hold the pregnancy. Some doctors, who suspect this is happening, give progesterone support in the second half of the cycle while you are trying to get pregnant. Some women may suspect this drop in progesterone is happening because they get breakthrough bleeding or spotting a few days before the period actually happens.

Assisted conception

These procedures can increase the number of eggs released during your cycle: in intra-uterine insemination (IUI) two or three eggs are normally released; in in-vitro fertilisation (IVF) between two and eight eggs can be released. They can also reduce the distance that the sperm has to travel to reach your eggs by inserting the sperm in a closer position. Fertilisation can take place inside or outside the body, depending on which procedure is used.

IUI (intra-uterine insemination)

IUI is a procedure that puts your partner's sperm directly into your womb using a fine catheter. The sperm is inserted at a much higher point than it would be during intercourse, which should improve the chances of fertilisation.

Stimulatory drugs (such as clomiphene) are usually taken to encourage two or three eggs to mature and to increase the chance of the technique working. If you have been given a diagnosis of unexplained infertility, you are under the age of 35 and there seems to be no medical or physical reason why you and your partner are not conceiving, IUI should be the first assisted conception treatment offered. The success rate is around 15 per cent.

IVF (In-vitro fertilisation)

IVF is a technique for fertilising your eggs with your partner's sperm outside your body – hence the use of the phrase 'test-tube babies'. The fertilised egg is then implanted back into your womb. In order to prepare your body for this procedure, drugs are used to put your body into a temporary menopause. This stops your own hormones interfering with the IVF treatment. Other drugs are then used to stimulate several follicles (eggs) to develop. Between 34 and 38 hours later the eggs are collected through your vagina using an aspiration needle that is guided by ultrasound. You may be sedated for this procedure or have a general anaesthetic. Some women may find this process painful; others do not.

Your partner provides a fresh semen sample and up to 100,000 sperm are mixed with each egg. The aim is to collect about 20 eggs. Those that are fertilised and start to divide well will be chosen to go back inside the womb. According to UK law, a maximum of only three embryos can be implanted in the womb. In the US, there is no limit to the number of fertilised eggs that can be put back. If too many 'take', they selectively reduce the number, meaning they terminate some of babies to make the pregnancy a manageable number. Success rates in the UK are about 15 to 20 per cent.

FROZEN EMBRYOS

Fertilised embryos from IVF treatment can be frozen if they are of good quality. Under the Human Fertilisation and Embryology Authority Act of 1990 these embryos can only be kept in storage for five years. It's worth noting, however, that frozen embryos do not always thaw well, and many will have to be discarded.

GIFT (gamete intra-Fallopian transfer)

In this procedure your unfertilised egg is mixed together with your partner's sperm and put back into the Fallopian tubes so that fertilisation takes place where it would naturally occur. GIFT can only be used when your Fallopian tubes are open and healthy. The same drugs used in IVF (see above) are used, but in this case the eggs are retrieved by a laparoscope through an incision in your abdomen. For this reason, a general anaesthetic will be required. Once again, a maximum of three eggs can be put back in the Fallopian tube.

GIFT–ET (GIFT and embryo transfer)

This is a fairly new technique, which is only practised by a few clinics, but it is well worth considering because the take-home baby rate for this technique can be as high as 41 per cent. The procedure involves a combination of GIFT and IVF, in which both procedures are performed in the same cycle. One or two of the eggs collected are mixed with sperm and put back in the Fallopian tube and, at the same time, one fertilised egg is put back in the womb.

ICSI (intracytoplasmic sperm injection)

ICSI is performed if your partner's sperm count is so low that IVF is not possible, if he is unable to ejaculate or if he has an obstruction that prevents sperm being released. This technique involves injecting a single sperm directly into the egg in order to fertilise it. The embryo is then implanted in the womb. The procedure involves much the same drugs as IVF (see page 339).

RISKS OF INFERTILITY TREATMENT

Infertility treatments are not without their risks, and these should be considered carefully before going ahead with any form of treatment. For one thing, many of the procedures take place under general anaesthetic, which has its own effects. Furthermore, many of these treatments require a large number of different drugs to control or change your cycles. It's worth considering the effects of these drugs when assessing the risks of each specific treatment.

Although it may be difficult to accept, it is important to consider the fact that you may not be able to conceive for a reason. Everyone and anything in the natural world is governed by a mechanism designed to protect the population – in other words, to ensure that the fittest survive. Today we have the technology to over-ride this natural order and many experts are concerned that there may be cases where this is inappropriate. Certainly the technology is there, but there may be consequences that will affect your baby's health, and these must be thought through carefully. Anyone considering assisted conception treatment must carefully assess what these risks may be, and how they will affect your life and that of any baby you may conceive.

In IVF treatment, a number of sperm are mixed with the egg. It is believed that the egg has an ability to 'favour' healthy sperm over those that may be defective, which is yet another safeguard measure nature has to offer. However, in ICSI, the egg is not given the opportunity

---

to 'choose' appropriate sperm because only one sperm is used and then directly inserted. For this reason, and because of the fact that immature sperm or even sperm cells are used instead of healthy, active sperm, there have been concerns that ICSI could result in babies being born with problems. It has been found that babies born after ICSI are twice as likely to have a major birth defect and 50 per cent are more likely to have a minor defect.[2]

When assisted conception techniques such as IVF are used, the body is put under great pressure to mature a large number of eggs in one cycle, when normally only one or two would ever be released at the same time. Not surprisingly, there is concern about the long-term effects of taking these drugs. Furthermore, some research suggests an increased risk of ovarian cancer. The scientific results are not conclusive and more long-term research needs to be undertaken; however, some studies show that there is an increased risk of ovarian cancer for women who have undergone fertility treatment.[3] Others show no risk.[4]

In the light of this confusion, it is better to err on the side of caution and to follow the advice on page 349 to maximise the chances of conceiving on your own. If you do decide to opt for assisted conception procedures, these suggestions will help increase the chance of the treatment working more quickly, thereby reducing the number of attempts that will be necessary.

My book, *Natural Solutions to Infertility*, has more detailed information on the different techniques available.

Before you start fertility treatment

Embarking on IVF treatment is a big step, both financially and emotionally, so it needs to be thought through carefully. Many couples are unaware of the implications. For example, it can take years to conceive and it can involve a great deal of regular treatment and attendance at clinics. If you work full-time, it can be difficult to fit it all in. Quite apart from that, it's important to consider the physical effects of the drugs on your body and the emotional roller-coaster on which you may find yourself. Remember that the average success rate for assisted conception procedures is only around 20 per cent. That means that 80 per cent of treatment cycles will fail, and it can be emotionally devastating when that occurs. Consider also the financial cost. At present it costs between £2,000 and £3,000 per treatment cycle. It's not unusual to need several to become pregnant. You'll need to be prepared for that.

It is not easy to get fertility treatment on the NHS or other health services and sometimes only drug treatments are available. In the UK all clinics offering assisted conception have to be licensed by the Human Fertilisation and Embryology Authority (HFEA)(see page 508). The HFEA produces 'league tables' showing how successful the clinics are, and these are essential reading for all couples deciding where to go for treatment.

What Natural Treatments Could Be Effective?

The natural approach to fertility is and has been enormously successful, largely because fertility is multi-factorial, meaning that there are many, many elements that can be at the root of your fertility problems. A study conducted by the University of Surrey in the UK showed that couples with a previous history of infertility who made changes in their lifestyle, diet and took nutritional supplements had an 80 per cent success rate.[5] Given that the success rate for assisted conception is around 20 per cent, it's worth considering these natural options.

Natural treatment plans are, by their nature, extensive and really do need to be adjusted to suit your individual needs. I will, however, go through the most important points below. Remember that it takes at least three months for immature eggs (oocytes) to mature enough to be released during ovulation. It also takes at least three months for sperm cells to mature, ready to be ejaculated. This means that when you are trying to improve your fertility, you need to have a four-month period before conceiving. This is called 'preconception' and it's as important to take care during this time as it is during a pregnancy itself.

If you are going for IVF treatment or another assisted conception procedure, you should also follow the recommendations listed below in order to increase the chances of the procedure working.

Diet

Both you and your partner should follow the dietary recommendations described in Chapter 1 (see page 16). Although it goes without saying that a healthy diet is crucial to a successful pregnancy and a healthy baby, many people are unaware of the fact that diet can help to correct hormone imbalances that may affect your ability to conceive. There are also certain foods and drinks that are known to lower fertility.

Alcohol

Alcohol will affect both you and your partner. In fact, drinking any alcohol at all can reduce your fertility by half – and the more you drink, the less likely you are to conceive.[6] One study showed that women who drank fewer than five units of alcohol a week (equal to five glasses of wine) were twice as likely to get pregnant within six months compared with those who drank more.[7]

Research has also shown that drinking alcohol causes a decrease in sperm count, an increase in abnormal sperm and a lower proportion of motile sperm.[8] Alcohol also inhibits the body's absorption of nutrients such as zinc, which is one of the most important minerals for male fertility.

As difficult as it may seem, you and your partner should eliminate alcohol from your diets for at least three months in order to give yourself the best possible chance of conceiving.

Caffeine

There is plenty of evidence to show that caffeine, particularly in the form of coffee, decreases fertility. Drinking as little as one cup of coffee a day can halve your chances of conceiving.[9] One study showed that problems with sperm – sperm count, motility and abnormalities – increase with the number of cups of coffee consumed each day.[10] Once again, it's important to eliminate all caffeine-containing food and drinks for at least three months before trying to conceive. That includes colas, chocolate, black teas and coffee, among other things.

Xenoestrogens

Xenoestrogens are essentially environmental oestrogens, coming from pesticides and the plastics industry. When you are trying to conceive, one of the most important things you need to do is to balance your hormones. It is extremely important to avoid anything that might cause an imbalance, and one of the main culprits is the xenoestrogens. On page 40 I discuss the ways in which your intake can be controlled. Follow these instructions as closely as you can. One of the best ways to eliminate an excess intake of xenoestrogens is to buy organic produce (see page 19) for the preconceptual period.

SMOKING

Smoking has definitely been linked with infertility in women.[11] It can even bring on an early menopause, which is a particularly important consideration for older women who may be trying to beat the biological clock.[12] Smoking can decrease sperm count in men, making the sperm more sluggish, and it can increase the number of abnormal sperm. With men, the effects on fertility are increased with the number of cigarettes smoked.[13]

Supplements

There is now a great deal of scientific knowledge about the use of nutritional supplements and their beneficial effects on both male and female fertility. As you will see, these supplements can be very effective in rebalancing your hormones, as well as improving you and your partner's overall health, which is so vital for successful conception.

Supplements are necessary because even the best diet in the world will not contain all the nutrients you need to give you the best chance of conceiving (see page 14).

Folic Acid

It is now known that folic acid can prevent spina bifida in your baby, and it is essential that you get plenty both before and during pregnancy. And that's not all: folic acid is undoubtedly crucial, but it is just part of the very important B-complex family of vitamins that are necessary to produce the genetic materials DNA and RNA. Together with vitamin B12, folic acid works to ensure that your baby's genetic codes are intact.

To sum up, it's not enough to take folic acid alone when you are trying to become pregnant. All of the B vitamins are essential during the preconceptual period. Research has shown that giving B6 to women who have trouble conceiving increases fertility[14] and vitamin B12 has been found to improve low sperm counts.[15]

Zinc

Zinc is the most widely studied nutrient in terms of fertility for both men and women. It is an essential component of genetic material and a zinc deficiency can cause chromosome changes in either you or your partner, leading to reduced fertility and an increased risk of miscarriage for you. Zinc is necessary for your body to 'attract and hold' (utilise efficiently) the reproductive hormones, oestrogen and progesterone.[16]

And it's equally important for your partner: zinc is found in high concentrations in sperm. Zinc is needed to make the outer layer and tail of the sperm and is, therefore, essential for the health of your partner's sperm and, subsequently, your baby. Interestingly, several studies have also shown that reducing zinc in a man's diet will also reduce his sperm count.[17]

Selenium

Selenium is an antioxidant that helps to protect your body from highly reactive chemical fragments called free radicals (see page 17). For this reason, selenium can prevent chromosome breakage, which is known to be a cause of birth defects and miscarriages. Good levels of selenium are also essential to maximise sperm formation. Blood selenium levels have been found to be lower in men with low sperm counts.[18]

Essential fatty acids (EFAs)

These essential fats have a profound effect on every system of the body, including the reproductive system and they are crucial for healthy hormone functioning. For men, essential fatty acid supplementation is crucial because the semen is rich in prostaglandins, which are produced from these fats. Men with poor sperm quality, abnormal sperm, poor motility or low count, have inadequate amounts of these beneficial prostaglandins.[19]

Vitamin E

Vitamin E is another powerful antioxidant and has been shown to increase fertility when given to both men and women.[20] Men going for IVF treatment with their partners have been given vitamin E, and fertilisation rates have, as a result, increased from 19 to 29 per cent.[21] It has been suggested that the antioxidant activity of vitamin E might make the sperm more fertile.

Vitamin C

Vitamin C is also an antioxidant, and studies show that vitamin C enhances sperm quality, protecting sperm and the DNA within it from damage.[22] Some research has indicated that certain types of DNA damage in the sperm can make it difficult to conceive in the first place, or it can cause an increased risk of miscarriage if conception does take place. If DNA is damaged, there may be a chromosomal problem in the baby, should the pregnancy proceed. Whether or not DNA damage does have these effects has not been conclusively proven, but it's worth taking vitamin C and the other antioxidants (see page 17) as a precautionary measure.

Vitamin C also appears to keep the sperm from clumping, making them more motile.

One study has shown that women taking the drug clomiphene to stimulate ovulation (see page 234) will have a better chance of ovulating if vitamin C is taken alongside the drug.[23] Clomiphene does not always work in every woman, but the chances are always increased when vitamin C is supplemented.

L-arginine

This is an amino acid found in many foods and the head of the sperm contains an exceptional amount of this nutrient, which is essential for sperm production. Supplementing with L-arginine can help to increase both the sperm count and quality.[24]

> ### Note
> People who have herpes attacks (either cold sores or genital herpes) should not supplement arginine because it stimulates the virus.

L-carnitine

This amino acid is essential for normal functioning of sperm cells. According to research, it appears that the higher the levels of L-carnitine in the sperm cells, the better the sperm count and motility.[25]

Vitamin A

This vitamin needs to be mentioned because there is a lot of confusion about its use before and after pregnancy. Many health practitioners now advise that *no* vitamin A is taken during pregnancy. This advice is incorrect, and it can be dangerous to assume that any vitamin or other nutrient should be avoided during the gestational period. Vitamin A has important antioxidant properties, and the consequences of Vitamin A deficiency during pregnancy can be devastating. For one thing, vitamin A is essential for healthy eyes. Animal studies show that vitamin A deficiency during pregnancy has produced newborn animals with no eyes, eye defects, undescended testes and diaphragmatic hernias.[26]

It is only when the vitamin A is in the form of retinol (in other words, the animal form of vitamin A) that there is a problem. It has been found that retinol can cause birth defects if taken in excess of 10,000iu a day.[27] Beta-carotene, which is one of the vegetable forms of vitamin A, does not carry any risks.

Herbs

Herbal treatment is aimed at restoring hormone imbalances, and encouraging ovulation if it is not occurring. It will also give you the best possible chance of maintaining a pregnancy, should you conceive.

Agnus castus (vitex/chastetree berry)

This is the herb of choice for helping to restore hormone imbalance and increasing fertility. In one study 48 women diagnosed with infertility took *Agnus castus* daily for 3 months, 7 of them became pregnant during that time and 25 of them regained normal progesterone levels.[28]

Agnus castus is particularly helpful for those women who have a luteal phase defect (shortened second half to the cycle) or those with high prolactin levels, because it stimulates the proper functioning of the pituitary gland, which controls the hormones.

Agnus castus works to restore hormonal balance and can be used where there are hormone deficits as well as excesses. It:

- regulates periods
- restarts periods that have stopped
- helps with heavy bleeding
- increases the ratio of progesterone to oestrogen by balancing excess oestrogen.

Saw palmetto (*Seronia serrulate*)
This is one of the best herbs for the male reproductive system. It acts like a tonic, toning and strengthening.

USING HERBS

The herbs listed above provide the most general course of herbal treatment and are effective in many cases. However, if fertility problems persist, you may need more individual treatment, from a qualified practitioner.

The Treatment Plan

The aim is to follow the recommendations for four months to optimise fertility. This means:

- eating a healthy diet
- taking the correct nutritional supplements (see below)
- adopting a healthy lifestyle
- being screened for infections
- avoiding environmental hazards
- timing your fertility investigations.

I suggest that you follow this four-month plan and do not try to conceive within that time. Why? Because when you follow the plan, your fertility will begin to increase. Everything needs to be working at optimum level before you conceive, both to prevent a miscarriage, and to give you the best possible chance of having a healthy baby.

If you have been trying to conceive for six months or more

If you are *under* the age of 35 and have been trying unsuccessfully to conceive for six months, follow the dietary and supplement suggestions given below for four months. At the end of this period, begin trying to conceive again. Give yourself six months before embarking on any fertility treatments or investigation by your doctor or a gynaecologist.

If you have been trying for six months and are *over* 35, follow the recommendations but visit your doctor and ask for tests to begin during that first four-month period. If you are given a diagnosis of unexplained infertility, then try for six months on your own before going for medical treatment.

The Integrated Approach

If you are already taking clomiphene or drugs to help you conceive, it is well worth taking four months off the drug treatment (you need to tell your doctor you are doing this) in order to optimise your fertility naturally. Then you can ask for a re-test of the investigations that determined you needed the drugs. If the situation is the same, resume the drug treatment but continue to take the vitamins and minerals. If things have improved, try for about six months, without any drugs, to become pregnant. Continue to take the supplements over this time.

If you have already been told that IVF (or ICSI) is your best option, you should still take the time to follow the four-month plan first. Those four months are crucial, no matter what age you are. Both you and your partner need to be in optimum health before you go for the IVF treatment, to give it the best chance of working. You want to produce good-quality eggs that will be fertilised easily with good-quality sperm, and your body must be as healthy as possible to increase the possibility that those fertilised eggs will implant and stay in place. Continue to take the vitamins and minerals throughout assisted conception.

Your Supplement Plan

Nutrients	You	Your partner
Folic acid	400mcg	–
Zinc	30mg	30mg
Selenium	100mcg	100mcg
Linseed (flaxseed) oil	1,000mg	1,000mg
Vitamin B6	up to 50mg	up to 50mg
Vitamin B12	up to 50mcg	up to 50mcg
Vitamin E	300–400iu	300–400iu
Vitamin C	1,000mg	1,000mg
Vitamin A	up to 2,300iu	–
Manganese	5mg	5mg
L-arginine	–	1,000mg
L-carnitine	–	100mg

To avoid having to purchase single supplements for all of the above, and to make the process easier, I have formulated two supplements that contain the most important nutrients for fertility. They are called Fertility Plus for Women and Fertility Plus for Men. These are available in most good healthshops, but if you have trouble finding them, please contact me directly (01892 750511).

You	Your partner
Fertility Plus for Women (1 capsule, twice a day)	Fertility Plus for Men (1 capsule, three times a day)
Linseed oil (1,000mg, once a day)	Linseed oil (1,000mg, once a day)
Vitamin C (1,000mg, once a day)	Vitamin C (1,000mg, once a day)

Herbs

Take 1 teaspoon of *Agnus castus* three times every day over the four-month plan. Your partner can take saw palmetto at the same dosage.

In Summary

- Always investigate the cause of fertility problems before taking any drugs.

- Ensure that you and your partner are screened for infections, if you are unable to conceive (see page 332).

- Begin the hormone balancing diet (see page 16).

- Avoid caffeine, which decreases fertility in men and women.

- Avoid smoking, which has been linked with both infertility and premature menopause in women, and with sperm problems in men.

- Avoid xenoestrogens (see page 40).

- Both you and your partner should avoid alcohol during the pre-conceptual period.

- If you are under 35, follow the treatment programme for four months (the preconceptual period), then try on your own to conceive naturally for six months before going for fertility investigations. Continue with the supplement programme over that time.

- If you are over 35, follow the programme for four months (the preconceptual period) *while* seeking tests from your doctor. If you are given a diagnosis of unexplained infertility, try on your own for the next six months. If you are told you need treatment (either drugs or IVF), finish the four-month preconceptual plan and stay on the supplements, but embark on the treatment at the same time.

Susan

Susan and her partner were 30 and 31 respectively, and they'd been trying to have a baby for four years before coming to see me. They had been diagnosed with 'unexplained fertility' and had had four unsuccessful attempts at IUI (see page 339). Susan had many problems with her periods: she had a regular cycle, but bled heavily with spotting and headaches before her period. At ovulation, her abdomen swelled up and she felt nauseous.

I asked them to arrange screening for infections and the tests came back positive to one infection, which was easily cleared up by antibiotics. Susan was deficient in a number of nutrients, including zinc, selenium, calcium and magnesium, and her partner had low zinc and high aluminium levels. I therefore recommended that he cut out canned soft drinks (see page 428) and switch to an aluminium-free deodorant. Because I was concerned that the imbalance causing the problems with Susan's cycle could also be a factor in her inability to conceive, I also used a combination of balancing herbs, including *Agnus castus*, to alleviate Susan's spotting and heavy bleeding. Susan and her partner followed the four-month programme (outlined on page 349) and waited until their mineral levels were back to normal. Nine months from their first appointment day, they conceived, and, not surprisingly, had a baby another nine months later.

CHAPTER 11

Pregnancy

Like the menopause, pregnancy is not an illness but a natural event. I have included it in this book because there can be complications and uncomfortable symptoms that can be distressing and even debilitating for some women. It's also very important that you know how to reach and maintain a state of optimum health in order to prepare for a comfortable pregnancy and the delivery of a healthy baby.

PROBLEMS IN PREGNANCY

Now, more than any other time, you will be considering what you eat when you are pregnant. The responsibility of feeding (indeed, growing!) another human being should never be taken lightly. You need to know what foods are beneficial for your baby's health and development, but you'll also need to know what should be avoided and what supplements you should be taking, if any.

Many women experiment with natural approaches to health for the first time when they are pregnant, largely because so many drugs are inappropriate for use during pregnancy, but also because it simply feels right to let nature take its course. During the early weeks and months of pregnancy a baby's cells divide and multiply rapidly and its organs are formed. For the remainder of the pregnancy, everything that will eventually make up your baby is formed. I cannot stress too much the importance of nutrition during pregnancy.

For many years, we have believed that babies in the womb are insulated from the external environment, and that they are protected from anything that could cause them harm. It makes sense that nature would protect the next generation. However, we now know that this is only true to a point. If there is little food, for example, your baby is more likely to benefit from it than you are. That's one of nature's protective mechanisms. However, it appears that what an expectant mother eats – or doesn't eat – can have a profound effect on a baby's health in the womb, after it is born and even when the baby becomes an adult.

Your Diet During Pregnancy

It is important to eat as well as you can from the moment you discover that you are pregnant. However, it is even more beneficial to prepare for pregnancy by changing your eating and drinking patterns up to four months before conception. If you are considering having a baby, then take a four-month 'preconception' break, and follow the recommendations outlined in Chapter 10. You may be alarmed to find this information in the infertility section of the book, but let me reassure you that the recommendations are the same, whether you are trying to conceive, or simply getting yourself into peak condition before having a baby.

If you are already pregnant, start straightaway with the nutrition recommendations in Chapter 1 (see page 16). Eat a healthy, varied diet, including fruits and vegetables, wholegrains, nuts, seeds, beans and pulses, eggs and fish. Where possible buy organic. What's the reason? Organic food does not contain chemicals in the form of pesticides, herbicides or other toxic substances. When you are pregnant it is essential that you reduce your exposure to all types of chemicals in order to protect yourself and your developing baby. If you take in chemicals, your baby does too. Furthermore, there is some evidence that organic food is more nutritious (richer in key vitamins and minerals).

Make sure you get enough essential fatty acids (EFAs; see page 27) from oily fish, nuts and seeds. They are crucial for brain, eyes and central nervous system development in a growing baby,[1] and they are even more vital in the last trimester (last three months) of pregnancy, where the intellectual development is as its most critical point. Because EFAs are so important, I would advise that you take them in supplement form (linseed oil is your best bet; see page 30). Early research indicates that these essential fatty acids are important not only for the brain development of your baby, but they can also help prevent low birthweight and decrease the risk of a premature birth.[2]

FOODS TO AVOID DURING PREGNANCY

- liver and cod liver oil (which can provide too much vitamin A in the animal form, retinol)

- meat pâtés (which can contain food-borne illnesses, and which are normally made of liver; see above)

- peanuts (in excess these can cause allergies in your baby)

- unpasteurised soft or blue cheese, such as Camembert, Brie and Stilton (there is a risk of food-borne illnesses, such as listeria)

- raw eggs, including mayonnaise (which can contain salmonella)

- raw meat and raw fish (which can contain food-borne illnesses)

- ready-to-eat-salads in bags (because of the risk of listeria; see page 365)

- sweets, chocolates and fizzy drinks (which provide unacceptable levels of toxins and/or caffeine that can harm your baby's development)

- too much undiluted fruit juice (which can cause blood sugar swings and unnecessary weight gain)

Problems You Might Experience During Pregnancy

Although pregnancy is not an illness, there are a number of different problems that may cause concern or discomfort during this time. These can include morning sickness, faintness, headaches, piles, constipation, heartburn, pre-eclampsia, concerns about your weight, premature labour and infections.

What Treatment Can You Be Offered By Your Doctor?

Because of the difficulties encountered in the past with drugs such as thalidomide, which was given for morning sickness, doctors are usually extremely careful about prescribing medication during pregnancy. Many of the problems, such as morning sickness, are left untreated unless they become extreme, at which point anti-nausea medication may be used or hospitalisation advised. Antibiotics may be needed when an infection is present, particularly something like bacterial vaginosis (see pages 250 and 251), which can bring on a premature labour.

Antacids may be recommended for heartburn, as they are safe in pregnancy; however, the natural alternatives should be tried first because antacids can reduce the absorption of iron.

Stimulant laxatives for constipation are not recommended during pregnancy because they can increase womb activity in some women. The general advice for constipation will always be to make dietary changes and ensure that you are getting plenty of fluids.

Conditions such as pre-eclampsia will be monitored, and hypertensives (drugs that lower blood pressure) may be prescribed. If untreated, pre-eclampsia can lead to eclampsia (see page 362), which can be life-threatening. The only course of action is the immediate delivery of the baby and anti-convulsant medication for you.

Natural Treatments For Pregnancy Problems

One of the keys to a healthy pregnancy is your diet. So many of the problems associated with pregnancy are directly caused by diet or nutritional deficiencies. If you take steps to address these well before conception, you are much less likely to experience discomfort or worrying symptoms. Eat a good diet, and supplement with some extra nutrients (see page 16) to ensure that you and your baby have everything you need. There is evidence that vitamins can prevent one of the most dangerous conditions that can occur in a pregnancy – pre-eclampsia – which gives an idea of just how important diet can be. And it's not just in the early days that your nutritional status will make a difference. You need to eat well and take appropriate supplements all the way through pregnancy and to help post-natal depression (see page 381).

Cravings

Your body can tell you a lot about what it needs and it is important to listen to the messages it is sending out through pregnancy. Some women will instinctively go off certain foods or drinks and may not be able even to stand the smell of them (coffee is a common dislike).

Sometimes a craving can give you a clue about particular requirements your body has. Try to choose the healthiest food you can in order to satisfy cravings. A craving for pickles, for instance, may be telling you that you need salt or calcium, whereas a craving for ice-cream may indicate a need for fat, protein or calcium. If you crave sweets, try adding more protein to your diet, or choose a healthier 'sweet' option, such as raisins or fruit.

Morning sickness

This is a very common complaint in pregnancy and although it is known as 'morning' sickness, it can occur at any time of the day or night (for some women, all of both). Some women experience only mild nausea, while others will vomit once or more each day. In a small minority of women, however, this can be extreme, causing dehydration, malnutrition and terrible discomfort, requiring admission to hospital. This condition is known as 'hyperemesis', and in some cases it can be prevented by using the correct elements of nutrition alongside other natural therapies, such as homeopathy or herbal medicine.

Morning sickness usually, but not always, stops by the 14th week of pregnancy. Although an uncomfortable symptom, it has been associated with fewer miscarriages, probably because the levels of certain hormones are relatively high.

There are several factors to take into consideration if you suffer from morning sickness, or if you want to prevent the condition from occurring.

Blood sugar

Morning sickness can definitely be eased by regulating your blood-sugar levels. Make sure that you eat little and often, using complex carbohydrates as snacks to keep your blood–sugar levels up. Suitable choices include rice cakes, wholemeal bread, rye crackers and any whole, unrefined products.

Vitamin B6

This vitamin has been found to be very helpful in reducing the attacks of nausea and vomiting.[3] One theory is that morning sickness may be caused by high oestrogen levels, and vitamin B6 is helpful in clearing excess oestrogen from the body by optimising liver function.

Ginger

This a traditional remedy for morning sickness, and it can be extremely effective, as confirmed by a 1991 double–blind clinical trial.[4] It can be taken in the form of supplements, capsules or herbal tea. One of the most effective ways I have found is grating the fresh root and then simmering it in water for about ten minutes. Add tamari (or soya sauce) for flavouring if you wish and drink as a tea. Another good method of taking ginger is in lemon and ginger tea. If you are having trouble keeping fluids down, sweeten the tea with a little honey or maple syrup and freeze as ice–cubes to suck as required.

Apple cider vinegar

Add two to three teaspoons of apple cider vinegar to warm water as your first drink of the morning. This has helped some women.

Natural medicine

Aromatherapy can also be used for morning sickness, and adding essential oils of peppermint, rosewood or chamomile to bath water can help to relieve nausea.

Acupuncture has been found to be extremely helpful in treating morning sickness and so has homeopathy. One of the most commonly used homeopathic remedies for this symptom is Ipecacuanha. It's always advisable to see a qualified practitioner for individual treatment, particularly during pregnancy.

Constipation

This is a common complaint during pregnancy because of hormone changes that can soften the smooth muscles of the bowel, and slow up the passage of food. The result can be both constipation and wind.

Make sure that you are eating enough natural fibre in your diet, including vegetables, fruits and wholegrains. Don't be tempted to take bran, which can add to the problem and irritate your gut. Bran contains substances called 'phytates', which can block the uptake of valuable minerals such as iron, calcium, magnesium etc. It is better to get your fibre from other sources.

If you need extra help, sprinkle 15ml (1 tablespoon) of linseeds on to your breakfast cereal in the morning or soak 15ml (1 tablespoon) of linseeds in a small amount of water and then swallow. Ensure that you are drinking plenty of fresh water, particularly if you are taking linseeds.

Iron in the form of ferrous sulphate (an inorganic iron) can also give you constipation, so change to organic iron if this is a problem. Your doctor may have prescribed iron supplements for anaemia during pregnancy, so check that the brand you are taking is not making your constipation worse.

Act quickly if you begin to suffer from constipation, which can cause straining that will lead to haemorrhoids (piles). (If you do get piles, use cold compresses to reduce the pain and swelling, and increase circulation in that area.)

Heartburn

Digestive disturbances are common in pregnancy because the pregnancy hormones relax the muscles in the valve between the food pipe (oesophagus) and the stomach. The result is that gastric juices flow upwards causing irritation and, often, fairly debilitating pain. These symptoms can become worse as the pregnancy progresses because the growing baby can 'concertina' your digestive organs, moving everything upwards.

Try not to eat large meals, particularly at night or when you are planning to lie down shortly afterwards. Eat little and often, and stay upright for as long as possible following a meal or even a snack.

Avoid foods that can cause an acidic reaction, such as sugary foods, spicy foods and coffee. Use peppermint tea after a meal to aid digestion, and to relieve heartburn and wind. Try taking digestive enzymes with your meal to aid digestion. Taking digestive enzymes in supplement form can help the digestion of fats, proteins and carbohydrates.

Weight

You may be worried about gaining weight during pregnancy, or you may have begun the pregnancy at a heavier weight than you would have liked. In Chapter 13 weight is discussed in some detail, and the aim with the natural approach is always to find your natural weight by eating well. Under no circumstances should you diet during pregnancy. If you crash diet you will deprive yourself and your baby of valuable nutrients. Your body may also start to detoxify (losing toxins stored in fat throughout your body) and these toxins will pass though the baby before they are excreted.

If you eat a good, nutritious diet (see page 16), you will lose any unnecessary weight naturally. The way to lose excess weight during pregnancy is to eat more healthily and any unnecessary kilos will come off. A healthy weight gain during pregnancy is considered to be not more than 15kg (33lb) and also not less than 5kg (11lb). If you find that you are well above or below this range, talk to your doctor. Some women find that they gain a great deal of weight, but lose it after the pregnancy with ease. If this is the case for previous pregnancies, and you know that it has not presented problems, don't worry. Every woman is unique.

The most important thing you can do to maintain a healthy weight is to ensure that your blood sugar is balanced by eating regularly. If you miss meals in an attempt to restrict calories, you may end up craving sweets and chocolates because your blood sugar has dropped too low.

Reduce your intake of concentrated fruit juices, even unsweetened brands. These juices may have some nutritional value, but they lack fibre and many women have found that they can lead to weight gain because they cause the blood sugar to fluctuate. Juice should always be diluted (half and half) with water.

Eat slowly and chew well. It takes 20 minutes for your brain to register that you are full, so if you eat slowly you can avoid overeating before you get that message.

STRETCHMARKS

You may also be concerned about stretchmarks which can appear as you begin to put on weight during pregnancy. Use a mixture of wheat-germ oil and vitamin E to massage into the skin once a day to improve its elasticity.

Pre-eclampsia

This is a condition that can affect women in late pregnancy. It is characterised by high blood pressure, protein in the urine, and swelling in the hands and feet. If the pre-eclampsia is allowed to continue unchecked, headaches can develop and your blood pressure can increase even further.

Bed-rest is required if this condition is diagnosed, which can help to lower your blood pressure. However, if symptoms continue to get worse, your doctor may decide to induce an early birth, or perform a Caesarean section.

Untreated pre-eclampsia may develop into eclampsia, which can be fatal. In fact, 10 per cent of women who develop eclampsia will die. The risk to the baby is even greater – 25 per cent of affected babies will die.

The medical cause of this condition is unknown, but certain nutrients have been found to be helpful in preventing pre-eclampsia.

In 1999 the *Lancet* published results of the first trial into whether vitamin supplements were effective in preventing pre-eclampsia.[5] Half of a group of pregnant women, some with a history of the condition and others with an abnormal blood flow to the placenta, were given vitamin E and vitamin C supplements. The other half were given a placebo (dummy tablet). The group who took the vitamins had a 76 per cent reduction in pre-eclampsia, compared to those taking the placebo. At least four other studies over the last few years have confirmed the link between low levels of antioxidants and a higher risk of pre-eclampsia.

Antioxidants are the nutrients that fight free radicals (see page 17). Interestingly, vitamin A (women are often told to avoid this vitamin during pregnancy; see page 375) is an antioxidant and it has been found that women who develop pre-eclampsia are deficient in vitamin A.[6]

Other research has shown that women with the lowest levels of Omega 3 fatty acids (which come from fish and linseeds) are more likely to have pre-eclampsia.[7] Both vitamin E and the Omega-3 essential oils help to prevent blood clotting and abnormal blood flow to the placenta .

Supplementing with 1.5 to 2g of calcium a day is also known to be effective in preventing pre-eclampsia[8] and also a lack of zinc can be connected with a risk of developing pre-eclampsia.[9]

Premature labour

A good diet can decrease the risk of having a premature baby. It has been found that essential fatty acids (EFAs; see page 27) can decrease the likelihood of giving too birth too early. Other research shows that women who are deficient in zinc can go into labour prematurely. It's important that you are getting enough of these nutrients.[10]

Low birthweight

Once again, eating well and looking after yourself can prevent problems from occurring. Any baby weighing less than 2.5kg (5.5lb) will be classed as 'low birthweight'.

In our mothers' generation, women longed for larger babies because they were considered to be stronger. In baby competitions of that era, the babies who won first prize were usually bigger and classed as 'bonny babies'. The trend then shifted in the other direction, and women began to think that 'smaller' babies were 'cuter'. The misconception that a smaller baby would mean an easier labour also gained credence. Before explaining the reasons why low birthweight is unhealthy – and even dangerous – I'd like to point out that a smaller baby does not affect the delivery to any great extent. Difficult deliveries are often the result of factors such as the shape of a woman's pelvis, the position of the baby and, interestingly, the size of the baby's head, not his body. It is perfectly possible to have a big baby with a normal head size, and a correspondingly easy birth. The opposite is also true.

A good birthweight has been found to be a strong predictor of an infant's chances of survival and subsequent health not only in infancy and childhood but into adulthood. Adults who were a normal weight at birth have a reduced risk of cardiovascular disease and diabetes.[11]

Pioneering work by Professor David Barker, at Southampton General Hospital in England, has also confirmed that what we weigh at birth can have an immense effect on our health later on in life. Low birthweight has been linked to an increased risk of high blood pressure,[12] a higher risk of coronary heart disease[13] and a greater risk of non–insulin dependent diabetes[14] when we are older.

Unfortunately, according to the World Health Organisation, the UK shares the astonishing and unenviable record of ranking equal with Albania as having one of the worst statistics in Europe for producing seriously underweight babies. Seven per cent of babies in England and Wales are classed as low birthweight, which puts them at an increased risk of stillbirth, mental handicap, dying within a month, blindness, deafness, cerebral palsy and autism. Only Hungary (9 per cent) and Poland (8 per cent) have worse statistics than we do in the UK.

One study showed that women who had babies with low birthweight were deficient in 43 out of the 44 nutrients tested.[15]

Infections

Infections can cause a number of different problems. They may be passed on to your baby during delivery, they can cause a miscarriage or, in extreme cases, they can cause malformations. It is important that you follow the recommendations below to try to avoid picking up an infection, but it's even more important that you get some medical treatment if you suspect that there is something wrong.

Chlamydia trachomatis

An infected pregnant woman can pass on Chlamydia trachomatis to her baby during delivery causing conjunctivitis, failure to thrive, gastro-enteritis, and respiratory problems. It can also increase her baby's risk of getting otitis media with infusion (otherwise known as 'glue ear'). This infection will need to be treated as soon as it is diagnosed.[16]

For more on chlamydia, see pages 253–4.

Listeria

Listeria is a bacteria that is present in animals and soil. In men and non-pregnant women the infection is mild, but if a pregnant woman acquires listeria, she can have a late miscarriage. Listeria can be found in soft cheeses such as Brie, Camembert and blue-veined cheeses, meat pâtés, undercooked meat, ready-to-eat poultry (unless thoroughly reheated), soft whipped ice-creams that come out of machines, unpasteurised dairy products and ready-prepared salads in sealed bags. Avoid these foods throughout pregnancy.

Salmonella

One of the most common causes of food poisoning is salmonella, which can cause severe diarrhoea and vomiting. It does not seem to harm a developing baby, but the fever accompanying a salmonella infection may cause a miscarriage. Make sure that all poultry and eggs are thoroughly cooked, and avoid eating anything that contains raw eggs, such as mayonnaise.

Some other infections such as Group B haemolytic streptococci or bacterial vaginosis (see page 251) can cause a premature birth, so do have a check-up if you suspect an infection. If you notice any unusual or smelly discharge, any soreness or redness around the vagina, or any burning sensation when passing urine, see your doctor.

TIPS TO AVOID FOOD POISONING

- Wash your hands before preparing food and in between handling raw and cooked food.

- Keep your worktops clean and wash chopping boards in hot soapy water between jobs.

- Wash utensils used for raw foods in hot soapy water before they are used on other foods.

- Keep the temperature of your refrigerator set at less than 5°C and your freezer set at below minus 18°C.

- Prepare and store raw and cooked food separately.

- Keep pets away from food.

- Do not prepare food for other people if you have symptoms of food poisoning.

- Don't overfill the refrigerator as it can stop air circulating, which could increase the temperature inside the refrigerator.

- Put leftovers back in the refrigerator as soon as possible after they have cooled.

- Heat any leftovers thoroughly.

- Thoroughly cook meat and poultry so there are no pink bits.

Toxoplasmosis

One of the reasons why it is recommended that you do not eat raw or partially cooked meat and meat products is because toxoplasmosis can be acquired from these foods. Toxoplasmosis is a parasite infection. This parasite (*toxoplasma gondii*) grows and reproduces in cats, which is why it is also important that you avoid any contact with cat litter throughout pregnancy. Other than meat, toxoplasmosis can be acquired by drinking contaminated water and eating unpasteurised dairy products.

If a woman acquires toxoplasmosis during pregnancy, her baby has a 45 per cent chance of getting the disease. This is a very serious condition. The risk to the baby is greater in the first three months of pregnancy, when toxoplasmosis can cause hydrocephalus (accumulation of fluid on the brain), eye problems, convulsions, blindness and brain damage.

If you have to handle cat litter during pregnancy, wear disposable gloves and wash your hands carefully. Gloves should also be worn while gardening and your hands should be washed thoroughly afterwards. Take extra care if you are handling raw meat. All meat should be served well cooked, your vegetables and fruit should be washed thoroughly to remove all traces of soil, dairy foods such as milk and cheese should be pasteurised, and you should always wash your hands carefully before eating.

Thrush

A mild discharge is normal during pregnancy and you may experience more than usual because the cervix excretes more mucus at this time. But vaginal secretions during pregnancy may be a breeding ground for the yeast *Candida albicans* and thrush is often a common problem. Follow the dietary recommendations from Chapter 8, and take acidophilus capsules by mouth to help with or even to prevent thrush if you are susceptible to frequent attacks. Do not insert yoghurt or any of the vaginal acidophilus creams into the vagina when you are pregnant.

What To Avoid During Pregnancy

Alcohol

You may be told by your doctor to avoid drinking alcohol for the first three months only. Many women are advised that drinking the odd glass or two after that is acceptable. This advice is not only wrong, but it can be dangerous.

Even a little alcohol may be too much, and here's why. During the first 12 weeks, the highest rate of cell division takes place and all the major organs are formed, so there is more risk if a toxin like alcohol reaches your baby during these weeks. After the third month your baby grows and matures. Even though most of your baby's crucial organs will be fully formed, they are unable to function on their own and they will be maturing at a steady rate. Your baby's heart, lungs and brain are all in key developmental stages during the whole pregnancy, and they can be vulnerable to damage after these first 12 weeks. The brain in particular is at risk.

It has been known for centuries that drinking during pregnancy can cause problems with the health of the baby. In the 1720s 'gin epidemic', the Royal College of Physicians stated that parental drinking was a cause of 'weak, feeble and distempered children'.[17]

Alcohol is classed as a 'teratogen', which literally translates as 'monster-forming'. A teratogen is an agent or drug that can cause malformation of an embryo or foetus. Professor David Smith from Washington in the US points out that 'there is no known teratogen yet studied in man which clearly shows a threshold effect where the substance is quite safe to a particular level, beyond which it is teratogenic'.[18] In effect, he is saying that the experts cannot provide a safe limit because there probably is not one. As the World Health Organisation states, 'no alcohol during pregnancy is the only safe limit'.

By the 36th day of pregnancy, the neural tube (the embryological structure from which the brain and spinal cord grow) of the embryo develops and a rudimentary system is formed. If a teratogenic substance like alcohol is drunk at this most crucial time, it can result in various malformations in your baby, including a defective heart and muscular skeletal abnormalities.

Even though the first three months are the most critical, the teratogenic effects of alcohol continue throughout the whole pregnancy affecting, at the later stages, brain development and function. Low birthweight and congenital abnormalities have all been linked to the negative effects of alcohol, and studies show that there is almost twice the risk of abnormalities.[19]

In January 2000, research from Queen's University in Belfast, Northern Ireland, claimed that the UK Department of Health (which recommends that pregnant women can drink four units of alcohol a week) and the Royal College of Obstetricians and Gynaecologists (who say that seven units of alcohol a week is not harmful) were offering 'unsound and dangerous advice'. The study showed that even a tiny amount of alcohol (four glasses of wine a week) can affect an unborn baby's brain and central nervous system. Scientists concluded that women who drink throughout their pregnancy will produce children with shorter attention spans, and their children will also find it more difficult to do well at school. Britain is the only developed country where pregnant women are officially told that they can drink alcohol. Remember the problems associated with birthweight in this country? This is no coincidence.

FOETAL ALCOHOL SYNDROME

In its most extreme form, the effects of alcohol can cause a condition called foetal alcohol syndrome (FAS).[20] The characteristics of this syndrome include growth problems, craniofacial, musculoskeletal, cardiac, nervous system and neuro-developmental delay or mental deficiency (with an average IQ of 65). In a nutshell, that means that your baby will not grow normally, the face and skeleton may be unusual, and there will be problems with the nervous system, the heart and the brain.

Babies born with FAS will look visibly different from other babies. They can be smaller and thinner, and their head circumference will be less than that of a healthy baby. They may also fail to thrive. The bridge of the nose can be poorly formed and a baby can have large ears that are 'simply formed', which means that they will lack the intricate detail of a healthy ear. An FAS baby may also have a cleft palate. Limb defects are also common, including such defects as congenital hip dislocations. Congenital heart disease is also a concern. Because a baby will effectively be an alcoholic, there may be signs of withdrawal once out of the womb, including fretfulness, nervousness and irritability.

FOETAL ALCOHOL EFFECTS

It is now recognised that there are children who do not bear the severe physical characteristics of FAS but who have subtle mental or behavioural difficulties caused by being exposed to alcohol in the womb. These characteristics are now identified as foetal alcohol effects.[21] And we are talking about effects that are being produced merely by 'social drinking'.

One study looked at the effect of consuming two or more drinks most days during the pregnancy or binge drinking (drinking five or more drinks in one go, at a party for example) before a woman realised she was pregnant. The babies born from these mothers were followed over seven years to see how they progressed. From the beginning, the babies had a lower than average birth weight and were more jittery. They had difficulty establishing a good sucking pattern and had disrupted sleep patterns. From eight months, their co-ordination was not good and they still had disrupted sleep patterns. A follow-up study at 7 years old showed that those children whose mothers had been drinking two or more drinks a day were seven points lower in their

IQ scores than the average seven-year-old. Children of mothers who had been binge drinking before they realised they were pregnant were approximately one to three months behind in reading and arithmetic. Other tests from this study showed a poor attention span, problems with memory and negative behaviour patterns.[22] In fact, some of the classic symptoms of hyperactivity, now called attention deficit hyperactivity disorder (ADHD), are associated with drinking during pregnancy.

Instead of focusing attention on drugs such as Ritalin to control hyperactivity, perhaps funding should be ploughed into preventative measures. Something as simple as recommending that women do not drink at all during pregnancy may make an enormous difference.

Alcohol is also a diuretic, which means that it causes valuable vitamins and minerals to be excreted in your urine. Zinc, a very important mineral during pregnancy (see page 378) is known to be depleted with alcohol consumption[23] and studies show that when zinc levels are reduced, low birthweight and foetal malformations can follow.[24] Folic acid deficiency can also result from the diuretic effect of alcohol and this is the nutrient that we know can help to prevent spina bifida.[25]

Smoking

Smoking is known to cause a wide range of serious health problems including lung cancer, emphysema and heart disease. Thankfully most people are now aware of the detrimental effects of smoking during pregnancy, and it has actually become socially taboo to do so.

Tobacco smoke contains more than 4,000 compounds and these pass directly into the baby's blood supply. These chemicals have different effects on the developing baby:

- Nicotine causes the foetal heart rate to accelerate, it decreases blood flow to the placenta and can affect placental amino acid (the building blocks of all our cells) uptake, resulting in serious growth problems (retardation).

- Carbon monoxide affects the flow of your baby's blood to the brain, heart and adrenal glands and can affect brain DNA (genes) and the way the body uses protein.

- Polycyclic aromatic hydrocarbons are mutagens and carcinogens (they affect genes and may cause cancer), and they can also interfere with the hormone activity of the placenta.

- Cyanide can retard your baby's growth in the womb.

No less than 45 studies have confirmed that smoking is a major cause of low birthweight, and lack of oxygen to the developing baby (called foetal hypoxia) from cigarette smoking during pregnancy also leads to a higher risk of prematurity and congenital abnormalities.[26]

Cadmium is a poison present in cigarette smoke, and when a pregnant woman smokes, it becomes concentrated in the placenta. Like alcohol, cadmium is classed as a teratogen (monster-forming) and it interferes with the absorption of many important minerals, including zinc. Cadmium is also a poison to a baby, which (together with low levels of zinc) has been associated with stillbirth, underweight and various forms of abnormalities.[27]

Pregnant women who smoke 30 cigarettes a day have a 33 per cent likelihood of having a premature baby, compared to only 6 per cent of non-smoking mothers. Studies have found that smokers (both male and female) are more likely to have children with all types of congenital malformations – in particular, cleft palate, hare lip, squints and deafness. Even if you don't smoke, having a partner who smokes over ten cigarettes a day can increase your risk of having a baby with congenital abnormalities (birth defects) by 2.5 times. If your partner insists on smoking, he should not smoke in the house or when you are with him. According to a Health Education Authority Leaflet, only 15 per cent of the smoke from a cigarette is inhaled – the remainder goes into the air and will be inhaled by those near to the smoker.

The same leaflet states that children of parents who smoke inhale amounts of nicotine equivalent to actively smoking 60 to 150 cigarettes a year. This results in an increased risk of asthma, chest infections, and ear, nose and throat infections. It is estimated that 50 children a day are admitted to hospital due to the effects of passive smoking.

Mercury

Mercury is a toxic metal that is found in dental fillings, so there are concerns about its effects on pregnancy. One study demonstrated how quickly mercury passes from a pregnant mother to her baby. Pregnant sheep were fitted with 12 molars filled with amalgam (a mixture of mercury and other metals used in dentistry). As early as three days after putting in the fillings, mercury accumulation was seen in both the mother's and baby's blood, and in the amniotic fluid. The mercury was also present in the baby's kidneys and liver (which had higher accumulations than those found in the mother). After the birth of the lambs, the mercury continued to be transferred to the lambs via the milk. In fact, the sheep's milk had eight times the normal level of mercury in her blood!

The Department of Health has suggested that women do not have mercury (amalgam) fillings during pregnancy and I would take that further and recommend that you avoid all dental work, if at all possible, during pregnancy.

Occupational hazards

Many occupations pose a risk during pregnancy. It has been found that pregnant women exposed to organic solvents have a 13-fold risk of having a baby with a serious congenital malformation (birth defect). Organic solvents can be present in the printing, graphic design, clothing, textile and healthcare professions. The suspected solvents include hydrocarbons, phenols, trichloroethylene, xylene, vinyl chloride and acetone.[28] If that sounds like a mouthful of jargon, ask to the see the labels of the chemicals with which you are in contact.

Normal office equipment, such as photocopiers, fax machines, computers and laser printers, can produce high levels of ozone. It is worth keeping your office stocked with plants to keep the air as fresh as possible. Some plants (such as peace lilies and spider plants) actively absorb toxic materials. Houseplants will also prevent the air from becoming too dry.

What to do about your job

You may be in a job that regularly exposes you to hazards and you will need to think about whether the risk can be minimised, or whether you may have to change your occupation. For example, women exposed to pesticides – such as sheep farmers during lambing – can have miscarriages, stillbirth and babies with malformations.[29] Take steps to find out what risks there may be at your workplace, and then consider carefully whether they can be avoided or whether you may have to leave.

Street drugs

The use of street drugs such as marijuana and cocaine has increased steadily over the years to the point where some people use them in their daily lives. As well having an adverse effect on your fertility, these drugs can also affect the development and health of your growing baby. Here's what the research is saying:

- In animals, marijuana has been linked to stillbirths and malformations.[30] In general the effects appear to be similar to those caused by tobacco smoking (see page 370).

- If women use cocaine once they are pregnant they are more likely to have a miscarriage, a stillbirth or a baby born with a malformation.[31]

- The number of stillbirths are increased in women who take heroin while they are pregnant and the rate of prematurity goes up.[32] Even more appallingly, perhaps, babies born to mothers who have taken heroin and cocaine suffer severe and even life-threatening withdrawal symptoms.

Medication

If you are taking tranquillisers and sleeping pills, talk to your doctor about gradually cutting down and then stopping. You'll need to find other ways of dealing with the problem and there are a wide variety of natural therapies designed to do just that. Homeopathy, aromatherapy, relaxation techniques and herbal medicine can all help to ease problems requiring conventional medication such as tranquillisers, and the majority are safe during pregnancy.

Even ordinary, over-the-counter drugs can have an effect on pregnancy. Taking analgesics or painkillers – the kind you buy at the chemist and in the supermarket – have been shown to increase the risk of miscarriage,[33] and paracetamol has been linked to causing mutations (cell changes) in both animals and humans.[34]

One kind of tranquilliser, called benzodiazepines (BZD) is often taken during pregnancy but could cause irreversible central nervous system and behavioural disorders. The UK drug reference books list suggest it can be given with 'special precautions' during pregnancy. The *American Physicians' Desk Reference*, however, states that these drugs should not be used in pregnancy. In the UK, as many as 35 per cent of pregnant women can be given these tranquillisers for insomnia and other nervous disorders.[35] Babies born from mothers who have taken these drugs have problems such as dyslexia and attention deficit hyperactive disorder.[36]

The Pregnancy Plan

The aim is to help you to have a comfortable, symptom-free pregnancy with a healthy baby as the end result. The most important steps to focus on when you are pregnant are:

1. Work on eating well for both you and the baby, by following the recommendations in Chapter 1.

2. Make sure that you avoid toxins where possible (such as alcohol, drugs, smoking and other chemicals from the environment).

3. Use nutritional supplements that can provide you with important nutrients while you are pregnant. These supplements are known to be beneficial to both you and your baby.

4. Use herbs to help with labour. If you require herbs to deal with stress or any other symptom of pregnancy, see a registered practitioner.

Supplements

Your baby gets first call on all the nutrients it requires, so you need to make sure that you are feeding yourself well and taking in enough nutrients to keep yourself healthy. These nutrients will also help to give you energy, and to prepare you for the birth and looking after your baby when it is born.

Apart from eating well, there are certain supplements that should be taken during pregnancy. I'm not suggesting megadosing anything – simply ensuring that you have adequate levels of everything that is now proven to be essential for your baby. Unfortunately much of the food we eat no longer contains adequate levels of vitamins, minerals and other nutrients, and unless you eat entirely organic, and a hugely varied diet, it unlikely that you will be getting enough.

Folic acid

You are normally told to take this vitamin for the 3 (or 4) months leading up to conception, then during the first 12 weeks of pregnancy. Your need for folic acid doubles when you are pregnant so it is a crucial vitamin to take supplementally. It not only helps to prevent spina bifida, but research has shown that women taking folic acid during pregnancy gave birth to babies who have a good birthweight, higher Apgar scores (the test given to a baby just after birth) and a lower incidence of foetal growth retardation.[37]

I recommend that you take folic acid throughout pregnancy. Research is now showing that the need for folic acid becomes even greater in the last trimester (last three months) of pregnancy, and that the amount taken in this period should increase to 540mcg per day.[38]

APGAR SCORE

The Apgar score, named after an American anaesthetist, evaluates a baby's condition by giving a score for heart rate, breathing, muscle tone, reflexes and colour one minute and then five minutes after birth.

B vitamins

Folic acid is a B vitamin, but I listed it first to draw attention to its importance. The other B vitamins are equally important during pregnancy, and levels of B1, B2, B6 and B12 are often deficient at this time. Studies have shown that supplementing with these vitamins is associated with babies who are healthier in terms of birthweight and the circumference of the head.

The B vitamins are known as the 'stress' vitamins, so they can be very useful during pregnancy, when stress levels can be higher. These vitamins can also help with the mood swings and tearfulness that often accompany pregnancy.

Vitamin A

There have been concerns about using vitamin A during pregnancy. These concerns came about for two reasons. One was the result of a woman eating vast and regular amounts of liver during her pregnancy. Liver contains large amounts of the animal form of vitamin A, which is known as retinol. The other instance was linked to the use of medications for acne during pregnancy. A number of these preparations contain synthetic vitamin A.

Research has shown that there can be a problem with high doses of retinol (the animal form of vitamin A) during pregnancy. A study in the *New England Journal of Medicine* found that pregnant women who take high doses of retinol on a daily basis increase their risk of having a handicapped baby. The danger threshold appeared to be daily doses in excess of 10,000iu, which gives you a 1 in 57 chance of having a baby with birth defects. Interestingly, the study also supported the fact that beta-carotene (the plant form of vitamin A) is a safer alternative to vitamin A. Apparently the retinoids (in the animal version) and not the carotenoids (in the vegetable version) are the cause of birth defects. Even at high doses beta-carotene does not raise vitamin A levels in the body sufficiently to cause defects in an unborn baby.[39]

Unfortunately, this type of information causes women to swing from one extreme to the other. Doctors have recommended that *no* vitamin A be taken during pregnancy, the consequence of which is that deficiency is becoming a problem. Vitamin A deficiency during pregnancy can have devastating effects. Vitamin A has antioxidant (see page 17) and protective properties similar to those found in the mineral selenium (see page 346), which can protect against cell mutation. It is essential for healthy eyes, and animal studies show that a deficiency of vitamin A has produced animals with no eyes, eye defects, undescended testes and hernias of the diaphragm, which means that breathing can be a problem.[40]

Even worse, women who develop pre-eclampsia have been found to be deficient in vitamin A *but not beta-carotene*.[41] How can this occur? If there is a retinol deficiency, it's possible that the body isn't converting beta-carotene properly.

Magnesium

Magnesium is a mineral that your body needs to form bone, protein and fatty acids. It relaxes your muscles and helps your blood to clot appropriately. This is a useful mineral if you suffer from leg cramps. Studies show that magnesium levels are lower in women who have had a premature labour.[42]

Furthermore, it can help to prevent premature contractions by relaxing the muscles of the womb. Scientists have investigated the effect of giving magnesium during pregnancy and found that women taking magnesium supplements had less chance of having low birth-weight and premature babies, and their babies had better Apgar scores (see page 375).[43]

Magnesium is known as 'nature's tranquilliser', so it can be invaluable if you are suffering from tension and/or stress. It's also a good basic treatment for insomnia. Take it as a separate supplement (apart from what is contained in your multivitamin and mineral supplement) for best effect. A total of 200mg per day is the optimum dosage. If you need help with sleeping, take it about an hour before going to bed.

Calcium

For many years it was believed that pregnant women have additional calcium requirements because the calcium needed for a baby's growing bones would be 'leached' from the mother's bones if there wasn't enough available. However, recent research has shown that a mother's body changes to meet this requirement by making sure that calcium is more efficiently absorbed from the food you eat.[44]

Obviously it is important that there is calcium available in your diet to meet your baby's needs, but it is not necessary to take extra during pregnancy. A good multivitamin and mineral will contain calcium.

Iron

Years ago iron supplements were routinely offered during pregnancy, regardless of whether or not a woman was iron deficient. Thankfully, this practice has now stopped. Iron is a strange mineral. Until recently, scientists believed that we really couldn't have too much. Our bodies need iron to make red blood cells and to transport oxygen around the body. Without iron, new cells cannot be produced and our organs would be starved of oxygen. Iron deficiency is characterised by fatigue because the body is, literally, being starved of oxygen.

However, too much iron is not a good thing. Any iron that is not used is not eliminated from the body, but stored as something called 'ferritin'. The only time we actually lose iron from our bodies is during our periods, during childbirth, when we donate blood, or when we suffer blood loss through an accident. In other words, we have to lose blood to lose iron.

Iron supplements should, therefore, *only* be taken if you have a deficiency. Most women are routinely tested for iron deficiency during pregnancy.

NOT ALL IRON SUPPLEMENTS ARE THE SAME

If you are found to be deficient in iron, you will probably be given a supplement. Unfortunately, some iron supplements can be largely ineffective depending on the form in which they are given. Inorganic iron – such as ferrous sulphate and ferrous gluconate, which are the standard irons given medically – are very difficult to absorb and can cause problems in the digestive system, resulting in constipation or black stools (which shows that the iron is not being absorbed). Inorganic iron or chelated forms of iron (which are combined with an amino acid) are much more easily absorbed and do not usually cause any bowel changes.

There are ways to help increase your iron intake (or uptake by your body), which do not involve using supplements. For example, drinking black tea, which contains tannins, during a meal can block the uptake of iron (and other vital minerals). Leave a gap of at least 30 minutes between eating and drinking tea. If you are prescribed iron, it should be taken with a vitamin C supplement on an empty stomach, to ensure that it is properly absorbed.

Zinc

This mineral is very important for the health of your growing baby, and low levels have been linked to low birthweight, spina bifida and other abnormalities. Your zinc levels can go down by about 30 per cent during pregnancy, so it is important that you have adequate supplies.[45]

Herbs

Herbs can be very helpful during pregnancy. Many can help with unpleasant symptoms such as morning sickness, while others will help your body to prepare for the birth. Some herbs can be extremely useful for sleep problems. Always see a registered practitioner if you have a health problem during pregnancy, so that the most appropriate herbs are used. Remember always to stick to the recommended dosage. Herbs can be enormously powerful healing agents and although they are natural, there are some that should be avoided during pregnancy.

Red raspberry (*Rubus idaeus*)

This is the herb most often used to prepare for labour because it helps to strengthen and tone the womb. It is rich in vitamins and minerals, and also helps to increase the flow of milk. It is usually recommended from the 34th week of pregnancy and can be taken as a tea.

NATURAL THERAPIES DURING PREGNANCY

There are many therapies that can be extremely helpful during pregnancy, such as acupuncture, homeopathy, reflexology and osteopathy. Some women respond better to some therapies than others, so it's worth experimenting to find a therapy or combination therapy that appeals and works best for you. Always check that your practitioner is registered, and has experience treating women during pregnancy.

Your Supplement Plan

- A good multivitamin and mineral supplement designed for pregnancy. This multi should contain the B vitamins (including folic acid), vitamin A (at less than 2,500iu), vitamin E, calcium, magnesium, zinc, selenium and chromium

- Linseed oil (1,000mg per day)

If you have had a previous episode of pre-eclampsia then add an extra:

- Vitamin E (300iu per day)
- Vitamin C (500mg per day)

Note

If you are concerned that you may be deficient in certain nutrients, you can arrange a test by post (which involves using a hair sample). This will ensure that you are taking everything you need. For details, see Chapter 4, on page 70.

In Summary

- Begin the dietary recommendations listed in Chapter 1 at least four months before you plan to conceive, and continue throughout your pregnancy.

- Ensure that you get plenty of essential fatty acids (EFAs; see page 27).

- Avoid foods known to cause problems with pregnancy and the health of your baby, including peanuts, liver, unpasteurised foods, meat pâtés, raw fish, meat or eggs, sweets, chocolate and caffeine.

- Ensure that you eat little and often, with meals based around complex carbohydrates, in order to balance your blood sugar levels.

- Eat wholefoods to avoid suffering from constipation.

- No matter how much you want to lose weight, don't be tempted to diet during pregnancy. You will lose excess weight naturally if you adopt a healthy eating plan.

- If you suspect that you may be suffering from a vaginal or other infection, ask for tests from your doctor.

- Do not drink *any* alcohol during pregnancy.

- Do not smoke during pregnancy, and ensure that you are not in the vicinity of smokers.

- Take note of occupational hazards and see if there is anything you can do to ensure that you are not in contact with them.

- Do not take recreational drugs while pregnant.

- Cut down on non-essential medication with the help of your doctor.

- Take supplements at least four months before you plan to conceive, and continue taking them throughout the pregnancy and while breastfeeding.

POST-NATAL DEPRESSION

The 'baby blues' is very common and may occur on the day of the birth, the day after or 3 days later or not at all. Crying and confusion are experienced by most women and are partly due to the hormone changes experienced during the labour and can also be connected to when the milk comes through. But for some 15 per cent of women, this despair and tearfulness continues and develops into post-natal depression. Symptoms can include:

- mood swings
- comfort eating
- inability to cope with the baby
- feeling inadequate as a mother
- low self-esteem
- tearfulness
- despair
- feeling exhausted
- increase or decrease in appetite.

It is important that you make sure that you are eating little and often. Keeping your blood sugar in balance is crucial for helping you through this time. Follow the recommendations on page 39 for which foods and drinks will cause mood swings and worsen the symptoms.

Make sure that you are taking a good multivitamin and mineral, the one you took during pregnancy such as the Fertility Plus is fine and then add in some extra zinc, so that you have in total 50mg of zinc a day.

Herbs, such as St John's wort, can be very useful for post-natal depression but they need to be given by a qualified practitioner if you are breastfeeding. Other hormone balancing herbs such as *Agnus castus* can be beneficial but a practitioner can tailor-make a remedy for your own individual needs.

Homeopathy can also be helpful and remedies such as sepia and pulsatilla are often used and again these will depend on your symptoms.

You may need to ask for help with the housework and other chores so that you can have time to rest, sleep, eat properly and also spend time getting to know the baby. You may also need to get out of the house on your own because, especially with the first baby, the feelings of this new person being totally dependent on you 24 hours a day can feel so overwhelming that you feel you can't cope.

Giving birth may bring up unresolved emotional issues from the past which need to be dealt with and counselling may be very helpful if this has happened.

GIVING YOUR BABY THE BEST CHANCE

It has become increasingly clear from recent research that a number of problems experienced during pregnancy and even throughout your baby's life can be prevented. If you do the best you can to have a healthy diet and lifestyle, and to remove environmental dangers, you will give your baby the best possible chance of being healthy both at birth and long into the future.

Taking the time to make changes before conception and carrying them through pregnancy may seem like a lot of effort. However, science is now showing us that this effort is well rewarded. In the first place you'll find it easier to become pregnant, and you will be less likely to experience a miscarriage. Most importantly, however, you and your baby will be healthy throughout the pregnancy, and after the birth.

It has been recognised that the environment in your womb has an enormous impact on the future health and even the intellectual development of the baby. A year or so of taking care of yourself will reap rewards both for you and any children you go on to have.

MISCARRIAGE

Suffering a miscarriage is one of the most devastating things that can happen to a woman, and to her partner. Many women conceive easily and are not emotionally or physically prepared for the shock of losing a baby. To make it worse, there are often complaints that the medical profession lack sympathy, and investigations into the cause are normally not even considered until you have suffered three miscarriages. It may seem a callous approach, but the reason for this response is simply that miscarriage is extremely common. In fact, one in four pregnancies end in miscarriage, usually before the 12th week of pregnancy. Many women miscarry without having been aware that they were pregnant. Nevertheless, if you do suffer a miscarriage, no amount of reassurance that it is 'normal' or 'common' can ease the pain.

What Is a Miscarriage?

A miscarriage, which is also known as 'spontaneous abortion', occurs when a baby (foetus) is lost spontaneously before the 24th week of pregnancy. After this time, the death of a baby is called a 'stillbirth'.

Many women feel well and will not notice anything untoward before a scan confirms that the baby has stopped developing and has died. In this situation, the miscarriage is called a 'missed abortion' because the baby has died, but has not been expelled from the womb. In some cases, a fertilised egg will not have developed, or developed poorly. On a scan, this would show as a pregnancy, but there would be no embryo because the foetus will have stopped growing early on. This is known as a 'blighted ovum'. Unfortunately, you may not know anything is wrong until you have the first routine scan, which is a great shock to an expectant mother.

Are There Any Symptoms?

In the case of a threatened miscarriage, where the risk of losing your baby is increased, you may experience:

• bleeding from the vagina, often containing clots

- blood in the vaginal mucus
- abdominal pain and/or cramping
- back pain

What Causes a Miscarriage?

This question is still largely unanswered. There are medical reasons for miscarriage (see below), and a series of tests will establish whether or not there is a cause. Other women miscarry but have completely normal test results. If you know there is something that can be done to prevent it happening again, you'll feel much more confident about embarking upon another pregnancy. When the diagnosis is 'unexplained', women are more likely to blame themselves and may be frightened to try again.

The greatest risk of miscarriage takes place before the 12th week of pregnancy. Until that time, the embryo floats unattached in the womb. At week 12, it becomes attached to the placenta and the pregnancy becomes more firmly established. If a miscarriage takes place after this date, the reasons are normally quite different from those that occur before.

NATURAL SELECTION?

Scientists believe that in many cases these early miscarriages are nature's way of dealing with an abnormal foetus that could not succeed in becoming a healthy baby.

Some of the most common causes of miscarriage are as follows.

Fibroids

Fibroids are discussed in detail in Chapter 6. If fibroids protrude into the womb (called submucosal fibroids), they increase the risk of miscarriage because they may make it difficult for the implanted embryo to develop properly.

Chromosomal abnormality

This is the most common reason for a miscarriage. It is normally the result of a one-off genetic abnormality in the baby, which means that it is unlikely to recur in future pregnancies. In other words nature is working according to the law of survival of the fittest.

Inherited genetic problems

This is a much less common reason for a miscarriage, and you might be unaware that you carry problematic genes. If you suffer repeated miscarriages, it will probably be suggested that you and your partner undergo chromosome (karyotype) analysis. This detects whether there are any defective genes, in either you or your partner. Some gene defects can cause miscarriage, but it is more likely that a genetic problem will cause abnormalities in the baby, such as cystic fibrosis or muscular dystrophy.

Infection

There are two possible scenarios here: you may have caught a severe infection during the early part of pregnancy, which has caused damage to the foetus and then a miscarriage. In this case, you are highly unlikely to miscarry again for this reason. Alternatively, the miscarriage could be caused by a genito-urinary infection, which could possibly lead to further miscarriages unless it is treated. For a list of all infections that need to be checked, see pages 364–7.

Bacterial vaginosis

It has been known for a number of years that an infection called bacterial vaginosis (see page 250), can increase the risk of a late miscarriage (between 16 and 24 weeks) or bring on a premature labour.[46] But researchers have now found that bacterial vaginosis may also cause an early miscarriage (before 12 weeks).[47]

Weight problems

We now know that obesity increases the risk of miscarriage.[48] Furthermore, women with PCOS (polycystic ovary syndrome; see Chapter 7), who often have a weight problem as well, are more likely to suffer a miscarriage. In a study of women with PCOS who were asked to change their diet, the rate of miscarriages dropped from 75 per cent to 18 per cent in those women who had lost weight.[49]

Hormonal problems

Luteinizing hormone (LH) controls the development and release of the egg from the ovary. Women who have high levels of this hormone in the first half of their menstrual cycle seem to have a greater risk of miscarriage. In addition, women with polycystic ovary syndrome (PCOS; see Chapter 7) have raised levels of LH.

Progesterone is the hormone that is responsible for maintaining a pregnancy during the first few weeks. After the egg has been released from the ovary, the ruptured follicle then develops into the corpus luteum, which produces progesterone. If the egg is not fertilised, after 14 days the corpus luteum withers, progesterone levels fall and a period occurs. If the egg is fertilised and the embryo implants successfully, and starts to produce another hormone HCG (human chorionic gonadotrophin), then the corpus luteum gets the message to continue producing progesterone. Without sufficient levels of progesterone, the pregnancy cannot continue, and that is why anti-progesterone drugs are now used to terminate an early pregnancy without the need for an operation.

Ultrasound can be useful for those women with a history of recurrent miscarriages, as it can pick up an indication of corpus luteum failure before any drop in progesterone is seen in the blood. At this point, progesterone supplementation can be beneficial. It is offered in the form of an injection, or as a pessary, to prevent a miscarriage.

Auto-immune disorders

An auto-immune condition occurs when you produce antibodies against your own cells. Normally, antibodies are produced by the body to fight off invaders. In this case, however, they fail to recognise cells as being normal, and set up defences against them. These antibodies are believed to cause blood clots in the placenta, preventing the baby from getting adequate blood and nutrition. Treatment involves drugs, such as aspirin or heparin, that thin the blood.

This blood–clotting syndrome can be detected though the presence of antiphospholipid antibodies in the blood. Tests will determine if the two main antiphospholipid antibodies, lupus anticoagulant and anticardiolipin antibodies, are present. Women should have two tests performed at least eight weeks apart and they must test positive on both occasions. If these tests are both positive, blood-thinning drugs are given.

Incompetent cervix

In a healthy pregnancy the neck of the womb (the cervix) remains closed until near the birth. However, when the cervix is 'incompetent', the neck of the womb painlessly dilates without contractions, resulting in miscarriage or premature birth. The condition may be congenital (in other words, you may have been born with an incompetent cervix) or it may be the result of a previous pregnancy.

When an incompetent cervix is the cause, miscarriage normally takes place later, often well into the second trimester of pregnancy. The usual treatment is to hold the cervix together with a stitch (called a cervical stitch). Some doctors put the stitch in before conception (particularly in women who have suffered miscarriage for this reason in the past), others in early pregnancy and others only in the third month. It's difficult to diagnose an incompetent cervix, and research has not led to any clear-cut conclusion about how beneficial cervical stitches really are. Furthermore, if it is inserted too early there is a possibility it could stop nature from miscarrying an abnormal baby.

Anatomical abnormalities

An unusually shaped womb may cause problems with implantation. Some women can be born with anatomical problems, such as a double uterus (two wombs), and still go on to have a healthy pregnancy, while others, with exactly the same condition, can repeatedly miscarry. Surgery is an option if you suffer from an abnormal womb.

Abnormal sperm

Because it is the woman who miscarries, greater emphasis has been placed on problems with the female reproductive system. However, if you continually miscarry, and there seems to be no medical cause, it is logical to consider that the problem may be caused by your partner's sperm. Early studies have shown that there is an increased risk of miscarriage where there are sperm abnormalities.[50] It is, therefore, essential that you and your partner are in optimum health before trying to conceive (see page 349).

Smoking

A study published in the *British Journal of Cancer* showed that men who smoke run the risk of fathering children who develop cancers such as leukaemia and brain tumours.[51] The theory is that chemicals in tobacco smoke can damage the DNA in the sperm. Taking this one step further, it's easy to see that any changes in DNA in the sperm could lead to a possible increase in the miscarriage rate. DNA damage cannot be picked up in a normal semen analysis so this problem would not be seen during routine fertility investigations.

If you smoke, there is an undoubted and proven increased risk of miscarriage.[52]

Alcohol

It is well known that alcohol can alter a man's sperm count and cause an increase in abnormal sperm.[53] Therefore, it follows that if an abnormal sperm fertilises an egg, nature will try to 'get rid' of that embryo.

Alcohol is a substance that is known to cause mutations. For example, studies have shown that alcohol given to female mice immediately after mating caused severe damage to the chromosomes of one-fifth to one-sixth of the embryos.[54] This chromosomal damage led to a higher rate of miscarriage or death shortly after birth in these mice. Chromosomal damage is a recognised cause of miscarriage.

It is also known that even moderate alcohol consumption during pregnancy works as a reproductive toxin and increases the risk of miscarriage.[55]

Caffeine

Caffeine is a stimulant and has been found to increase the risk of a miscarriage.[56] Some studies suggest there is twice the risk of miscarriage when as little as one to three cups of coffee are consumed a day.[57] Caffeine can also increase the probability of chromosomal abnormalities, which could lead to a miscarriage.[58]

Even decaffeinated coffee has been linked to an increased risk of miscarriage,[59] partly because some caffeine remains in the coffee after the decaffeination process, but also because decaffeinated coffee contains two other stimulants: theobromine and theophylline, which are not removed when the coffee is decaffeinated. Furthermore, most decaffeinated coffee has been decaffeinated by a chemical, and this can remain in the product.

And it's not just women who are affected by caffeine. Problems with sperm health (such as count, motility and abnormalities) seem to increase with the number of cups of coffee men drink each day.[60]

Radiation

Visual display units (VDUs) on computers emit non-ionising radiation. Microwaves, televisions, electric blankets, mobile phones and other electrical appliances do the same. A number of studies have looked at the effects on women who work in front of computers, but the results are not conclusive.

One 1984 study showed that out of 55 pregnancies in VDU users, 14.5 per cent ended in miscarriage, as compared to 5.3 per cent in women without exposure to VDUs. A further 22 per cent of the pregnancies had resulted in a malformation, compared to 11 per cent in non-VDU users. And 6.7 per cent had suffered a stillbirth, compared to only 1 per cent in the other group.[61] However, the Royal College of Obstetricians and Gynaecologists in the UK suggests that VDUs are not a hazard.

This type of controversial research is not without some basis, and because we simply do not know the long-term effects on a developing baby, I feel it is sensible to limit time spent working on VDUs during pregnancy. This is not only because of the possibility of unknown risk factors, but also because working for long, uninterrupted periods in front of VDUs is stressful and can cause other symptoms such as headaches, nausea, fatigue, insomnia and menstrual disturbances.[62]

What Treatment Can You Be Offered By Your Doctor?

The treatment will be determined by the cause of the miscarriage, if one can be found. If all the tests are normal, no treatment will be given and it will be suggested that you try to conceive again.

Drugs

Progesterone

If you have suffered repeated miscarriages, you may be offered progesterone as soon as you become pregnant. Progesterone is prescribed in either pessary or injection form. Some doctors may begin progesterone therapy even before you are pregnant, normally in the second half of your cycle.

It appears that if progesterone levels are not maintained during the second half of the cycle, then conception can take place but it will not result in a successful pregnancy. Progesterone levels need to reach a certain level in your body before you are able to sustain a pregnancy. You may experience a period without ever having known that you were pregnant.

If your doctor suspects that this is happening, progesterone support may be offered in the second half of the cycle, while you are trying to become pregnant.

Some women may suspect a drop in progesterone because they experience breakthrough bleeding or spotting a few days before the period actually happens. This drop in progesterone can be assessed by a simple saliva test (see box).

MONITORED CYCLE USING SALIVA

This is a very simple test that is done at home and then sent to the lab for analysis. A total of 11 saliva samples are collected over one cycle at specific times. The level of the hormones oestrogen and progesterone are mapped for that month to provide a pattern that can show whether you have problems maintaining progesterone levels or whether you have a very short luteal (second half) phase of the cycle, which can make it difficult to stay pregnant.

You can arrange to have this test sent to you by post (please see Staying in Touch, page 507).

Aspirin and heparin

If you have tested positive to the antiphospholipid antibodies (see page 386) on two occasions, at least eight weeks apart, you will be offered treatment for an auto-immune condition.

The treatment of choice for this 'sticky blood' condition is aspirin, which is prescribed at a low dose (about 75mg), normally prior to conception.

Trials using both aspirin and heparin (a drug used to thin the blood) have shown that a combination of these drugs works more effectively than just aspirin alone. As with any drug treatment, it is important to weigh up the benefits against the risks. It has been reported that women taking heparin during pregnancy may have an increased risk of osteoporosis (thinning of the bones), which means that you will be subject to monitoring throughout your pregnancy and probably thereafter.

If you have not tested positive to the antibodies on two separate occasions, it is not a good idea to go down this drug route. There is no evidence to show that taking aspirin 'just in case' has any benefit in terms of miscarriage, and it is always best to try to avoid any unnecessary medication during pregnancy.

What Natural Treatments Could Be Effective?

If you have suffered a miscarriage, it is natural to be very concerned about why it happened, and to want to prevent a recurrence. Like many women, you may have been subjected to a number of tests, all of which have been inconclusive. There may simply be no medical reason why you are miscarrying. Many women are told to 'go away and try again', which is a confusing and often frightening proposal. You may be concerned that because nothing has changed between one miscarriage and the next pregnancy, there is a possibility that it could happen again.

It is believed that up to 50 per cent of miscarriages are due to a chromosomal abnormality. Only a small portion of chromosomal abnormalities are inherited and you can be tested (screened) to see if there is a problem that needs to be addressed. Other chromosomal abnormalities occur before, during and after fertilisation, as the chromosomes divide. For this reason, it is extremely important that both you and your partner are in optimum health before you conceive in order to make sure that the egg and sperm are as healthy as possible before fertilisation.

You can achieve optimum health and minimise the risk of a miscarriage by following the recommendations below.

The natural approach to miscarriage, particularly when there is no medically diagnosed cause, has proved to be very effective. A study conducted by the University of Surrey in England showed that 83 per cent of couples, with a previous history of miscarriage, who made changes in their lifestyle and diet, and took nutritional supplements, conceived and had a baby within the three years of the study without experiencing another miscarriage.[63] The national average for miscarriages is one in four, so one would have expected to see some in the study, particularly in those couples who had already experienced a miscarriage. However, none of the couples who became pregnant during the study suffered a miscarriage. Those statistics speak for themselves.

It takes at least three months for immature eggs (oocytes) to develop to maturity. At this point they are ready for ovulation. As a result, there is a four-month period in which you can take steps to ensure that all of the factors necessary for a healthy conception and pregnancy are present. This is called the preconceptual period, and it is essential that you look upon this period as one that is as important as the pregnancy itself in terms of your lifestyle and diet.

It also takes at least three months for sperm cells to mature, ready to be ejaculated, so your partner needs to follow the recommendations below over four months as well.

So take four months off. Don't even try to conceive over that time and spend those months achieving optimum health before you try to get pregnant again. Make sure that you and your partner have corrected any vitamin and mineral deficiencies, and that toxins (see below) are avoided as much as possible.

Natural treatment is designed to work on a number of factors at the same time:

1. Improve your diet, based on the recommendations in Chapter 1 (see page 16).

2. Use nutritional supplements that are known scientifically to help prevent miscarriages.

3. Look at your lifestyle to avoid any environmental hazards such as VDUs, household chemicals and others.

4. Stop unnecessary toxins or drugs, such as smoking, street drugs and over-the-counter medication.

5. Use herbs to help prevent a miscarriage.

Dietary changes

Both you and your partner should follow the dietary recommendations given in Chapter 1 of this book. They will help to correct any hormone imbalances you have been experiencing and because the diet is extremely healthy, it will help to optimise the health of your partner's sperm and your own eggs. It will also ensure that your body is rich in the types of nutrients that a growing baby needs.

There are certain aspects of your diet that will need particular attention when trying to prevent a miscarriage.

Saturated fats

Both red meat and dairy produce contain arachidonic acid, which encourages the production of PGE2, a prostaglandin that leads to abnormal blood flow and blood clotting.

When you are trying to prevent a miscarriage, the aim is to reduce any abnormal blood clotting. So reduce your intake of saturated fats by cutting down on animal foods. Fish, however, should be top of your list. Fish contains certain unsaturated fats, called essential fatty acids, that encourage the production of healthy prostaglandins (see page 27). It is these prostaglandins that help to reduce abnormal blood clotting. Good sources of essential fatty acids (EFAs) are found in seeds, nuts, oils and oily fish (salmon, mackerel and kippers, for example).

Alcohol

There is no doubt that alcohol can cause miscarriages, so it is crucial that both you and your partner eliminate alcohol in the four months leading up to the next pregnancy. Alcohol is a toxin (which is why we talk about being 'intoxicated'), so it needs to be removed completely.

Smoking

This is another toxin that affects the health of both partners. In order to minimise the chance of miscarriage, you both need to stop smoking and to have four clear, smoke-free months before you get pregnant again.

You may need help to give up smoking and there are a variety of different natural therapies you can try. Acupuncture, homeopathy, flower essences and hypnotherapy can all be very effective (see page 57). If you are going to use nicotine replacement therapy, such as nicotine patches or gum, you will need to have given these up before beginning your four-month preconceptual period. Do not try to conceive while you are using nicotine patches or gum, because nicotine is effectively a drug that will be entering your bloodstream.

Caffeine

As mentioned on page 388, caffeine can increase the risk of a miscarriage. To improve your chances of carrying a pregnancy, eliminate it from your diet. Remember that caffeine comes in a variety of forms apart from tea and coffee, so watch out for colas, soft drinks, chocolate and even pain-relieving remedies, such as those designed to ease headaches.

Furthermore, because decaffeinated coffee has also been linked to an increased risk of miscarriages, it is important to eliminate decaffeinated products from your diet as well.

Caffeine can also affect the quality of the sperm, which can ultimately affect the quality of the developing baby. The quality of the embryo needs to be as good as possible in order to avoid a miscarriage, so your partner should avoid caffeine for the four-month period.

Environmental hazards

Try to minimise the amount of time you spend on the computer, under an electric blanket or using a mobile telephone. Reduce the number of household chemicals you use at home, and assess what, if any, chemicals to which you may be exposed at work. Certain chemicals have been linked to miscarriages, so aim to reduce your exposure to as many as possible. For more information on the effects of environmental hazards and how to avoid them see my book *Natural Solutions to Infertility*.

Supplements

Your diet will be supplemented in order to ensure that both you and your partner have all the nutrients required to create healthy eggs and sperm. Below you'll also find nutrients that are vital for preventing miscarriage.

Folic acid

Any woman trying to become pregnant now knows about the importance of folic acid, which has been proven to prevent spina bifida.

What you may not know is that it is extremely important for women who experience miscarriage.

Research into heart disease suggests that folic acid and vitamin B12 together might be beneficial in controlling an amino acid called homocysteine that is found in the blood. In high quantities, homocysteine causes damage to the lining of the blood vessels. Interestingly, high levels of homocysteine have also been found in women who experience recurrent miscarriage. It is, therefore, important that both folic acid and vitamin B12 form a part of your supplement plan.

Vitamin E

Aspirin and heparin are given to women who have blood clotting antibodies in order to thin the blood. Another possibility – and certainly the natural alternative – is to take vitamin E. This vitamin can help thin the blood and prevent clots. A study published in the *Lancet* in 1996 found that taking a daily dose of vitamin E reduced the risk of having a heart attack by an astonishing 75 per cent.[64] The scientists heading this study commented that the results were even more 'exciting than aspirin'.

Zinc

Zinc is an essential component of genetic material and a zinc deficiency can cause chromosome changes in both partners, leading to an increased risk of miscarriage. Zinc is found in high concentrations in the sperm, and adequate levels are needed to make the outer layer and tail. It's fairly obvious that it is a crucial nutrient for healthy sperm.

What's more, zinc plays a vital role in normal cell division, so it is particularly important that adequate levels are available at the time of conception in order to prevent a miscarriage.

Selenium

Researchers have found that women who miscarry have low levels of selenium in their blood compared to women who don't miscarry.[65] Selenium is a powerful antioxidant and it can prevent chromosome breakage and DNA damage, which are known to be a cause of miscarriages and birth defects.

Selenium is also needed for healthy sperm formation, so I strongly suggest that your partner supplements with selenium if the semen analysis shows a high percentage of abnormal sperm. As an antioxidant, selenium can also protect against possible DNA damage to sperm.

Essential fatty acids (EFAs)

Essential fatty acids produce beneficial prostaglandins which can reduce abnormal blood clotting. In order to make sure that you are not deficient in these fatty acids it is preferable to take them in supplement form over the four-month preconception period and during the pregnancy itself. I would recommend linseed (flaxseed) oil or fish oil capsules to help reduce any abnormal blood clotting.

Herbs

There are a number of herbs that can be very helpful in the prevention of miscarriage, and they should be taken during the four-month preconceptual period. Once you are pregnant, herbs can be used to stop a threatened miscarriage, but you will need to see a qualified practitioner to ensure that you are given the right ones. In fact, it is essential that you find a registered and qualified practitioner before taking any herbs during pregnancy. Remember, however, that herbs will not prevent a miscarriage if there is something wrong with your baby. Sometimes nature has to be allowed to take its course.

Agnus castus (vitex/chastetree berry)

This is a very helpful remedy for women who experience miscarriage because of a luteal phase defect (shortened second half of the cycle) or insufficient progesterone levels. It stimulates the function of the pituitary gland, which controls and balances our hormones by producing luteinizing hormone. This increases progesterone production and helps regulate a woman's cycle.

In one study on women with corpus luteum deficiency, 25 out of the 35 women normalised their serum progesterone levels after three months of taking *Agnus castus*.[66]

Blue cohosh (*Caulophyllum thalictroides*)

Blue cohosh is an important herb for the reproductive system. It tones and strengthens the whole system, and is particularly indicated for prevention of miscarriages.

False unicorn root (*Chamaelirium luteum*)

This herb is particularly recommended for those women who have been subject to recurrent miscarriage. It is believed to be a tonic for the womb and the whole of the reproductive system. False unicorn root is usually used in combination with the other herbs mentioned here in order to prevent a miscarriage.

Black haw (*Viburnum prunifolium*)
Black haw helps to relax the womb and to prevent it contracting inappropriately, which can be a feature of miscarriage.

The Treatment Plan

First have some investigations to find out if there is a reason for the miscarriage. This is more important if you have experienced a number of miscarriages. While these investigations are ongoing, put into place the natural recommendations, with the following exceptions:

The Integrated Approach

If you have been given progesterone by your doctor, follow the dietary and supplement recommendations, but do not take herbs at the same time.

If you have been told that your miscarriage was due to a blood-clotting problem and have been given aspirin and/or heparin, do not take vitamin E or essential fatty acids (EFAs) in supplement form (linseed or fish oil, for example), as these will also thin the blood.

Your Supplement Plan

- A good multivitamin and mineral supplement designed for pregnancy (it must contain 400mcg of folic acid, plus the following nutrients at these levels)

- Vitamin B12 (20mcg per day)

- Zinc citrate (30mg per day)

- Selenium (100mcg per day)

- Vitamin E (300iu per day)

- Linseed (flaxseed) oil (1,000mg per day)

To make this easier I have formulated two supplements (Fertility Plus for Women and Fertility Plus for Men), which contain all of these nutrients in the correct quantities. The only additional supplement required is linseed oil. I would also suggest adding vitamin C at 1,000mg per day, which is the generally recommended level for the preconceptual period.

You would take	Your partner would take
Fertility Plus for Women (one capsule twice a day)	Fertility Plus for Men (one capsule three times a day)
linseed oil (1,000mg per day)	linseed oil (1,000mg per day)
vitamin C (1,000mg per day)	vitamin C (1,000mg per day)

Fertility Plus supplements should be available from any good health-food shop, but if you have any difficulties please contact me (see Staying in Touch, page 507).

Continue taking supplements throughout your pregnancy.

Herbs

Blend the following herbs in equal parts, using the tincture form: *Agnus castus*, blue cohosh, false unicorn root and black haw. Take 1 teaspoon three times a day over the four-month preconceptual period while you are not trying to conceive and stop when you have a period.

Stop taking the herbs when you are trying to conceive or pregnant.

In Summary

- Always investigate the cause of miscarriage before taking any drugs, or beginning a natural treatment programme.

- Begin the hormone balancing diet (see page 16), and follow the dietary recommendations in Chapter 1.

- Ensure that you work towards optimum nutrition for at least four months before trying to conceive again. This is called the preconceptual period and it is crucial to the health of your pregnancy and your baby.

- Try to find your natural weight – miscarriage has been linked to overweight.

- Avoid smoking, caffeine, alcohol and animal fats, all of which are linked to miscarriage.

- Avoid radiation in the form of VDUs and anything else that emits low-level radiation, such as mobile phones, microwaves and electric blankets.

- Watch out for chemicals at home or at work.

- Take supplements (see page 397) throughout the preconceptual period, and pregnancy.

- Take herbs (see page 398) throughout the preconceptual period, stopping when you have a period, or when you become pregnant.

CHAPTER 12

The Menopause

The menopause is not an illness. If you subscribed to the standpoint currently taken by the conventional medical profession, you'd be forgiven for thinking it was.

In conventional terms the menopause and its symptoms are viewed as a disorder caused by falling hormone levels. So, by giving menopausal women hormones in the form of hormone replacement therapy (HRT), the deficiency can be corrected and we have a 'cure'. This argument is supported by the supposed similarity between the menopause and diabetes. When insulin levels are insufficient to maintain normal blood glucose levels, then insulin is supplied from outside and the balance is corrected. But diabetes is different from the menopause in one important respect: diabetes is not a natural event. It is not expected that everyone will get diabetes; but all women will pass through the menopause. It is a natural stage in our lives and there is a wealth of scientific evidence that there are alternatives to HRT.

THE MENOPAUSE

Women in many other cultures do not experience the menopause as a crisis demanding medical intervention. Many of them simply do not suffer the physical and emotional symptoms that women in the West are programmed to accept as inevitable. In our society the focus of the menopause is one of loss. Women are programmed to dwell on loss – the loss of periods, the loss of the ability to create life, the loss of hormones, the problems of the 'empty-nest' syndrome. In other societies, this time in a woman's life is seen as one of gain, a time of great wisdom.It is a time when the emphasis shifts away from doing the chores and working in the fields, to the role of lawmaker and counsellor to younger couples, where maturity and experience make a significant and valuable contribution to the family and society.

My approach is to take the menopause as a natural event. HRT is always there as the last resort, and it should only be used as such. Try the natural approaches first, and then assess whether you really do need HRT. The odds are that you won't.

What Happens At the Menopause?

We saw in Chapter 5 that the monthly cycle is governed by a number of reproductive hormones, the main ones being oestrogen, progesterone, follicle-stimulating hormone (FSH) and luteinizing hormone (LH).

At the menopause women literally run out of eggs. Each woman has a supply of eggs (approximately two million) from the moment she is born and over the years they are used up and die off. She finally reaches a certain age when there simply aren't any more. What the body does then to try to get that woman to ovulate is to release the hormone FSH. This hormone is released every month in a normal cycle but during menopause, a woman's body registers that ovulation is not taking place, so even more FSH is pumped out.

The interesting thing is that as the ovaries decline their production of oestrogen, nature has something else up her sleeve. We are also able to produce a form of oestrogen (called oestrone) from our adrenal glands in order to compensate for the decline from the ovaries. This makes it all the more important the adrenal glands are healthy in order for you to ensure that this other form of oestrogen is being produced.

We also produce oestrogen from fat cells, so being ultra-slim will not have health benefits in the long run, particularly if you are going through the menopause. Overweight isn't the answer, either, but from an oestrogen-production point of view, you are better off being slightly overweight than slim.

Are There Any Symptoms?

These vary from woman to woman. Some women sail though the menopause without any symptoms and the only thing they notice is that their periods have stopped. Some of the women I have seen in my clinic report being completely drenched in sweat day and night, and getting up to change their nightclothes two or three times a night, or even taking a shower in the middle of the night.

Symptoms of the menopause can include hot flushes, night sweats, vaginal dryness, mood swings, declining libido, osteoporosis, ageing skin, lack of energy, joint pains, weight gain, headaches and changes in hair quality. Interestingly, men also experience a lot of these symptoms, with irritability, a declining libido, changes in weight, ageing skin and hair, depression and anxiety. These symptoms are apparently part of the Western ageing process for both men and women, so it's important not to blame every symptom that you experience on the menopause.

Unfortunately, if a woman around the age of 45 goes to her doctor with any of these symptoms, it will immediately be put down to 'hormones', and you can guess what the first line of treatment will be. I have seen more women than I can count who have been put on HRT because of 'hormone' problems, only to find that they were not menopausal at all. There are a variety of other health conditions that throw up symptoms similar to those of the menopause, so don't assume – or, more importantly, let your doctor convince you – that there may not be another cause. What's important is working out what symptoms are due to the menopause, and what are simply symptoms of ageing.

Leading up to the menopause, ovulation becomes less likely because oestrogen levels decline during the first two weeks of the cycle, which means that progesterone will not be produced in the second half. Without the rising levels of oestrogen in the first two weeks to send a message back to the ovaries to produce smaller amounts of FSH, the levels of

FSH in the bloodstream keep rising. So a period can still happen without ovulation occurring. At this time, the adrenal glands begin to produce a form of oestrogen to compensate for the decline from the ovaries, and body fat also kicks into action as a manufacturing site.

There are three distinct phases of the menopause:

1. **Pre-menopause** – periods are still regular but the first symptoms, such as hot flushes and mood changes, may appear

2. **Peri-menopause** – the function of the ovaries declines, the periods can become irregular and symptoms may be more severe

3. **Post-menopause** – this stage runs from the last period onwards

Medically speaking, the passage through the menopause is termed the 'climacteric'. Your last period is known as 'the menopause'.

How Do You Know You Are In the Menopause?

If you see your doctor because you suspect you may have entered the menopause, he or she will measure your FSH levels. As a woman goes through the menopause FSH levels rise higher. Therefore, the level of FSH in your body is a relatively good measure of what stage you may be at (although levels can vary from month to month).

What Treatment Can You Be Offered By Your Doctor?

For the main symptoms of the menopause, such as hot flushes or vaginal dryness, you will be offered HRT. You can also be offered HRT to prevent or treat osteoporosis (this is covered in more detail later in this chapter). Newer 'designer' drugs called SERMS (selective oestrogen receptor modulators) are being developed for the menopause, but they do nothing for hot flushes, so they are discussed in the section on osteoporosis (see page 432).

Hormone replacement therapy (HRT)

Everyone has heard of HRT, and you will find advocates and critics wherever you go. Some women swear by it, and if their claims are to be believed, HRT has been the wonder drug of the 20th century. But is it so wonderful? Here's the HRT story. Work it out for yourself.

The idea for HRT was sparked when scientists decided that if oestrogen drops at the menopause, it should be replaced – hence hormone replacement therapy. Oestrogen therapy has been around since the 1930s, when injections of oestrogen were given for menopausal symptoms. Because of the inconvenience of this form of treatment, implant pellets of oestrogen were introduced in 1938. HRT was originally called oestrogen replacement therapy because only oestrogen was given as the treatment.

HRT has been seen as a universal panacea, a solution to all menopausal problems from osteoporosis to ageing skin. However, it soon became clear that giving oestrogen alone could increase the risk of cancer of the womb and breasts.[1] Research studies appeared to demonstrate that this increased risk could be up to seven times higher for endometrial cancer.[2] Oestrogen builds up the lining of the womb ready to receive a fertilised egg. Without the other main hormone (progesterone) to cause a bleed, cell mutations were taking place in the lining of the womb. The risk of that was too great. The scientists realised that they had to add in the other hormone. So, progestogen, the synthetic version of progesterone, was added to the therapy. This is called 'combined HRT', because it combines the two main hormones. Since then only women who have had a hysterectomy will be given just oestrogen.

The sex hormones, oestrogens and progesterone, are steroids. HRT contains the same combinations of oestrogens and progestogen that make up the Pill. The difference between the Pill and HRT is the chemical structure of the oestrogens they contain, and, of course, the dose! HRT can now be taken in a variety of different ways including implants, tablets, skin patches, creams, vaginal pessaries and gels.

SIDE-EFFECTS OF HRT

In the US, doctors use a manual called *The Physician's Desk Reference,* which is much more detailed than anything to which we have access in the UK. It lists the possible side-effects for HRT as:

• endometrial (womb) cancer

- undesirable weight gain/loss
- breast tenderness/enlargement
- bloating
- depression
- thrombophlebitis (inflammation of a vein)
- elevated blood pressure
- reduced carbohydrate tolerance
- skin rashes
- hair loss
- abdominal cramps
- vaginal candidiasis (thrush)
- jaundice
- vomiting
- cystitis-like syndrome.

Womb cancer

Even with the combined HRT (oestrogen and progestogen together), there is still over twice the risk of developing endometrial cancer compared to women who don't take HRT at all. This was confirmed by a meta-analysis (an overview of all the studies into HRT) of the effects of HRT on womb cancer.[3]

Breast cancer

The first inkling of the risk of breast cancer came in 1976 when the *New England Journal of Medicine* reported a study linking menopausal oestrogens to an increase in breast cancer.[4] Numerous studies since then have confirmed this finding. In 1997, a large meta-analysis (again, an overview of all the relevant studies) co-ordinated by the Collaborative Group on Hormonal Factors in Breast Cancer looked at more than 50 previous research projects involving more than 160,000 women and found a statistically significant increase in breast cancer for women on HRT.[5] What does that mean in layperson's terms? The research showed that HRT is undoubtedly linked to breast cancer.

In the early part of 2000 two studies have come out showing an increased risk of breast cancer in women on HRT. One from the *Journal of the American Medical Association* studied over 46,000 women and found a 40 per cent increase in breast cancer risk in women taking HRT.[6]

Blood clots

A number of studies have shown that women taking HRT have an increased risk of venous thromboembolism (in other words, blood clots). In addition, the risk appears to be greater during the first year or so of taking HRT.[7] Why are blood clots dangerous? They can cause stroke and heart attacks.

Heart disease

Apart from the prevention of osteoporosis, protecting against heart disease is the main reason why many women are encouraged to begin taking HRT. HRT supposedly decreases the risk of heart disease, even though heart disease is not a 'symptom' of the menopause. It is true that as women get older their risk of cardiovascular disease changes. By the time women reach 50, they have half as much risk of heart disease as men. It is not until they get to the age of 75 that they have an equal risk to men. The study that first seemed to show that HRT could have a protective effect on cardiovascular health, was reported in 1985 with a follow-up in 1991.[8] It followed a group of nurses taking HRT over a period of years and compared them with another group not taking HRT. Those taking HRT were found to be less susceptible to heart attacks.

Unfortunately, the study was flawed. The nurses were assigned a group depending on whether or not they were already taking HRT. This was not a double-blind placebo-controlled trial (where a group of women were randomly split into two groups and one-half given HRT and the other a placebo, which is a type of 'dummy pill', with neither the women nor the scientists knowing which group was actually taking the drug).

There are contraindications to HRT (see page 407) and some include history of thrombosis (clotting) and high blood pressure. It is, therefore, unlikely that any of the nurses with a history of either of those problems would have been prescribed HRT in the first place. So these 'high risk' nurses would be counted in with the group of women who were not taking HRT.

I voiced my concerns about this in my book *Natural Alternatives to HRT*, which was published in 1997, and since then other findings have emerged.

Results from the only published randomised, double-blind, placebo-controlled trial (the type that we should note) on the effects of HRT and cardiovascular disease, which had been started when I wrote the book, have shown that there is *no* benefit in taking HRT for heart disease. The women in this study had experienced heart problems already and the HRT was given to see whether it would prevent a second attack. There was no difference in the deaths caused by a heart condition whether the women were taking HRT or not. Unfortunately, those women taking HRT were nearly three times more likely to have a clot in a vein.[9]

Another clinical trial run by the Women's Health Initiative in America, which began in 1992, is the largest-ever study on women's health. Among other issues, it is looking at the effects of HRT on heart disease over a period of nine years. However, in the first two years of this trial, there were increasing numbers of women on HRT who experienced cardiovascular problems such as heart attacks, strokes and clots – that's in comparison to those women given a placebo (dummy pill). A press statement was issued in April 2000 to support those findings.[10] Because this has only happened to a small number of the women in the study, the trial has not been stopped.

The conclusion at the moment is definitely the following: 'HRT should not be prescribed solely for this purpose of secondary prevention of coronary heart disease.'[11] In other words, do not be talked into taking HRT to protect your heart because it doesn't.

CONTRAINDICATIONS FOR HRT

If you suffer from a particular medical condition – or are part of a group that may be at higher risk of getting a medical condition – there will undoubtedly be drugs that are not suitable for you. HRT is no exception. The British National Formulary suggests that HRT is not suitable for women who currently suffer from, or are in the 'high risk' category, for:

- liver disease
- breast cancer
- history of thrombosis.

Cautions (where doctors should think carefully before prescribing HRT) are:

- hypertension
- benign breast disease
- fibroids
- migraine
- endometriosis.

Fibroids and endometriosis are both oestrogen-dependent conditions (see Chapter 6) and as women reach the menopause these conditions actually start to sort themselves out because oestrogen levels are naturally declining. Adding HRT (oestrogen) means that these conditions will be kicked into action again.

One woman recently came to see me because her fibroid, which had been perfectly manageable, had grown to an enormous size when she began taking HRT. She is now scheduled for a hysterectomy because the fibroid has become so large, there is no other choice.

Progesterone

This drug is available on prescription, but it is unlikely that you will be offered this form of hormone therapy by your doctor, although women are taking it themselves for the menopause because of the media hype.

The idea of using progesterone at the menopause has been made popular by an American called Dr John Lee who extolled its virtues at the menopause and its benefits on osteoporosis (see later in this chapter).

As I explained in my book *Natural Alternatives to HRT*, 'natural' progesterone is not natural at all and that complementary practitioners had been hoodwinked into thinking that it was a natural alternative to HRT.

The logic behind giving progesterone at the menopause was based on the premise that we are living in an industrialised world where we are being bombarded with foreign oestrogens (xenoestrogens). These xenoestrogens have an oestrogenic effect on the body, which means that they can increase the risk of breast cancer, for example. Xenoestrogens are nearly all petrochemically based and can come from packaging, plastics, foods and pesticides (see page 40). The suggestion is that many of us are suffering from oestrogen dominance because of the increased amount of xenoestrogens we encounter daily. So, according to the pro-progesterone camp, the answer is to balance all this unwanted oestrogen with progesterone – 'natural' progesterone.

The production of both oestrogen and progesterone decline at the menopause. And while we go on making some oestrogen all our lives, the production of progesterone will stop completely. So are we seriously suggesting that nature has got this all wrong? Progesterone is needed to maintain a pregnancy so we can see logically why the body doesn't need it at the menopause. Why replace it?

This 'natural' progesterone is normally accepted to be an extract from the wild yam plant. In fact, progesterone itself is not found in wild yams. It is synthesised from the plant by a number of chemical steps, which means that it is not 'natural' at all. The assumption has been if we ate wild yams our bodies could convert it into progesterone. This is simply not true. Progesterone can only be synthesised from wild yams by a chemist in a laboratory. And the fact is that these progesterone creams do not contain any wild yam at all.

You need to be aware that progesterone creams contain a powerful pharmaceutical hormone that is made in a laboratory. My main concern has been that women are being duped into thinking they are using a natural herbal remedy containing wild yam. They are not: they are using a hormone replacement – just a different hormone. Progesterone is termed 'natural' because it is identical to the hormone you produce from the ovaries.

'Natural' progesterone is being touted as a 'natural' alternative to HRT. But there is nothing natural or alternative about it. The theory behind it is the same as the theory behind HRT – that menopausal women are suffering from a hormone deficiency disorder.

My argument is that we need to aim to get our bodies back into a *natural* balance, using *natural* means. Adding any kind of direct hormone to our bodies may address *symptoms*, but it will do absolutely nothing for the fundamental cause of the problem. If you stop using progesterone cream, you are back to square one: and your body will not have become any healthier in the process.

Natural Treatment

The natural treatment programme below aims to encourage optimum health, so that your body can manage this natural event with ease.

Colleen

Colleen, aged 49, came to see eight months after she had suffered haemorrhaging during her period. She had been given a D&C to stop the bleeding, but after that she started to experience irregular bleeding. She'd seen her doctor who had checked her over and then recommended HRT. Because she had had several benign breast lumps in the past, she refused to take it.

Colleen then took progesterone cream for three weeks, but when she started to bleed constantly, she stopped taking it. By the time I saw Colleen, she had been bleeding on and off for three weeks, with some clots. Her greatest fear was that she was going to haemorrhage again. We talked through her diet, and came to the conclusion that her three cups of coffee and one cup of tea a day meant that she was taking in too much caffeine, which was likely to make the bleeding worse. I put her on a programme of supplements, asked her to make changes in her diet and suggested some herbs to take to control the bleeding. It took three weeks for the bleeding to stop and by the time I saw her again she'd had no bleeding for eight weeks.

There are a number of stages to the treatment plan:

1. Improve your diet, based on the recommendations outlined in Chapter 1

2. Use nutritional supplements that are known scientifically to help to control menopausal symptoms

3. Use certain foods such as phytoestrogens that are particularly beneficial around the menopause

4. Control excess oestrogens absorbed from your environment, and make sure that your body is excreting any 'old' hormones

5. Use herbs that are known to help with menopausal symptoms such as hot flushes, vaginal dryness etc

Dietary changes

A well-balanced diet is essential during the menopause as it enables the body to adjust automatically to the hormone changes, naturally maintaining oestrogen from the adrenal glands and fat deposits. It is important that you put into practice the suggestions about diet from Chapter 1 and pay particular attention to the following points:

1. Stabilise blood sugar levels by reducing the amount of sugar and refined foods (anything with white flour) and make sure that you eat complex carbohydrates on a 'little and often' basis. This prevents your adrenal glands from working overtime, which is important because they should be producing oestrogen as your ovaries produce less.

2. Avoid tea and coffee, which contribute to the blood sugar problem, and also deprive the body of vital nutrients and trace elements.

3. Reduce your intake of dairy products and red meat as these are animal proteins·and can increase the amount of calcium you excrete (see section on osteoporosis, later in this chapter).

4. Ensure your diet contains sufficient essential fatty acids such as oily fish, nuts and seeds. They help to lubricate the joints, skin and vagina, as well as performing other functions, such as keeping cholesterol in check and ensuring healthy metabolism.

5. Make sure that you are eating enough fibre from good sources (not bran; see page 34). Eat plenty of fresh fruit and vegetables (cooked and raw) and wholegrains such as brown rice, wholemeal bread, wholemeal pasta and oatmeal, for example. Fibre binds oestrogen so that it is excreted more efficiently, it helps to keep your blood sugar stable and it encourages the elimination of toxic waste products.

Elizabeth

At 55, Elizabeth had entered the menopause, and her periods had stopped three years before her visit to me. She had, however, been experiencing hot flushes for quite some time. I recommended that she take *Agnus castus* and dong quai, both useful

---

herbs for menopausal symptoms. When she returned, she confirmed that the hot flushes had stopped almost immediately.

Margaret

Margaret, aged 55, had had a hysterectomy six years before her visit because she'd had terrible flooding and a number of ovarian cysts. She was pleased that she had agreed to the hysterectomy because she was relieved not to have any more periods.

She was put on HRT (oestrogen only because she didn't have a womb) immediately after the operation and had stayed on it for two years. Margaret had gained 2 stone (12.5kg) in weight while she was taking the oestrogen and was not happy about this. Recently she'd had trouble sleeping – she found it difficult to get off to sleep, and then woke in the middle of the night, tossing and turning. She felt her energy was low and that her memory was poor. As well as these symptoms, she was concerned that she was crying too easily and felt depressed. She'd already bought my *Natural Alternatives to HRT Cookbook*, and had started to change her diet. A hair mineral analysis showed that she was deficient in magnesium, zinc and chromium. I suggested what supplements she should take and I received a letter from her two months later. 'Everyone agrees I am much happier now, and apart from the (very) odd day, the family don't get their heads bitten off or come home to find me in tears. Much, much better. I know you will see a different person this time.'

Phytoestrogens

One of the questions that most perplexes scientists is why and how the menopause is experienced so differently around the world. There are other cultures where women experience minimal and often no menopausal symptoms. Also linked to this issue is the fact that in some parts of the world, notably the Far East, breast cancer is not the major killer that it is here in the West. For example, the UK seems to have a breast cancer death rate that is about six times higher than that of women in Japan. The interesting thing is that as soon as Japanese women move to the West their breast cancer rate is the same.[12]

It is clear then that there is no genetic disposition protecting Japanese women. There has to be something different about the Japanese lifestyle that changes when they move to Western countries. Many experts think that the main factor is diet and this is borne out by the fact that as the traditional Japanese diet becomes more Westernised, cases of breast cancer are increasing among Japanese women in Japan itself.

There are a number of differences between the traditional Japanese diet and our own. They eat a good quantity of unsaturated fats in oils and fish, and they do not eat much dairy food. The other main difference is their large consumption of soya bean products, including tofu, miso (soya bean paste), tamari (wheat-free soy sauce), tempeh and soya milk.

As a result of this theory, scientists have begun to study the benefits of a group of plant hormones known as phytoestrogens. These hormones naturally occur in certain foods such as soya. Soya contains two flavonoids, genistein and daidzein, and studies have shown that they are chemically similar to Tamoxifen, which is the drug used to prevent a recurrence of breast cancer.

These very weak plant oestrogens latch on to the oestrogen receptors in the breast and they stop the more powerful carcinogenic oestrogens getting through. So they have a protective effect, as well as helping to balance hormones, which are responsible for menopausal symptoms such as hot flushes. Phytoestrogens have also been studied extensively for their effect on lowering cholesterol, so they can have protective effects in terms of heart disease, which is important around the menopause.

A study published in the *British Medical Journal* in 1990 took a group of post-menopausal women and then gave them soya, linseed and red clover.[13] Ten per cent of their diet was changed, and the remaining 90 per cent of their food intake was left exactly as it was before the study. Within six weeks there was a rapid and noticeable effect on the cells of the vagina – vaginal dryness and irritation were both reduced. Another interesting observation was that the diet lowered the FSH levels of the women who changed their diets. This is the hormone that goes up during the menopause.

At the moment there are more than 4,000 articles about phytoestrogens being published every year. One 1998 study published in

Obstetrics and Gynaecology looked at the effects of soya capsules against a placebo (dummy tablets given to part of the group). Within four weeks there was a significant reduction in hot flushes in women taking soya.[14]

Although the scientists have concentrated on soya, which is an important source of phytoestrogens, there are other forms, which include linseeds, wholegrains such as brown rice, oats and legumes, including chickpeas and lentils. Garlic, fennel, celery, rhubarb, parsley and hops are also phytoestrogens.

These are the types of foods that traditional cultures would have eaten on a daily basis from childhood. What's even more exciting is the news that these phytoestrogens can also have a protective effect on men. In Japan the death rate from prostate cancer is far lower than it is in the West. It appears that these foods have a balancing effect on the hormones in both men and women.

Soya research

What is the research showing? Soya beans, for instance, contain phyto-chemicals known as isoflavones which make up about 75 per cent of the soya protein. In the human gut, bacteria convert isoflavones into compounds that can have an oestrogenic action. And yet, soya can have a balancing effect on oestrogen. One study showed that soya increased oestrogen levels when they were low and reduced them when they were too high.[15] It seems to explain why soya beans can reduce hot flushes (which are thought to be due to a lack of oestrogen) and also reduce the incidence of breast cancer (which is thought to be linked to an excess of the hormone). For more information on soya and the confusion surrounding it, see pages 24–7.

These phytoestrogens appear to fit into oestrogen receptors on breast cells. Although they are a source of oestrogen, they are probably too weak to stimulate the cells to produce cancer. What seems to happen is that these weak oestrogens *block* the oestrogen receptors and prevent cancer from developing. The flavonoid compounds that have this mild oestrogen activity also help to reduce cholesterol and decrease LDL (the 'bad' cholesterol).[16]

Supplements

Supplements are beneficial during the menopause in order to ensure that you have adequate nutrients for maintaining healthy bones (see page 420). Many of the following supplements are also known to help with the symptoms of menopause.

Vitamin C

Vitamin C is known for its beneficial effect on the immune system, strengthening blood vessels and also for its role as an antioxidant in the body (see page 15). So not only is vitamin C important for preventing illness, and for encouraging your health in general, but it also has specific benefits at menopause. Giving women vitamin C with bioflavonoids has been shown to help reduce hot flushes.[17]

Vitamin C helps to build up collagen, giving skin its elasticity. It is therefore helpful in the prevention and treatment of vaginal dryness (which can cause discomfort when the vagina loses some of its 'stretch'). It can also help retain the elasticity in the urinary tract and so prevent leakage or stress incontinence, which is common at the menopause (see pages 209–11). Collagen is also important for your bones.

Vitamin E

This is an important vitamin to consider at the menopause. Over many years clinical studies have shown its effect on reducing hot flushes.[18]

Vitamin E is also helpful for vaginal dryness and one study showed that just 400iu taken daily for between one and four months helped 50 per cent of the women given supplemental vitamin E. It can also be used internally inside the vagina every night for about six weeks to help relieve dryness.

Although most women fear breast cancer, our biggest killer is heart disease. There is now such a wealth of information on the effects of nutrition on heart disease that taking HRT to prevent this condition is illogical and, in fact, has not been proved (see page 406). In 1996 a study published in the *Lancet* showed that 2,000 patients with arteriosclerosis (fatty deposits in the arteries) had a 75 per cent reduction in their risk of heart attack when given vitamin E. At the time, researchers claimed that vitamin E was even more effective than aspirin in reducing heart attacks.[19]

B vitamins

These are called the 'stress' vitamins because they are enormously beneficial when you are under a great deal of pressure. Symptoms of

B-vitamin deficiency include anxiety, tension, irritability and poor concentration. Therefore, supplementing them in the form of a good B-complex supplement can be useful if you have any of these symptoms of stress. During the menopause it is extremely important that you give your adrenal glands (which will be called into action to produce oestrogen) a break. B vitamins will help to do this. They can also be useful if you are suffering from reduced energy levels.

Essential Fatty Acids (EFAs)

Signs of an EFA deficiency are dry skin, lifeless hair, cracked nails, fatigue, depression, dry eyes, lack of motivation, aching joints, difficulty in losing weight, forgetfulness, breast pain – all symptoms that could be 'blamed' on the menopause. If you have also tried to lose weight by going on a low-fat or no-fat diet, you are likely to be deficient in these essential fats. They need to be supplemented around the menopause because they can help with many of the symptoms. Furthermore, because they help to 'lubricate' the body in general, they can help with vaginal dryness.

Magnesium

Magnesium is an important mineral for your bones at the menopause (see page 438) so it is important that you have enough in your body. Magnesium is also known as 'nature's tranquilliser', so it will help with symptoms such as anxiety, irritability and other mood changes.

Herbs

There are a number of herbs that have traditionally been used at the menopause. The main ones are termed 'adaptogens', which have a balancing effect on the body.

Agnus castus (vitex/chastetree berry)

This is by far the most potent remedy for hot flushes as it contains the chemical precursors of the sex hormones. It stimulates and normalises the function of the pituitary gland, which controls and balances the hormones in the body. This is one of the most important herbs you can take at the menopause because it works as an adaptogen, generally balancing all hormone production.[20]

Black cohosh (*Cimicifuga racemosa*)

Black cohosh, a herb used by the Native North Americans, is very effective in restoring female hormonal balance and helps to relieve menopausal symptoms, such as hot flushes and vaginal dryness.[21]

Dong quai (*Angelica sinensis*)

This is a herb used in traditional Chinese medicine (TCM) as a tonic for the female reproductive system. It is used both for relieving hot flushes as well as vaginal dryness.

Milk thistle (*Silymarin marianum*)

This is an important herb for the liver, which is useful at the menopause to make sure that all 'old' hormones are being excreted efficiently.

It is often more effective to have a remedy that contains a combination of herbs to help with menopausal symptoms than just one herb on its own. In the clinic, I use a mix of about seven herbs to help with the symptoms. Please see page 510 (Staying in Touch) if you need extra help with taking a herbal programme

---

Warning

You should not take any of the above herbs if you are already taking HRT or any other hormonal treatment unless they are recommended by a registered, experienced practitioner.

Ginkgo biloba

As people get older, both men and women can find that their memory and concentration is not as good as it was. This is often a problem to do with age rather than hormones. The herb ginkgo biloba has been found generally to have a rejuvenating effect on the brain. A number of clinical trials have shown that it improves learning ability, memory and concentration. Studies are also being undertaken at present to establish whether ginkgo may slow down the progression of Alzheimer's disease.

A common feature of heart disease and strokes is the formation of blood clots (thrombosis) within the circulatory system. Underlying these clots can be an excess of platelet activating factors (PAFs). We now know that excess PAFs are at least partly responsible for blood clots (thrombosis) and bronchoconstriction (as occurs in asthma). Excess PAFs can be stimulated by chronic stress, a diet high in processed hydrogenated fats and exposure to allergens. Numerous studies have confirmed that ginkgo biloba extract is an extremely effective agent for inhibiting PAFs.[22]

Valerian

If you are finding it difficult to sleep, night sweats may be at the root of the problem. If the herbs and supplements listed above don't make a difference, you may want to consider valerian. This herb has been used for centuries to help with insomnia and to improve sleep quality.

Lack of sex drive

Loss of libido is very common around the menopause, but it can also affect women of any age. Sometimes it is just connected with basically not having enough energy so that when you get to bed all you really want to do is sleep. It is the ovaries that produce testosterone, the 'male' hormone, that gives us some of our drive and motivation, so women who have had their ovaries removed will often complain about lack of libido. It is important that your adrenal glands are not being overworked through stress or blood sugar fluctuations (see page 38), because they produce androgens, which are the male hormones.

Herbs can be particularly helpful for increasing sex drive. It has been noticed that St John's wort (Hypericum), which is used to help with depression, can also be helpful with libido. Damiana (*Turner aphrodisiacal*), a herb which is grown in Central America and Mexico, has been used traditionally by women and is best taken as a tincture, about 1 teaspoon half an hour before sex or once a day for a while to generally increase your sex drive. Also make sure that you are getting enough of the essential fatty acids in your diet (see page 27) or take a linseed oil 1,000mg capsule. Our hormones are manufactured from cholesterol, so a low-fat or no-fat diet can contribute to a low sex drive.

Natural medicine

Both acupuncture and homeopathy can be particularly helpful around the menopause, to deal with underlying imbalances and to control menopausal symptoms, such as hot flushes. In general terms, they will help you to cope with this stage in your life. Both therapies can be used successfully alongside the treatments outlined here.

The Treatment Plan

The aim is to eat as healthily as possible throughout the menopause, to encourage your body to balance itself. Choose foods that are known to have beneficial effects at the menopause and take herbs to help with the menopausal symptoms. Along with this, make sure that you get plenty of exercise. This is not only beneficial for your heart and weight, but it plays an important role in protecting your bones (see page 440).

There are some tests that you may find useful around the menopause, including those that assess nutritional deficiencies and bone turnover. These are described in Chapter 4.

The Integrated Approach

The dietary and supplement recommendations are important whether or not you are already taking HRT. Whatever choices you have made regarding HRT, you will need to take care of your body, so that you feel well (mentally and physically), have good levels of energy, sleep well and, in the long term, prevent heart disease and osteoporosis. If you are on HRT, there will usually be a time when you decide to stop. Whenever that time may be, you will want to be as healthy as possible.

If you are not taking HRT

Follow all the dietary recommendations, take the nutritional supplements and make sure that you are exercising regularly. If you are experiencing menopausal symptoms, use the herbs to help with the hot flushes and other problems, and add in all of the other supplements that might be useful for you. For example, if you are suffering from vaginal dryness, take vitamin E.

If you are taking HRT and want to stop

There may be many reasons why you want to stop taking HRT. You may feel that you have been on it long enough, or you may be experiencing side-effects. I see many women at the clinic who want to come off HRT for the side-effects alone. They can gain up to 2 stone (12.5kg) in weight, which doesn't seem to shift, no matter how little or well they eat. Many women also go up a couple of bra sizes, which makes them feel uncomfortable. Others have had problems with hair loss or skin rashes.

The best way to come off HRT is to take a gradual approach. Often women are simply told to 'stop'. This sudden stop can be uncomfortable and there can be something called 'rebound' effects. The symptoms such as hot flushes and night sweats can actually be worse than when starting HRT because of the sudden drop in hormones.

You need to speak to your doctor about giving up HRT. He or she may be able to give you a lower dose of the same HRT, or change the drug to another make with a lower dose. Allow yourself three months to ease yourself off HRT (taking a lower dose if possible). Then put into place the nutritional recommendations, add phytoestrogens to your diet, start taking the supplements and begin a good exercise programme. At the end of the three months, stop the HRT and use herbs if you are getting hot flushes or night sweats.

If you are taking HRT and wish to continue taking it

All women need to be as healthy as possible in order to cope with the demands on us, and the menopause is no exception. Whether or not you are taking HRT, you need to eat well and to take nutritional supplements. Take the herbs recommended for the menopause alongside HRT.

Your Supplement Plan

- A good multivitamin and mineral supplement designed for women, which includes boron, e.g. the Healthy Woman by the Natural Health Practice

- Vitamin C with bioflavonoids (1,000mg per day)

- Vitamin E (400iu per day)

- Vitamin B complex (providing 50mg of most of the B vitamins per day)

- Magnesium (300mg per day)

- Calcium citrate (500mg per day)

- Linseed oil (1,000mg per day)

Note

Each nutrient represents the total intake for one day, so if your multivitamin and mineral already contains 100mg of magnesium, for example, you only need to add in a separate magnesium supplement containing 200mg per day.

Herbs

Take a mixture of equal parts *Agnus castus*, black cohosh, dong quai and milk thistle, 1 teaspoon three times a day. If you need help with sleeping then you can take a mixture of valerian and passionflower to aid restful sleep.

To make this simpler, I have formulated a supplement called The Natural Menopack, which contains those nutrients and herbs that are known to be helpful. If you can't get this locally then call 01892 750511.

In Summary

- The menopause is not an illness, but a collection of symptoms showing a hormonal imbalance. The best way to address these symptoms is to balance your hormones naturally.

- Always investigate the cause of symptoms before taking any drugs (including HRT!), or beginning a natural treatment programme.

- Begin the Hormone Balancing Diet (see page 16).

- Stabilise blood sugar levels by reducing the amount of sugar and refined foods in your diet.

- Increase your intake of complex carbohydrates and eat them in the form of small meals, taken frequently.

- Avoid tea and coffee, and reduce your intake of dairy products and red meat.

- Ensure your diet contains sufficient essential fatty acids such as oily fish, nuts and seeds.

- Make sure that you are eating enough fibre from good sources.

- Increase your intake of phytoestrogens (see page 20), including soya.

- Make sure you are getting good levels of exercise to protect your bones (see page 440).

- Think carefully about HRT, and make a choice that suits you as an individual, carefully considering the risks versus the other benefits.

- Continue taking supplements, no matter how well you feel.

- Take herbs for three months, and if the symptoms do not improve, see a registered practitioner.

OSTEOPOROSIS

In 1993, the *Lancet* medical journal reported that the remains of an 18th-century woman were found beneath a church. Studies showed that these bones were stronger and more dense than the bones of any modern woman, either pre-menopausal or post-menopausal. Something in our modern lifestyle is clearly affecting the density and strength of our bones, and only now are we beginning to understand what that might be.

While traditionally considered to be a women's disease, osteoporosis is also found in men, although normally to a lesser degree. In this chapter, I'll examine why women are more likely to get osteoporosis and take a look at why this condition has become so prevalent. Lifestyle is one of the main factors that is within your control, and adopting a few simple changes can go a long way towards protecting the health of your bones.

What Is Osteoporosis?

The word osteoporosis literally means 'porous bones'; in other words, bones that are filled with tiny pores, or holes. Our bones change constantly – breaking down and being rebuilt as part of the living process. Two kinds of cells are important for this process, and they are known as osteoclasts and osteoblasts. Osteoclasts renew old bone by dissolving or resorbing it, leaving an empty space. The osteoblasts then fill this empty space with new bone.

If the rate of renewal does not equal the rate of breakdown, bone loss occurs. If this continues over years, the result is osteoporosis.

Are There Any Symptoms?

Unfortunately, the answer to this question may be no. Osteoporosis is often called a 'silent disease', because the first sign of the condition can be a fracture resulting from a minor accident. One patient told me that she discovered she had osteoporosis after breaking her ribs while sneezing. It has even been suggested that the majority of osteoporosis-related accidents are the result of the bone breaking, causing a fall, rather than the reverse.

This is one of the reasons why testing – and prevention – are so important.

What Is the Cause?

There are a number of factors that can contribute to the development of osteoporosis. These include:

- heredity
- premature menopause
- lack of exercise
- smoking
- certain medication
- irregular menstrual cycles
- weight
- digestive problems
- certain foods and drinks.

Heredity

It is now believed that heredity plays a major part in osteoporosis, so it is important to look back to your mother and even your grandmother to see if there are cases of osteoporosis in the family. Remember that the condition may not have been diagnosed, so consider whether there were any obvious signs, such as a dowager's hump (medically known as kyphosis; an outward curving of the spine) or height shrinkage.

Premature menopause

If your menopause takes place before you reach the age of 40, you will be at a much greater risk of developing osteoporosis. Premature menopause may have been caused by radiotherapy given to treat cancer or by surgical removal of the ovaries because of disease. Alternatively, there may be no definite cause. Menopause brought on by surgery or radiotherapy occurs suddenly, and oestrogen levels fall off sharply instead of undergoing the gradual decline you normally expect at the menopause. The suddenly low levels of oestrogen may be linked to a greater risk of osteoporosis because women who have their ovaries removed have a very rapid rate of bone loss for about five years after the surgery. Oestrogen helps to protect the bones from being dissolved (or resorbed) too quickly.

Lack of exercise

It's 'use it or lose it' for your bones when it comes to osteoporosis. Placing demands on your bones (through weight-bearing exercise, for example) encourages them to maintain their density. It is well known that astronauts lose some of their bone density while they are in space. In that gravity-free environment the body does not have to support itself, so it stops maintaining bone density. Never underestimate your body: it's perfectly logical that it would stop producing something that was not required!

If you make few demands on your bones, you will be risking osteoporosis. Even moderate exercise has been shown to increase bone density in post-menopausal women.[23] Being fit also means that improved co-ordination and flexibility makes you less likely to fall, and strengthening your muscles means you are more able to absorb the force of a fall.

Smoking

Smoking can reduce bone mass by up to 25 per cent, so it is very important that you stop. Not only can it bring on an early menopause,[24] but it can also change the pattern of female hormones into one more normally seen at the menopause, with lower levels of bone-protecting oestrogen in the blood.

Certain medication

Some drugs are known to increase the risk of osteoporosis by accelerating bone loss. If you have taken corticosteroids (steroid medication) because of a chronic inflammatory disorder such as rheumatoid arthritis or ulcerative colitis then you should be monitored carefully. Frequent use of laxatives and diuretics can also put you more at risk of osteoporosis because valuable minerals like calcium are being flushed out of the body. If you are on thyroxine for an underactive thyroid, make sure that you are only taking the dose you actually need, as excess thyroid hormone can also increase the risk of osteoporosis.[25]

The blood-thinning drug, heparin, can also increase bone loss. This is used on an increasingly common basis for miscarriage (see page 390), so you should consider the additional risks if you are being treated for recurrent miscarriage with this drug.

Irregular menstrual cycles

If you have been prone to irregular cycles or had gaps with no periods before you reach menopause, you may have an increased risk of osteoporosis. Even something as simple as losing periods through under-eating (say, from anorexia as a teenager, or while crash-dieting as a 20-something) can cause problems. Without those circulating female hormones for a number of months you will be at a higher risk of developing osteoporosis.

Research has shown that women with a history of irregular menstruation before the age of 40 have an average loss in bone density of more than 8 per cent compared to women with regular periods.[26]

Weight

When your ovaries reduce their production of oestrogen at the menopause, your fat cells produce another form of oestrogen, known as 'oestrone', to supplement this loss. As a result, it has become increasingly clear that achieving and maintaining your natural weight is extremely important not only for other health benefits, but also because you need to ensure that there is enough fat available to produce this valuable oestrone. Body mass index (BMI) is one of the best ways to determine your body fat ratio. If you fall below the normal range, you can be at an increased risk of osteoporosis. To calculate your BMI, see page 447.

A number of studies have shown that the BMI is a reliable indicator of osteoporosis risk.[27] One study showed that women aged 45 to 59 who had suffered fractures had an average BMI of 22.5 while those without fractures had an average BMI of 25.3.[28]

So this idea of being ultra-slim — fostered by the media — will be seriously detrimental in the long run if they succeed in convincing women that skinny is in. It's particularly worrying for women around the menopause, when fat stores are required to produce a form of oestrogen. Obviously there are health risks associated with overweight, but it's clear that being underweight can be just as dangerous. The answer is to find and stick to your natural weight, which should fall within the 'normal' range of the BMI. It is possible to have a fatter, post-menopausal woman producing more oestrogen than a skinny, pre-menopausal one.

Digestive problems

How well your digestive system works is generally important, but it is crucial for the prevention of osteoporosis. If you do not digest and absorb your food correctly, you will be fighting a losing battle, no matter how well you eat or what supplements you take.

Unfortunately, as we get older we produce less stomach acid (hydrochloric acid) and this can interfere with the proper absorption of calcium and other nutrients that are essential for your health and for maintaining strong bones. If you have any of the risk factors for osteoporosis listed on page 424, you have been warned that your bone density is low and/or you have symptoms of digestive problems, such as bloating, flatulence, irritable bowel syndrome or food allergies, then you need to see a practitioner to assess your digestive function.

Food and drink

Some of the substances contained in food and drinks can have a negative effect on your bones. If you have any of the risk factors, or have been told that your bone density is low, it is well worth making some changes, as described below.

Protein
Protein is the basic building block for all our cells and bones, as well as our hair, skin and nails. It is made from 25 amino acids, 8 of which are called 'essential' because we must get them from our diet, while the other 17 can be made in the body. Protein causes an acidic reaction in the body and calcium acts as a neutraliser. When you eat too much protein, your reserves of calcium, which are contained in your bones and teeth, are summoned to correct the imbalance. The calcium is then eliminated from the body through your urine. It is estimated that for every extra 15g (0.5oz) of protein that you eat, 100g (3.5oz) of calcium is lost in your urine.

In 1996 scientists at the Harvard School of Public Health in the US investigated ideal quantities of protein in our diet. They found that women who ate more than 100g (3.5oz) of animal protein a day had an increased risk of forearm fractures, compared with women who ate less than 68g (2.75oz) per day. It's interesting that women who ate vegetable rather than animal protein had no increased risk of fractures, no matter how much they ate.

Studies have shown that vegetarians do have greater bone density in later life, although that may not be the case under the age of about 40. It seems that vegetarians lose bone much more slowly than meat-eaters as they age.[29] In the end, vegetarians have a lower risk of osteo-porosis.[30]

Caffeine, sugar and alcohol

I have put these three together because they have a similar effect on the bones. They all cause extreme changes in blood sugar levels, which in turn causes the release of adrenalin. At menopause it is especially important that your adrenal glands are not overworking because they will eventually be called upon to produce a form of oestrogen, once your ovaries begin to produce less. This oestrogen from the adrenal glands can then help to protect your bones.

Both coffee and sugar cause an acidic reaction similar to protein, which leaches the calcium from your bones. For example, we now know that menopausal or post-menopausal women drinking more than two cups of coffee a day can significantly increase their risk of hip fractures.[31]

Damage caused by alcohol is also connected with osteoporosis because it increases bone loss and the incidence of fractures.[31]

Soft drinks

Soft drinks contain high levels of phosphorus. Phosphorus is an inter-esting mineral because women should not have too much of it. When phosphorus levels in your blood rise, a message is sent to your brain, telling it that there is not enough calcium. The result is that the body draws calcium from the bones and teeth to balance the high levels of phosphorus. So if you are getting too much phosphorus, you will begin to lose calcium from your bones. Phosphorus is contained in soft drinks, such as colas and other 'fizzy' drinks. The main concern is that women reach their peak bone mass by the age of 35 and it starts to decline after that. If girls are loading themselves up with soft drinks there is a possibility of having an osteoporosis epidemic in years to come.

> **Warning**
> Stop now and think carefully about these risk factors. If you
> fall into any of these categories, you should arrange to be
> tested (see below). If you do find that your bone density is
> lower than it should be (this is called osteopenia; when bone
> density is low, it is not 'proper' osteoporosis), there is time to
> make the changes that can prevent the development of full-
> blown osteoporosis.

Getting a Diagnosis

Testing for osteoporosis is important for a number of reasons, but one
of the prime reasons is that you will find it easier to make a choice
about taking HRT if you know where you stand. This may seem like
a funny way to begin this section, but one of the main justifications
for taking HRT is alleviating the risk of osteoporosis. Tests are done
to give you information and to assess the best means of treatment.
Consider your results carefully, and then consider your options (see
page 431).

> **DO YOU NEED HRT?**
>
> If you can control the symptoms of the menopause naturally (see page
> 409) and your bones are good, HRT is probably not the best option
> for you. I can see little point in risking the side-effects without good
> cause. The same goes for any medication – you will always have to
> weigh up the risks versus the benefits. However, bone density is some-
> thing that can be monitored and measured regularly. If the situation
> changes and your bones aren't as strong as they should be, you may
> be in a position to make a different choice about long-term treat-
> ment. My advice is that healthy women with healthy bones simply
> don't need unnecessary intervention.

The other benefit of testing for osteoporosis is that you know where you stand. If your bone density is lower than it should be, you can do something about it, before it becomes a problem. If you find that you are suffering from osteoporosis, rather than reduced bone density, you can take action straightaway and choose a more conventional form of treatment.

Tests give you information and allow you to make choices according to what is most appropriate for you, in your own individual circumstances. The following tests are those that are most commonly used to assess your bone status.

Dual energy X-ray absorptiometry (DEXA)

This is the 'gold standard' for measuring bone density. It is a scanner that uses two simultaneous X-ray energy beams – one high energy and the other low energy. The low energy beam can pass through soft tissue but not bone. Bone density can be calculated from how much energy the bone and soft tissues absorb from the energy beam. The scanner can measure bone mineral density at many different points on the body. This is important because mineral density (in other words, bone density) at one part of the body does not necessarily reflect the situation at other points. With osteoporosis the earliest bone loss typically starts in the trabecular bones (bones such as the spine and hip), so these are important sites to test. The disadvantage of this test is that you are exposing yourself to X-rays; however, I think it is important as a baseline measurement to know where you stand at the present time.

Ultrasound

In this procedure, sound waves are passed through the heel bone in order to provide information about bone density. It is not as precise as the DEXA scan and only the heel is measured. The idea is that the bones tested are representative of your bone density at *all* sites. This may not be the case.

Bone turnover analysis

This is a simple, non-invasive test performed on a urine sample that you collect at home. The test measures bone breakdown (in other words, how quickly your bone is rebuilding itself). As bone is renewed, chemicals are excreted in your urine. These chemicals can be measured to work out what is happening in your body. If the level of the chemicals is high, you may find that new bone formation is not keeping up with bone destruction and therefore the turnover is higher than it should be, meaning more bone is being resorbed. If this continues, your bones can become porous. Because this test is done on a urine sample, X-rays are avoided. If you'd like to arrange for a bone turnover analysis, you can do so by post (see Staying in Touch, page 507).

The best way to measure bone health is a combination of both the DEXA scan and the bone turnover analysis. A qualified practitioner can then help you to plan your best course of action, depending on the results of both of these tests. They measure your bones in two different ways, and together provide valuable information. You may be able to get a DEXA scan on the NHS if you have a strong family history of osteoporosis.

The bone turnover analysis is also extremely useful for monitoring treatment. If you decide to take HRT, start exercising, or taking supplements, this test can be repeated regularly (six-monthly is the norm) to see whether your treatment is working. A DEXA scan is usually only repeated on a two-yearly basis (rarely after one), so the urine analysis will take its place in providing essential information about the health of your bones.

What Treatment Can You Be Offered By Your Doctor?

Women are at greatest risk of hip and wrist fractures around the age of 75. HRT really may not be required until that time, contrary to popular opinion. In fact, you may not need it at all. It's important to remember that pharmaceutical companies do have a stake in the early use of HRT. If you begin this form of treatment in your mid-40s, you'll have many years of 'paying out'. Don't fall into that trap. If you choose HRT, consider the reasons carefully, and remember that unless your tests show otherwise, bone loss is not an issue until much later in your life.

The enormous revolution in testing procedures now means that your bone density can be scanned regularly. It's easy to assess whether or not a woman is at risk of osteoporosis, and it gives you every reason to postpone your decision about HRT until much later. Why wait? HRT is associated with a host of health problems, such as an increased risk of breast cancer, and there's no need to risk these if you don't need to do so. Is it logical to take HRT to prevent osteoporosis, which usually does not happen until you are 70 or 80, but which could cause breast cancer in your 50s or 60s?

HRT

For a number of years doctors have recommended that women take HRT in order to prevent and treat osteoporosis. HRT is discussed in more detail on page 403, and it's worth reading this section to get the full picture. It is interesting to note that bone mass will *only* be preserved if women continue taking HRT for more than seven years.[33] Women who take HRT for ten years can still have fractures and, as soon as they stop the HRT, they will experience a rapid decline in bone density. Indeed, one study showed that by the time women who had taken HRT when they were younger reached 75 to 80 years of age, their bone mass was only marginally higher than that of women who had never taken HRT.

The conclusion from this is that for HRT to be effective at preventing osteoporosis women need to start taking it at menopause and literally take it for all their lives.

Selective oestrogen receptor modulators (SERMS)

Many women are reluctant to stay on HRT for extended periods of time because of the risks (breast cancer is one; see page 319). Therefore, scientists have been looking at ways of creating drugs that can stimulate the production of oestrogen while avoiding any negative effects on the breasts and womb. This drug would function as an oestrogen promoter in organs where oestrogen is needed, such as the bones, while acting as an 'anti-oestrogen' in organs where unnecessary oestrogen can be dangerous (for example, the breast and womb). This new generation of designer HRTs is called SERMS. One of the newest SERMS on the scene is raloxifene, but its full potential is still being investigated. At the moment, possible side-effects include increased risk of clots and even an increase in hot flushes! In other words, it seems to be useless in the treatment of major menopausal symptoms such hot flushes and night sweats, which are, of course, one of the main reasons why women are attracted to HRT. It is, however, aimed at women who want protection for their bones without running the risk of breast cancer.

THE PROGESTERONE DEBATE

I have written a whole chapter on this subject in my book *Natural Alternatives to HRT* and my views on the use of progesterone at the menopause have not changed. In fact, they are further confirmed by the research that has been published since I wrote that book.

There has been a lot of confusion over 'natural' progesterone (as it is known). Many people have bought into this theory because they assumed they were using a natural product. This so-called 'natural' progesterone is synthesised (basically, man made) from wild yam in the laboratory. It can also be synthesised from soya. Oestrogen can be synthesised from wild yam or soya. But is it natural? The word 'natural' in front of any product does not make it something that is attuned to nature. In other words, synthesising, or creating something that is chemically identical, does not make it 'natural'.

In these terms, natural simply means chemically identical – it is a product that is identical to the hormone that your body produces from your ovaries, but it is not natural in the real sense of the word. It is not a herb. Don't be fooled.

A woman cannot eat wild yam or put it on her skin and expect her body to change it into progesterone. The body is physically unable to perform this magnificent feat. Progesterone can be made naturally in the body, but no wild yam will do it for you. If you choose a natural progesterone product (for example, a cream), make sure you are clear about the facts. You are taking a pharmaceutical hormone which constitutes HRT (hormone replacement therapy); you are just replacing the other hormone progesterone instead of oestrogen. You are not taking a wild yam product.

You can ask a number of questions of the pro-natural progesterone camp. How much should a woman take? Will she end up with too *much* progesterone (as I have seen occur in some women)? When should she stop taking it?

Dr John Lee, one of the foremost advocates of progesterone, suggests that women take it until they reach the age of 85, after which they should be reassessed. That's a long time to take any product. Dr Lee also claims that progesterone can help with osteoporosis, but the study he conducted into osteoporosis also involved women changing their diets, taking supplements and beginning an exercise programme. Alongside this, the progesterone cream was used. I suggest that it could well be factors other than the cream that were responsible for the health improvements in his patients.

There are ongoing studies into the effect of progesterone cream versus a placebo (a dummy cream), but it will be a number of years before we know the results. Right now things are uncertain, and I am concerned that women using progesterone are acting as guinea-pigs. Nobody knows yet whether it has any valuable effect on the bones. Perhaps studies will, in the long run, show this to be the case, but for the time being, remember this: progesterone is not a natural product, and by adding chemicals to your body on a daily basis you may well be taking an unacceptable risk. Do you actually need progesterone? Do you need oestrogen? Ask yourself if you need both of these hormones. Artificially adding a hormone (a drug) to the body will never address the fundamental cause of the problem. If you stop using the cream, you are back to square one, and your body will have become no healthier in the process.

What I aim to do with a more natural treatment is to use nutrition and/or herbs to encourage optimum health. This is a holistic approach, addressing all elements of your lifestyle, and it works by encouraging your body to do the work. In other words, your own body will find its natural hormone balance, which will encourage bone health and relieve a whole host of other symptoms at the same time.

It has also been suggested that progesterone can protect against breast cancer; however, at a higher level there are also concerns that higher levels of progesterone may actually be a risk factor for breast cancer.[34] We have both oestrogen and progesterone receptors in the breasts and womb. Too much oestrogen can be carcinogenic in the womb, and progesterone can protect against its effects. However, it has been shown that progesterone receptors in the breast respond differently to those in the womb,[35] and I have seen women who have had progesterone-receptor breast cancers as well as oestrogen-receptor breast cancers. What does this mean in real terms? If you are taking supplementary hormones, whether they be oestrogen or progesterone, you are increasing your risk of breast cancer. If you take oestrogen on its own, you may be increasing your risk of womb cancer and possibly even breast cancer, too.

Bisphosphonates

These are other non-hormonal drugs that are used specifically for osteoporosis. Two of the most commonly used ones are etridonate and alendronate. These drugs work by reducing the rate of bone turnover. Unfortunately, like most drugs, these have side-effects, including digestive disturbances. Alendronate seems to be the worst offender, and women are told to remain upright for at least 30 minutes after taking it because it irritates the oesophagus (the tube leading to the stomach).

Natural Treatments

If you have established osteoporosis there is no doubt that you will need some medical treatment. But don't write off the natural approach. Follow the recommendations below alongside your treatment in order to give your body the best chance of increasing bone density.

If you have been told that you do not have osteoporosis and that your bones are normal, or just below normal, it is worth following the recommendations in order either to maintain that good bone density or to prevent a minor problem from becoming a major one.

Your plan will comprise the following stages:

1. Improve your diet based on the recommendations outlined in Chapter 1.

2. Use nutritional supplements that are known scientifically to be beneficial to your bones.

3. Eliminate any foods or drink that will have a negative effect on your bones.

Dietary changes

It is important that you eat a wide variety of foods in order to get a good supply of nutrients for bone health. Follow the recommendations from Chapter 1 (see page 16) and pay particular attention to the foods and drinks mentioned under the risk factors on page 427. These are known to increase the risk of osteoporosis, and include coffee, sugar, alcohol, protein and soft drinks.

You need to be particularly careful if you are on a weight-loss diet. Some of the most popular diets of the moment focus on a high-protein intake. This is not suitable for women who are at risk of osteoporosis (nor, really, are they appropriate for anyone!). The higher your animal protein intake, the greater your bone loss. There are healthy ways to find your natural weight, and these are explained in Chapter 13, and in my book *Natural Alternatives to Dieting*.

Dairy foods

Remember that milk is an animal protein and you may be excreting more calcium than you are taking in if you eat too many dairy products. As you'll see below, calcium is not the most important aspect of osteoporosis treatment, and dairy foods are not the only source of calcium. It is interesting to note that breastfed babies absorbed more calcium from their mother's milk than from cows' milk, despite the fact that cows' milk contains four times the amount of calcium. What is crucial is how your body uses the calcium, and many people believe that our systems were not really designed to cope with cows' milk.

Tea

Tea contains caffeine, which will have an acidic effect on the body in the same way that coffee does (see pages 35–6). Fortunately, the effects are somewhat reduced with tea-drinking, so if you need your 'cuppa', take care to drink it away from mealtimes. Tannin in tea binds to important minerals such as calcium and iron, and prevents their absorption in the digestive tract. Leave a gap of at least one hour before or after eating if you are going to have a cup of regular black tea. Green tea is better, as it has antioxidant effects, but it still contains some caffeine. Therefore, it's best to keep it to a minimum, drinking mainly herbal teas, such as peppermint.

Bran

Bran is a refined food that contains substances called 'phytates'. These bind valuable minerals such as calcium and many others, including zinc and magnesium, that are essential for bone and general health. In other words, they attract these minerals, a bit like a magnet, and they are excreted with the bran from the digestive tract. Don't use bran on cereals. It is better to eat bran in the form that nature intended – in other words, as part of the wholegrain itself (wheat or oats, for example).

Supplements

The first supplement that comes to mind when considering osteoporosis is calcium. There's no doubt that calcium is important to build up and maintain the strength of our bones, but high levels in our diets or in supplements do not necessarily mean that the calcium is actually reaching our bones. When we consume calcium we need both stomach acid and vitamin D in order to absorb calcium properly.

Many other nutrients are equally crucial for healthy bones, and these include magnesium, vitamin C, vitamin D, zinc and boron. This is why it is important not to focus exclusively on calcium as a supplement for bone health, but to take a range of nutrients that are important for the bones.

Vitamin D

Vitamin D helps to regulate blood levels of both calcium and phosphorus. Without good levels of vitamin D you cannot absorb calcium from your food or your supplements. You may be getting plenty in your diet and from exposure to sunshine, but if your body thinks there is not enough in the blood, it will begin to leach it from your bones. Over time this will cause bone loss.

Vitamin C

This builds up collagen, the 'cement' that holds the bone matrix (the architecture of the bone) together, so it is as important as the minerals for prevention of osteoporosis.

Folic Acid

High homocysteine levels in menopausal women have also been associated with an increase in bone loss. Homocysteine comes from the breakdown of one of the essential amino acids (methionine) and should, under normal circumstances, be detoxified by the body. Giving women folic acid has helped to reduce the homocysteine in the blood.[36] It has been suggested that a B complex supplement that contains folic acid should be sufficient, and this will also contain vitamin B6, which is important for the bones. Vitamin B6 has been found to be deficient in people with hip fractures, and rats fed a vitamin B6–deficient diet developed osteoporosis.[37]

Calcium

You do need calcium for your bones, but you also need to be able to absorb the calcium you take. Not all calcium supplements are the same. Calcium carbonate is the cheapest form of calcium. It's literally that which is mined from the ground. This isn't a naturally occurring form of calcium, and no foods (either plant or animal) that we eat contain calcium carbonate. This is the most difficult form of calcium to absorb and you need a pretty efficient digestive system in order to manage it. If you have low levels of stomach acid (hydrochloric acid), you will struggle to absorb the calcium from a calcium carbonate supplement.

One study showed that of a group of post-menopausal women, 40 per cent were severely deficient in stomach acid. Those with the low levels only absorbed 4 per cent of the calcium from calcium carbonate, as compared to 45 per cent of the calcium from another form of calcium supplement, called calcium citrate. In another study, 500mg of calcium citrate was absorbed better than even 2,000mg of calcium carbonate.[38]

Blood-testing for calcium levels is not particularly helpful because your body has a fail-safe mechanism to take calcium from your bones if the level falls in the blood. In other words, your calcium levels might appear high even when they are not, because your body will have leached calcium from your bones. A hair mineral analysis is a better indicator because you can see high calcium turnover (the calcium level is higher than normal) in the results (see page 70 for details of how to arrange this type of test).

Excess calcium

Just as it is with everything else, balance is important. Too much calcium, especially in the wrong form (such as calcium carbonate), can lead to loss of appetite and abdominal pains. Too much calcium continually circulating in the blood means that it may be deposited in places other than in the bone, leading to painful kidney stones, for example.

Magnesium

Magnesium is just as important as calcium for your bones. It helps in metabolising calcium and vitamin C and helps to convert vitamin D to the active form necessary to ensure that calcium is efficiently absorbed by your body. A study conducted by Biolab in London compared different groups of women, some with osteoporosis, some post-menopausal but with no osteoporosis, and some on HRT.[39] They found that none of the women in any group had low levels of calcium. But the women with osteoporosis had low levels of other bone nutrients, including magnesium and zinc. They also had low levels of the enzyme alkaline phosphatase, which is an indication that the bone is not renewing itself adequately. Magnesium is required for normal levels of this enzyme.

Not having enough magnesium can stop bone growth, decrease bone cell activity and make the bones more fragile. Magnesium also prevents the build-up of unwanted calcium deposits elsewhere in the body. In a 1991 research project, one group of women took HRT plus magnesium. The other group took HRT alone. After nine months the bone mineral density of the women taking magnesium had increased by 11 per cent. The women taking only HRT showed no increase in bone mineral density. After two years the magnesium takers were still improving their bone density.[40] Good sources of dietary magnesium include dark green vegetables, apples, seeds, nuts, figs and lemons. Unfortunately, if you choose white bread instead of wholewheat, there can be as much as 82 per cent loss of magnesium from the refining process; the level of loss is 83 per cent between white and brown rice.[41]

Boron

Boron is another mineral that is being widely studied in relation to osteoporosis. Research conducted by the US Department of Agriculture demonstrated that giving post-menopausal women a short course of 3mg boron supplements daily resulted in a 44 per cent reduction in the amount of calcium excreted in their urine.[42] The conclusions of this study were that boron improved the metabolism (the way it is used by the body) of both calcium and magnesium. Boron is found in alfalfa, kelp, cabbage and leafy greens.

Zinc

Zinc helps vitamin D absorb calcium.[43] Zinc is needed for the proper formation of osteoclasts and osteoblasts, the two cells that are essential for bone turnover. Zinc has been found to be deficient in older people with osteoporosis.[44]

Ipriflavone

This is a derivative of soya that is taken in supplement form. Soya is discussed in detail in Chapter 1, but ipriflavone has been studied specifically in relation to osteoporosis. Two large clinical trials over a two-year period showed a significant difference in bone loss in those women taking the ipriflavone as compared to those on placebo.[44]

Exercise

Exercise is extremely important in the prevention of osteoporosis. You need to ensure that you are doing some weight-bearing exercise (such as brisk walking, running, tennis, badminton, stair-climbing and aerobics). Over the years our lifestyles have changed, and we have become more sedentary. We now have washing machines, most of us use the car to go shopping, and many of our jobs involve sitting behind a computer or another piece of technology. We need, therefore, to make time for exercise – to fit it into an already busy schedule. Don't be tempted to put it on the bottom of your to-do list. It's a priority for the prevention of osteoporosis, and a wide range of other health conditions. If you'd like some guidance about undertaking a good exercise programme, you'll find details in my book: *Natural Alternatives to HRT.*

Stress

Stress is bad for your bones. The reason for this is that when we are stressed we produce a hormone called adrenaline (see page 44), which should really only be brought into play in a life-threatening situation. Unfortunately, many of us live our lives under extremely stressful circumstances and adrenaline is pumped out on a daily basis. Our bodies believe we are in danger, and put us in 'alert' mode, ready to fight and flee. There are two issues here. First of all, the adrenal glands are not limitless. They can actually become exhausted and fail to function properly, which can be very dangerous in the case of osteoporosis. As you read on page 401, the adrenal glands are able to produce oestrogen when the body needs it (when our bodies reach menopause and our ovaries are no longer up to the job). If they are worn out, they won't be able to perform this crucial task. Secondly, when you are stressed, your energies are diverted away from everyday functions such as digestion, which means that you won't be getting the nutrients you need from your food. In the long run that can lead to severe malnutrition, which will undoubtedly affect the health of your bones.

Herbs

Herbs such as horsetail and alfalfa are often used alongside dietary recommendations, supplements and exercise for the long-term treatment of osteoporosis. Herbs that are rich in calcium and other minerals are required. A number of dried herbs can be made into a herbal tea and drunk on a regular basis. The best ones to choose (and you can blend these together) are: horsetail (*Equisetum arvense*), alfalfa herb (*Medicago sativa*) and nettles (*Urtica spp.*)

The Treatment Plan

The aim is to prevent osteoporosis, by ensuring that you are eating well, avoiding anything in excess that can cause you to lose bone, exercising and using supplements to ensure that you have all the nutrients your bones need to be healthy. Use a mix of herbs, taken in the form of herbal teas, to support the supplements.

The Integrated Approach

If tests show that you have osteoporosis, you will need to take medical advice. It may be more appropriate for you to take drugs that are particularly aimed at the treatment of osteoporosis, rather than HRT. This is something that will need to be discussed with your specialist.

Even if you do need to take medication, it is essential that you put into place all of the dietary recommendations listed here, that you get enough exercise and that you are taking supplements to boost your nutrient intake.

Your Supplement Plan

- A good multivitamin and mineral supplement containing boron, e.g. The Healthy Woman by the Natural Health Practice

- Vitamin B complex (50mg of most of the B vitamins per day; including the amount you get from your multivitamin and mineral supplement)

- Vitamin C with bioflavonoids (1,000mg per day)

- A combined magnesium and calcium citrate supplement (with up to 500mg of calcium citrate per day)

- Zinc citrate (15mg per day)

- Linseed oil (1,000mg per day, for general health)

> **Note**
> Each nutrient represents the total intake for one day, so if your multivitamin and mineral already contains 15mg of zinc citrate, for example, you would not need to add a separate zinc citrate supplement.

Herbs

If you have any of the risk factors above or have been told you have low bone density, take a cupful of herbal tea each day, with a mix of horsetail, alfalfa and nettles.

In Summary

- It's very important that you have your bones monitored regularly, particularly if you belong to the group of women who have a higher risk of osteoporosis (see page 424).

- If you find that you have osteoporosis, or even signs of severe bone loss, don't hesitate to take medical treatment. However, you should use the natural programme alongside to make it more effective. Have your bones reassessed regularly to ensure that everything is working as it should.

- If your bones are fine, or showing only minor signs of bone loss, follow the natural programme and have your bones reassessed to ensure that it is working.

- Make sure that you get plenty of weight-bearing exercise to improve bone health.

- Stop smoking. There's no doubt that this will negatively affect the health of your bones.

- If you are on regular medication, such as steroids, make sure you get your bones tested.

- Ensure that you are not underweight, which can reduce oestrogen levels in the body.

- Make sure you aren't eating too much animal protein. Stick to vegetable proteins whenever possible.

- Cut your intake of caffeine, sugar, alcohol and soft drinks as much as possible.

- Begin the hormone balancing diet in Chapter 1 (see page 16).

- Cut down on dairy produce.

- Don't drink tea with meals.

- Avoid using bran, except in its natural, whole form (see page 436).

- Take steps to reduce stress in your life. Consider a relaxation therapy, and make sure that you are getting enough rest.

- Take supplements (see page 441) and, if your bone density is low, see a qualified practitioner for extra help.

- Take one cup of herbal tea (see page 442) every day.

CHAPTER 13

Weight

Although both men and women can have weight problems, I have included this section in the book because it is an issue that affects so many women. Most women I see mention their weight in relation to their overall health, and on the basis of that concern, I have addressed the main issues that affect women.

OVERWEIGHT

Women form the majority of people dieting, joining a slimming club, trying the next 'quick-fix' solution to weight problems and they are the main purchasers of low-calorie and low-fat foods. It's also a fact that four times as many women as men will be diagnosed with an underactive thyroid (see page 450), which can affect your weight.

Overweight is the issue that concerns the most women, but there are some women who find it difficult to put on weight. In most cases there are health problems at the root of an inability to put on or keep on weight. It is these problems that need to be addressed. For this reason, I'll focus on the issues of overweight here, which can be successfully and permanently treated using natural means.

WOMEN HAVE MORE FAT CELLS THAN MEN

Excess weight is a bigger problem for women because we are built differently – and for a reason. A man has 26 billion fat cells (called adipocytes) in his body, while women have around 35 billion. Fat comprises 27 per cent of an average woman's total body weight, while men have only 15 per cent fat.

There are biological reasons for this. Fat is essential for reproduction and therefore fat stores are naturally laid down on women's bodies, in the event that there may be a pregnancy on the horizon. Fat is necessary for ovulation, and it's a well-known fact that girls do not begin to menstruate until their bodies are composed of at least 17 per cent fat. If a woman becomes too thin (in other words, loses too much body fat), her periods can stop and she will be unable to conceive.

So in a sense we already start at a disadvantage on the weight front. But remember, it's part of nature's survival mechanism for the human race.

Your Ideal Weight

How do you know what your ideal weight should be? According to the height and weight tables formulated for insurance companies, you'd think that everyone of the same height should weigh the same. Obviously this isn't the case!

All of us are built differently, and our body shapes can make a big difference to the amount of weight we can carry healthily. Furthermore, fit women will always look slimmer but weigh more, largely because muscle weighs so much more than fat. It's even possible to be underweight with unacceptably high levels of body fat.

It became clear that another method of assessing weight needed to be developed, and this is where the body mass index comes in.

Body mass index

If you want a rough idea of your 'ideal' weight then the body mass index (BMI) is the best indicator. It tries to identify the percentage of body tissue that is actually fat. It does have disadvantages in that it cannot allow for variations in fat, bone, organs and muscle, but it provides a broader range for what is considered to be normal.

Your BMI is the ratio of your height to your weight and is calculated as follows:

$$BMI = \text{your weight in kg divided by the square of your height in metres}$$

For example, if my weight is 63.5kg (10 stone) and my height is 1.68m (5ft 6in), my BMI is $63.5 \div (1.68 \times 1.68) = 22.5$

What does your BMI mean?

Under 20:	underweight
20–25	normal
25–30	overweight
30–40:	obese
Over 40:	dangerously obese

One of the best and most convenient ways to measure body fat is to use an electronic machine that uses bioelectrical impedance. Sound confusing? It's simple to understand. An electric current is passed though the body and the machine measures how long it takes for the current to come out, providing you with a measurement of your total body fat. Lean tissue is a much better conductor of electricity than fatty tissue, so the machine is able to measure the percentage of fat in the body.

stones	ft	4.10	4.11	5.0	5.1	5.2	5.3	5.4	5.5	5.6	5.7	5.8	5.9	5.10	5.11
	cms	147	150	152	155	158	160	163	165	168	170	173	175	178	180
	kgs														
6.11	43	20	19	19	18	17	17	16	16	15	15	14	14	14	13
6.13	44	20	20	19	18	18	17	17	16	16	15	15	14	14	14
7.1	45	21	20	19	19	18	18	17	17	16	16	15	15	14	14
7.3	46	21	20	20	19	18	18	18	17	17	16	16	15	15	14
7.6	47	22	21	20	20	19	18	18	17	17	16	16	15	15	15
7.8	48	22	21	21	20	19	18	18	18	17	17	16	16	15	15
7.10	49	23	22	21	20	20	19	18	18	17	17	16	16	15	15
7.12	50	23	22	22	21	20	20	19	18	18	17	17	16	16	15
8	51	24	23	22	21	20	20	19	19	18	18	17	17	16	16
8.3	52	24	23	23	22	21	20	20	19	18	18	17	17	16	16
8.5	53	25	24	23	22	21	21	20	19	19	18	18	17	17	16
8.7	54	25	24	23	22	22	21	20	20	19	19	18	18	17	17
8.9	55	25	24	24	23	22	21	21	20	19	19	18	18	17	17
8.11	56	26	25	24	23	22	22	21	21	20	19	19	18	18	17
9	57	26	25	25	24	23	22	21	21	20	20	19	19	18	18
9.2	58	27	26	25	24	23	23	22	21	21	20	19	19	18	18
9.4	59	27	26	26	25	24	23	22	22	21	20	20	19	19	18
9.6	60	28	27	26	25	24	23	23	22	21	21	20	20	19	19
9.9	61	28	27	26	25	24	24	23	22	22	21	20	20	19	19
9.11	62	29	28	27	26	25	24	23	23	22	21	21	20	20	19
9.13	63	29	28	27	26	25	25	24	23	22	22	21	21	20	19
10.1	64	30	28	28	27	26	25	24	24	23	22	21	21	20	20
10.3	65	30	29	28	27	26	25	24	24	23	22	22	21	21	20
10.6	66	31	29	29	27	26	26	25	24	23	23	22	22	21	20
10.8	67	31	30	29	28	27	26	25	25	24	23	22	22	21	21
10.10	68	31	30	29	28	27	26	25	24	24	23	22	22	21	21
10.12	69	32	31	30	29	28	27	26	25	24	24	23	23	22	21
11	70	32	31	30	29	28	27	26	26	25	24	23	23	22	22
11.3	71	33	32	31	30	28	28	27	26	25	25	24	23	22	22
11.5	72	33	32	31	30	29	28	27	26	26	25	24	24	23	22
11.7	73	34	32	32	30	29	29	27	27	26	25	24	24	23	23
11.9	74	34	33	32	31	30	29	28	27	26	26	25	24	23	23
11.11	75	35	33	32	31	30	29	28	28	27	26	25	24	24	23
12	76	35	34	33	32	30	29	28	28	27	26	25	25	24	23
12.2	77	36	34	33	32	31	30	29	28	27	27	26	25	24	24
12.4	78	36	35	34	32	31	30	29	29	28	27	26	25	25	24
12.6	79	37	35	34	33	32	31	30	29	28	27	26	26	25	24
12.8	80	37	36	35	33	32	31	30	29	28	28	27	26	25	25
12.11	81	37	36	35	34	32	32	30	30	29	28	27	26	26	25
12.13	82	38	36	35	34	33	32	31	30	29	28	27	27	26	25
13.1	83	38	37	36	35	33	32	31	30	29	29	28	27	26	26
13.3	84	39	37	36	35	34	33	32	31	30	29	28	27	27	26
13.5	85	39	38	37	35	34	33	32	31	30	29	28	28	27	26
13.8	86	40	38	37	36	34	34	32	32	30	30	29	28	27	27
13.10	87	40	39	38	36	35	34	33	32	31	30	29	28	27	27
	cms	147	150	152	155	158	160	163	165	168	170	173	175	178	180
	ft	4.10	4.11	5.0	5.1	5.2	5.3	5.4	5.5	5.6	5.7	5.8	5.9	5.10	5.11

Imperial measures given are only approximates

BMI = kg/m^2

Body Mass Index chart

These are available for use in the home, look just like ordinary scales and can also be used to weigh yourself normally. (If you have trouble obtaining one of these machines locally, please see Staying in Touch, page 507)

The Causes of Weight Gain

There are many reasons why you may gain weight and the cause may not be one factor but a combination of a number of different ones.

Dieting

Yes, one of the main causes of weight gain is dieting. Dieting makes you fat. As you reduce your food intake to lose weight, your body put itself on 'famine alert'. It gets the impression that food is scarce and therefore it slows down your metabolism to get the best use of the small amount of food it is receiving.

When you say you want to lose weight, what you actually want to lose is fat. If you lose weight rapidly, almost 25 per cent of that weight loss can be made up of water, bone, muscle and other lean tissue.

The reason for this is that your body is actually programmed to hold on to fat. So in times of what your body considers to be 'famine', it will actually go as far as breaking down muscle and losing water in order to hold on to its fat reserves. Faddy diets suggest that you can lose up to 4.5kg (10lb) in a week, but remember this: it is physically impossible to lose more than 900g (2lb) of body fat in a week.

Furthermore, if you lose weight quickly by restricting your intake and then go back to eating normally, a much higher percentage of the food you eat is laid down as fat. Why? Because your body wants to build up *extra* fat stores, in case this type of famine occurs again. There's also the question of metabolism. When you crash-diet, your metabolism slows down to conserve energy and make the most out of the small amounts you are eating. So, what happens when you go back to eating normally? Well, everything you eat is being dealt with at a much slower rate and more fat is stored.

It's a pretty vicious cycle, too. You go on a diet, then put on *more* weight. You are forced to diet, and it happens again. So you can be fatter after dieting than you would ever have been if you'd left things well enough alone. This is the yo-yo syndrome, and it's a common feature of weight problems.

Too much food and not enough exercise

This is the obvious reason, because if you eat more than you burn off then you are going to gain weight. The idea has been that if the number of calories going into your body is less than the calories being used up by bodily activity and exercise, then you will lose weight. Nowadays, we know that the type of calories is also an important factor in this equation. In other words, you need to consider what type of calories you are eating – whether they come in the form of fat, carbohydrates or protein.

The type of food you eat

Researchers have found that fat and thin people can eat roughly the same number of calories, but it seems that the *type* of food they are eating is different.

This is a very popular theory that goes something like: too much fat makes you fat. This may be right in principle (large amounts of saturated fat in the diet are not healthy), but it's important to remember that some fats are absolutely essential, hence their name: essential fatty acids. These EFAs, as they are known, are discussed in detail in Chapter 1, but what you need to know here is that they are important for overall health and, interestingly, weight loss. In fact, EFAs are absolutely crucial for keeping your metabolism working at optimum level.

The result of this theory is that women go on low-fat and no-fat diets, which are dangerous. Furthermore, no-fat and low-fat food tends to be high in sugar and salt, which is required to make it palatable. This is the type of thing that makes you fat. In fact, it's sugar and other foods that are 'fast-releasing' (see page 38) that will encourage weight gain, and here's why: the speed with which a food increases blood sugar (in other words, whether it is 'fast-releasing' or 'slow-releasing') determines whether or not it will cause you to gain weight. If your blood-sugar levels rise very quickly your body has to secrete more insulin in order to control it.

Every time you eat, your body has a choice: it can either burn that food as energy or store it as fat. Researchers have found that high insulin levels cause you not only to change your food into fat, but they also prevent your body from breaking down previously stored fat.

These fast-releasing foods include anything that contains sugar and refined flour, such as cakes, biscuits, pastries and other 'treats'.

If you crave sweet or starchy foods, feel tired during the afternoon, light-headed, dizzy or shaky if you miss a meal or wake up feeling tired after a full night's sleep, then your blood-sugar levels are probably fluctuating too much It's important that you pay particular attention to the recommendations on page 458.

Underactive thyroid

An underactive thyroid can be at the root of gradual weight gain, and it should be checked out by your doctor. See the panel below for details of symptoms.

THYROID PROBLEMS

If you answer 'yes' to four or more of the following questions, your thyroid gland could be underactive. Visit your doctor for a blood test, which can establish how well your thyroid is functioning.

- Has your weight gone up gradually over months for no apparent reason?
- Do you often feel cold?
- Are you constipated?
- Are you depressed, forgetful or confused?
- Are you losing hair or is it drier than it used to be?
- Are you having menstrual problems?
- Are you having difficulty getting pregnant?
- Have you noticed a lack of energy?
- Are you getting headaches?

The thyroid gland situated in your neck helps control your metabolism. It produces two hormones, thyroxine and triidothyronine. These hormones are produced when a message is sent from the hypothalamus and the pituitary glands, which also produces thyroid-stimulating hormones (TSH) and thyrotrophin-releasing hormones.

The thyroid gland is like a thermostat that regulates your body temperature by secreting the two hormones that control how quickly the body burns calories and uses energy. An underactive thyroid, or hypothyroidism, is a deficiency of thyroid hormone caused by one of

---

two things: either your pituitary gland is not producing TSH; or your thyroid is not working properly.

If a blood test does not show that you have an underactive thyroid, you may only have a mild problem, which could go undetected in a blood test. The other way to test whether you have low thyroid function is to measure your temperature. If your temperature is too low, it may indicate that you have a sluggish metabolism caused by an underactive thyroid.

Take your temperature once a day for three days. If you are having periods, then take your temperature on the second, third and fourth days of the cycle. A woman's body temperature rises after ovulation so it would not give a clear picture if done later in the cycle. If you are not menstruating, take your temperature on any three consecutive days.

Put a thermometer by your bed before you go to sleep (a mercury thermometer is fine but there are some good electronic ones on the market). When you wake, lie still in bed and take your temperature before drinking or visiting the bathroom. Put the thermometer in your armpit and leave it until it bleeps. If you are using a mercury thermometer, leave it for ten minutes.

If your average temperature over the three days falls below 36.4°C (97.6°F), your thyroid may be under-functioning.

WHAT YOUR DOCTOR MIGHT SUGGEST

If a blood test shows that your thyroid is not functioning properly, you would normally be given the drug thyroxine. Side-effects are usually only a problem if it is given in excessively high doses and it is normal procedure for you to be monitored to ensure that you are taking the correct dose.

Unfortunately an underactive thyroid problem may not be accurately diagnosed because it has not been tested. Furthermore, because blood tests can look normal, a diagnosis may not be given. Someone with all of the symptoms of an underactive thyroid may have normal blood tests – which can occur when the thyroid gland is producing enough hormones but the cells that are supposed to latch on to the hormones are not picking them up. This is one reason why the temperature test (see above) can be so useful.

NATURAL SOLUTIONS
Key foods to consider

Some foods are termed goitrogens, which means that they can block the uptake of iodine and so worsen an underactive thyroid problem. These include turnips, cabbage, peanuts, soya, pine nuts and millet. These foods only seem to be a problem when they are raw and eaten excessively, so make sure they are cooked well and eaten in moderation.

On the other hand, foods such as seaweed, which are low in calories, have a very good mineral content including the trace minerals zinc, manganese, chromium, selenium and cobalt, and the macro minerals calcium, magnesium, iron and also iodine. Iodine is essential for the healthy functioning of the thyroid gland. Scientific studies have shown that the consumption of seaweed can also have anti-cancer benefits[1] and can reduce cholesterol and improve fat metabolism.[2]

If you would like to know how to use seaweed in your cooking then read my book *Natural Alternatives to HRT Cookbook*.

SUPPLEMENTS

Supplements can help to optimise the proper functioning of the thyroid gland.

Selenium

This is a very useful mineral for the treatment of an underactive thyroid as it helps to ensure the proper functioning of the thyroid hormones. Low levels of selenium have been linked to underactive thyroid problems.[3]

HERBS

The two hormones produced by the thyroid gland (called thyroxine and triidothyronine) are made from iodine and the amino acid tyrosine. Naturally rich sources of iodine are seafoods, especially saltwater fish, and seaweeds such as kelp. Herbalists have traditionally used bladderwrack (*Fucus vesiculosus*), which is a seaweed, to help with an underactive thyroid. This is normally taken as a supplement, but if you are lucky enough to be able to buy it fresh or dried, you can make an infusion by pouring a cup of boiling water on to 10–15ml (two to three teaspoons) of dried bladderwrack and leaving it for ten minutes. This infusion can be drunk three times a day.

> **Warning**
> If you take too much iodine, you can actually make an under-active thyroid condition worse. It is recommended that you see a qualified practitioner for help with thyroid problems.

Nutritional deficiencies

Food can be converted into fat or energy. You can either store what you eat, which means you will probably put on weight, or you can use it for energy. Whether food is burned or stored is determined by a number of chemical reactions that take place in your body. These are activated by enzymes, which are, in turn, dependent upon vitamins and minerals. Therefore, if you are deficient by even a little in certain vitamins and minerals, you will gain weight (see page 449).

Prescription drugs

Weight gain is often linked to certain medication, such as HRT, the contraceptive pill and steroids. Some antidepressants can also cause increased appetite and weight gain. If you have to take medication, discuss your weight problem with your doctor and ask if there are alternative drugs you could take. Never stop taking any drug without the advice and supervision of your doctor.

Food allergies

Could a food allergy be making it difficult for you to lose weight? A good clue would be whether you crave a particular food that you eat frequently. Once a food allergy exists the food becomes mildly addictive and you can feel compelled to eat it. If you are allergic to a food, your body can react by storing it away instead of using it for energy. If you eat a lot of foods to which you are allergic, there will undoubtedly be weight gain.

There are two types of allergic reactions:

- **Type A (classic allergy)** – In this type of allergy, you will experience a reaction immediately after contact with an allergen (such as shellfish or peanuts, for example).

- **Type B (delayed allergy or intolerance)** – Here the reaction can take place between one hour or three days after ingesting the food. Symptoms such as weight gain, bloating, water retention, fatigue, aching joints and headaches can all be due to a Type B allergy.

It is now possible to have a blood test that analyses the effects of 217 different foods and food additives. This test measures the release of certain chemicals that are responsible for the symptoms of food intolerance. Once you find out what foods are causing problems, they can be avoided for a short period of time. Unlike the foods implicated in Type A allergies, you do not have to avoid these foods indefinitely. Giving your body a rest from them, and then ensuring that they don't make up too large a percentage of your diet will probably do the trick. If you'd like more details of this blood test, see page 507.

Artificial sweeteners

You may be tempted to substitute sugar with artificial sweeteners in order to cut calories. Don't. If a food or drink is described as 'low sugar', 'diet' or 'low calorie', it will usually contain a chemical sweetener, such as aspartame. You may think that you are at least avoiding sugar (which is fattening) by adding in artificial sweeteners but, ironically, it has also been found that people who regularly use artificial sweeteners tend to gain weight because these sweeteners increase the appetite.[4] Aspartame is 180 times sweeter than sugar and using it can lead to binge eating disorders and obesity. The use of aspartame has been linked to mood swings and depression because it alters the levels of the brain chemical serotonin.[5] My advice is to avoid any foods or drinks which contain artificial sweeteners. You will need to read the labels, as they are found in fizzy drinks, yoghurts, desserts and many other foods.

As you give up sugar and artificial sweeteners your taste-buds will change, and you will start to taste the natural sweetness of foods such as vegetables and grains. If you need some sort of sweetener, use a small amount of honey, maple syrup, brown rice syrup, barley malt syrup or stevia (most of these will be available in healthfood shops).

Yeast overgrowth

Do you suffer from any of these symptoms?

- Sugar cravings
- Cravings for foods such as wine, bread, cheese
- Migraines or headaches
- Chronic thrush
- Inability to lose weight
- Tired all the time
- Often feel spaced out
- Feel drunk on a small amount of alcohol
- Feel bloated and have flatulence

If these symptoms seem familiar, then you may have a yeast over-growth such as *Candida albicans* (see page 263).

We all have the yeast candida in our gut, but it is usually controlled by other bacteria. When the immune system is compromised (because of illness, for example, or a poor diet), the proportion of 'healthy' bacteria can be altered, causing candida to grow out of control.

This overgrowth can be also be caused by overuse of antibiotics, the contraceptive pill, HRT, steroids and stress. You can be tested for yeast overgrowth (see page 265). In Chapter 8 on thrush, yeast infections are discussed in detail.

What Treatment Can You Be Offered By Your Doctor?

Most doctors would be conservative in treating overweight and the first line of approach would normally be dieting. They would be reluctant to prescribe drugs unless a woman was clinically obese and the weight was a threat to her health. The same would apply to surgery for weight problems.

However, there are private slimming clinics where drugs are given to help with weight loss even when a woman is not obese. Furthermore, surgery can be obtained from private clinics.

None of the drugs or surgical techniques address *why* someone is overweight. The dieter has not learned a new way of eating, so a return to 'old' eating habits once the drugs are stopped or the jaw unwired, for instance, can cause quite a rapid gain in weight. In the end your eating habits have to be a way of life, not a diet that you do for a short-term solution.

Drugs

On-going monitoring and supervision needs to be available when people are on any weight loss medication, but some slimming clinics sell these drugs without that back-up. These types of drugs are designed for clinically obese people, in situations where overweight is life-threatening. What's happening now is that such drugs have become the lazy approach to weight-loss, and perfectly healthy (and often slim) men and women are risking serious side-effects and long-term damage in search of a quick-fix solution. Do not consider these drugs unless your doctor suggests that they are essential.

Amphetamine-based drugs

These drugs work by reducing hunger and cause weight loss by stimulating the stress response (see page 44). Some can be addictive, as they provide a feeling of euphoria. But side-effects of phentermine, one of the most widely used, include restlessness, dry mouth, high blood pressure and hallucinations.

Orlistat

A drug containing orlistat is now available on prescription, and it works by reducing the body's capacity to absorb fat into the bloodstream. Instead of being digested, the fat is excreted. The drug prevents absorption of about one-third of fat (about 600 calories a day), which should lead to a weight loss of about 450g (1lb) a week. Because excess fat goes straight through the body, dieters are asked to eat a low-fat diet to prevent diarrhoea. However, there are other side-effects, including anal leakage, flatulence and bowel pain. This drug can prevent the absorption of vitamins A, D, E and K, which are fat soluble, as well as essential fatty acids, all of which are important for health.

The surgical approach

Surgery is the most drastic approach to weight loss and, not surprisingly, it does not actually address the root of the problem. Every one of us, regardless of shape or size, needs to change our eating patterns to keep our weight under control. Surgical methods may work in the short term, but the minute that you start eating 'normally', your weight will come back. Even worse, some of these procedures are downright dangerous.

Jaw wiring

This technique involves wiring the jaw so that only liquids can be taken. Once the weight loss is achieved the wiring is removed. Sadly, it has seldom worked in the long term as lost weight is usually regained once the jaws are unwired.

Stomach stapling

Under anaesthetic, the stomach is literally stapled to make it much smaller. You would feel full more quickly and stop eating sooner. Unfortunately, it doesn't always work because the stomach can be stretched by overeating, even when stapled. The staples can also burst, which requires major surgery to repair.

Two other techniques that work on the same principle as the staple are the lap band (where a giant silicone band is placed around the stomach) and the stomach balloon (where a silicone balloon is inserted into the stomach and then inflated). The balloon stays in place for up to six months before being burst and removed via the mouth.

Liposuction

In this procedure, fat is sucked out from under the skin while the dieter is fully conscious. (It is usually only performed around the hip and thigh areas.) Women have complained of being left with baggy skin, which has been excessive in some cases. In some cases, this operation has been fatal.

Stomach by-pass

This is an even more drastic surgical technique, which involves stapling the stomach, and creating a shortcut around the upper digestive tract and bypassing 1.5m (5ft) of small intestine. The name of this procedure is misleading – it is actually a section of the small intestine rather than the stomach that is bypassed! This technique reduces the number of calories absorbed and also makes you sick if you try to overindulge. Side-effects can be liver and kidney damage because of the interference with digestion.

Natural Treatments

There is no 'quick fix' to losing weight. It is easy to try one diet after another, but this will never be a long-term solution. The only way to lose weight safely and to keep it off is to change your eating habits, and then ensure that those new, healthier eating habits become a way of life.

There's no point in adopting strict measures that prevent you from living life to the fullest. After all, food is there to be enjoyed. You need a way of eating where you can eat out with friends, and socialise without having to forgo the meal. Real and permanent fat loss (not just weight loss) has to be gradual and it takes time. The important thing, however, is that this approach works, and your weight will stay off.

There are four stages to the treatment plan:

1. Improve your diet, based on the recommendations outlined in Chapter 1.

2. Make sure that your blood sugar is in balance, which reduces cravings.

3. Use specific nutritional supplements that are known to help with weight loss.

4. Follow an exercise programme that you enjoy.

Dietary changes

Follow the recommendations in Chapter 1 (see page 16). Pay particular attention to the section on complex carbohydrates, because these help to keep your blood sugar in balance. Reduce or eliminate foods made with white flour or white sugar, and avoid refined foods where the fibre and goodness has been stripped away. These are 'fast-releasing' foods (see page 38), and can have detrimental effects on blood sugar and then your weight.

Cut out all sugar and artificial sweeteners. You will have to become a label reader because sugar can be added to almost anything, including savoury foods such as baked beans, tomato ketchup and even bread. In order to make sugar content appear lower, manufacturers list all the different types of sugar separately (look for words ending in -ose, such as fructose, glucose and sucrose). Don't be fooled. They all have relatively the same effects on our bodies.

A very simple tip to help with weight loss is to chew well and to take your time when eating. It takes your brain 20 minutes to register that you are full, so if you eat more slowly, you will actually want to eat less.

When you eat matters

This idea is discussed in much greater detail in Chapter 1. What is important to know now is that skipping meals can slow down your metabolism because your body thinks there is a shortage of food. It's better to eat little and often, to keep your blood sugar levels (and your metabolism) steady.

Glycaemic index

This is a measurement of how 'fast-releasing' or 'slow-releasing' a food is. This is explained fully in my book *Natural Solutions to Dieting*, but the basic premise is described below.

Glucose is the fastest-releasing carbohydrate and it raises insulin to the highest level, so it is given a score of 100 on the glycaemic index. Everything else is measured against glucose. Why does this matter? As discussed on page 38, foods that raise insulin levels prevent your body from breaking down previously stored fat, and help to ensure that the food you do eat is laid down as fat rather than used for energy.

The simplest way to work out the glycaemic index of a particular food, without resorting to charts before every meal, is to consider how refined it is. The more refined the food, the faster it will be digested, and the bigger its impact on your insulin levels will be. The result? If it's highly refined, it's going to make you fat. Go for foods that are in their most natural state, and base your diet around fibre-rich foods such as brown rice. Fibre slows down the release of sugars and gives them a lower GI.

Exercise

The benefits of regular exercise cannot be exaggerated. Regular exercise has been linked to a lower risk of breast cancer and an improved immune system. It helps to keep your bowels working efficiently, which means you are eliminating waste products your body doesn't need. It stimulates your thyroid gland and it helps to improve thyroid function, which has a direct effect on your metabolism.

Which exercise?

Studies have shown that the best way to lose weight is to exercise for longer periods of time. This is because fat can only be mobilised in the presence of oxygen. If you exercise to the point of puffing and panting, your oxygen supplies will be low.

Sugars	GI Score	Fruit	GI Score
Glucose	100	Watermelon	72
Honey	87	Pineapple	66
Sucrose (sugar)	59	Melon	65
		Raisins	64
Grains and Cereals	**GI Score**	Banana	62
French baguette	95	Kiwi fruit	52
White rice	72	Grapes	46
Bagel	72	Orange juice	46
White bread	70	Orange	40
Ryvita	69	Apple juice	40
Brown rice	66	Apple	39
Muesli	66	Plum	39
Pastry	59	Pear	38
Basmati rice	58	Grapefruit	25
White spaghetti	50	Cherries	25
Porridge oats	49		
Instant noodles	46	**Vegetables**	**GI Score**
Wholegrain wheat bread	46	Parsnips (cooked)	97
Wholemeal spaghetti	42	Potatoes (baked)	85
Wholegrain rye bread	41	Potatoes (fried)	75
Barley	26	Potatoes (boiled)	70
		Beetroot (cooked)	64
Pulses	**GI Score**	Sweetcorn	59
Baked beans	48	Sweet potatoes	54
Butter beans	36	Potato crisps	54
Chickpeas	36	Peas	51
Blackeye beans	33	Carrots	49
Harricot beans	31		
Kidney beans	29		
Lentils	29		
Soya beans	15		

Glycaemic Index of common foods

This lack of oxygen causes an excess of 'lactic acid' in the muscles, and it provides that 'burning' sensation that you experience during high-impact exercise such as jogging. Lactic acid prevents your body from efficiently using fat as an energy source. Therefore, if there is not enough oxygen available, or you are exercising too intensely, your fat supplies will never be used up.

The best fat-loss exercise programme is a combination of both cardiovascular and resistance training (using weights). The less muscle you have, the harder it is to lose weight because muscle burns fat. And the more muscle you can build up, the more calories you will use up: 1lb of muscle burns off 42 calories whereas 1lb of fat burns 3 calories.

For a simple exercise programme to follow at home, see my book, *Natural Alternatives to Dieting.*

Pamela

Pamela, aged 48, came to see me because she was concerned about her weight. She was 5 ft 3½ins and weighed 14 stone 7 lb. She was also feeling tired, had a lot of bloating and flatulence and was always constipated. She was still having regular periods, but had a lot of PMS symptoms with headaches and mood swings. Her doctor had checked that her thyroid function was normal. Pamela was deficient in a number of minerals, including magnesium, zinc and chromium. We talked about what she should be eating and I also gave her a programme of supplements to take and suggestions for the constipation.

The chromium had helped with her sugar cravings, and she gave up chocolate straight after the consultation. I asked to reduce the amount of bread she was eating, which would help with the bloating.

By the end of six months, she had lost 2½ stones and was very pleased about this. She aimed to lose another 1½ stone, which she did over the next six months.

Supplements

If you have been yo-yo dieting for a number of years, either restricting your food intake or trying different diet drinks or pills, it is likely that you are deficient in a number of vitamins and minerals. Supplements could certainly help if you know you've been depriving yourself for a long time. You may want to find out if you are deficient and there are tests now available to do just that (see page 70).

B vitamins

These are important vitamins in terms of weight loss, and they are often known as the 'stress' vitamins. Vitamins B3 and B6 are especially important because they help to supply fuel to cells, which are then able to burn energy. Vitamin B6, together with zinc, is necessary for the production of pancreatic enzymes which help you to digest food. If your digestion is good, you will be much more likely to use your food efficiently, instead of storing it as fat.

Vitamins B2, B3 and B6 are necessary for normal thyroid hormone function production, so any deficiencies in these can affect thyroid function and consequently affect metabolism. B3 is also a component of the glucose tolerance factor, which is released every time your blood sugar rises.

Vitamin B5 is involved in energy production and helps to control fat metabolism.

As you can see, the B vitamins as a group are important and the best way to get them is in a good B-complex supplement.

Chromium

This mineral has been the most widely researched nutrient in relation to weight loss Chromium is needed for the metabolism of sugar and without it insulin is less effective in controlling blood sugar levels. This means that it is harder to burn off your food as fuel and more may be stored as fat. It also helps to control levels of fat and cholesterol in the blood. One study showed that people who took chromium picolinate over a ten-week period lost an average of 1.9kg (4.2lb) of fat, while those who took a dummy tablet lost only 0.2kg (0.4lb).[6]

Zinc

This is an important mineral in appetite control and a deficiency can cause a loss of taste and smell, creating a need for stronger tasting foods (which tend to be sweeter, saltier and more fattening). Zinc also functions with vitamins A and E to manufacture the thyroid hormone.

Manganese

This mineral helps with the metabolism of fats, and also works to stabilise your blood sugar levels. It also functions in many enzyme systems, including those enzymes involved in burning energy and in thyroid hormone function.

Magnesium

Magnesium aids in the production of insulin and helps to regulate blood sugar levels, so it is important that this mineral is in good supply.

Co-enzyme Q10

Co-enzyme Q10 is needed for energy production. It is found in all the tissues and organs in the body. As we get older we may become deficient, which results in a reduction of energy. It has been used to help heart problems, high blood pressure, gum disease and immune deficiencies.

It has also been shown to help with weight loss. A study showed that people on a low-fat diet doubled their weight loss when taking Co Q10 compared to those who used diet alone.[7]

Garcinia cambogia

A tropical fruit called Garcinia cambogia, used in Thai and Indian cooking, contains HCA (hydroxy-citric acid), which encourages your body to use carbohydrates as energy, rather than laying them down as fat. The HCA in this fruit seems to curb appetite, reduce food intake and inhibit the formation of fat and cholesterol.

Herbs

While you are beginning to eat well and take nutritional supplements, herbs can be useful to help with water retention and liver support.

Herbs for water retention

This is a problem for many women and it is often worse just before a period. Don't be tempted to limit your intake of fluids, which can actually cause bloating because your body thinks it has to conserve water. Water is a natural diuretic and it should be drunk as frequently as possible, particularly when you are retaining water. Cut down on your intake of salt, which can encourage water retention. It can be particularly high in foods aimed at dieters.

Many women who suffer from water retention turn to diuretics. These will certainly increase the rate at which fluid is lost, but important minerals will also be flushed from your body, including potassium, which is crucial for heart function.

The herb dandelion is a natural diuretic that allows fluid to be released without losing vital nutrients at the same time. It contains more vitamins and minerals than any other herb and is one of the best natural sources of potassium.

Herbs for liver function

Liver function is extremely important as part of the digestive process, and because of its ability to clear out toxins. There are a few good herbs, such as milk thistle, that can help with liver function. For more advice on how to use them, see pages 37–8.

The Treatment Plan

The basic plan involves following the dietary recommendations in Chapter 1, making sure that you eat little and often to keep your blood sugar balanced. This reduces sweet cravings and also keeps your metabolism working at optimum level. Follow the supplement programme over a period of three months to rectify any deficiencies and to help with the weight loss. If you have opted for drugs or surgery, you may have to follow specific dietary recommendations because of the nature of the treatment. However, once the drugs are stopped (or when surgery, such as jaw wiring and stomach balloons, has been reversed), you can put into place the natural recommendations to maintain the results of the treatment and to prevent the need to take such a drastic approach again.

Your Supplement Plan

- A good multivitamin and mineral supplement, e.g. The Healthy Woman by the Natural Health Practice

- Vitamin B-complex (containing 50mg of most of the B vitamins per day)

- Chromium polynicotinate or picolinate (200mcg per day)

- Zinc citrate (30mg per day)

- Linseed (flaxseed) oil (1,000mg per day)

Warning
Each nutrient represents the total intake for one day, so if your multivitamin and mineral already contains 15mg of zinc, for example, you only need to add in a separate zinc supplement containing 15mg per day

---

Herbs

I have used some excellent formulas from a company called New Spirit Naturals. They supply organic herbs that are simply dropped into a hot or cold drink. The ones I have found most helpful with weight loss are the Liver Enhancer, Meta Slim I and Meta Slim II. If you have trouble finding these remedies then get in touch with me (see page 507).

In Summary

- Follow the guidelines in Chapter 1, see page 16.

- Don't be tempted to diet! Dieting makes you fat.

- Replace all refined and sugary foods in your diet with complex carbohydrates and unrefined foods.

- Increase your intake of fibre.

- If you suspect a thyroid problem (see page 450), see your doctor.

- Increase the level of essential fatty acids in your diet.

- Eat slow-releasing foods rather than those that are quickly converted to sugar in your bloodstream (see page 37). The best way to do this is to avoid refined foods.

- Talk to your doctor if you are on medication that is making you 'fat'. There may be alternatives.

- Take steps to correct any nutritional deficiencies, which can be at the root of your problem.

- Check to see that food allergies are not causing weight gain.

- Check the symptom list on page 263 to see if you could be suffering from candida.

- Increase your intake of foods such as seaweeds.

- Ensure that you are getting plenty of exercise that will 'burn' fat. The best forms are resistance training (see page 461), taken alongside a good cardiovascular exercise programme.

- Take supplements (see page 465) for three months.

- Take herbs (see page 465) for one month.

UNDERWEIGHT

If you are underweight or have unexplained weight loss and yet have a good appetite then it is important to go to your doctor for a check-up. The weight loss could be due to a more serious problem and that needs to be ruled out.

What Can Cause You to be Underweight?

Overactive thyroid problem

The opposite of an underactive thyroid is an overactive thyroid (medically known as hyperthyroidism or thyrotoxicosis). In this situation the thyroid is functioning on overdrive and releases too much thyroid hormone. Symptoms of an overactive thyroid include:

- weight loss
- increased appetite
- frequent bowel movements or diarrhoea
- mood swings
- sweating
- rapid heartbeat
- irregular or absent periods
- bulging eyes
- swelling in the throat (goitre).

Testing for an overactive thyroid
Your doctor will use a blood test in the same way that the hormones are tested for an underactive thyroid.

You can also use the temperature method which is described on page 451. If you have an overactive thyroid your body temperature will be above 98.2F (36.7C).

What Treatment Can You Be Offered By Your Doctor?

An overactive thyroid is often treated with drugs which suppress hormone production or by removing part or all of the thyroid gland. The thyroid gland can also be shrunk with radiation and this is done by swallowing radioactive iodine.

The body's balance is very delicate and if the thyroid is overtreated, there is always the possibility of an overactive problem becoming an underactive one.

For dietary support you need to eat the goitrogens (see page 25) which women with an overactive thyroid should avoid. They should be eaten raw if they are going to work as a natural thyroid blocker so eat plenty of raw cabbage and peanuts. Be careful of using foods which are rich in iodine such as seaweed.

Digestive problems

If you have been checked out medically and given the all clear or told you have irritable bowel then it is worth seeking another approach.

It may be possible that you are malabsorbing or have an inherent problem such as a parasitic infection. Weight loss can be caused by difficulties in digesting and absorbing nutrients. It is possible to perform an analysis on a stool sample and find out how well you digest and absorb nutrients. The test also evaluates whether you have hidden yeasts or bacterial or parasitic infections and whether your intestinal flora are balanced i.e. do you have enough of the 'good' bacteria in the intestines.

You will need a nutritional therapist's help with this so please see Staying in Touch (page 507) for my contact details.

What Natural Treatment Can Be Effective?

The use of the natural approach is going to depend on what diagnosis you have been given. This is a situation where you are going to need individual help tailored to your needs so do see a qualified practitioner who can arrange the necessary tests.

Supplements

Weight loss itself especially if accompanied by diarrhoea or caused by malabsorption can cause nutritional deficiencies and these can be tested for. You may need help with not only supplements in terms of vitamins and minerals that may have been lacking because of the weight loss but also digestive enzymes in order to increase the absorption of nutrients.

Eating Disorders

Women today and especially young girls face a lot of pressure to look good. Every time we turn on the television or watch a film we see constant reminders of beautiful body-shape. There are endless magazine articles about weight loss, image make-overs, make-up, plastic surgery and anti-ageing creams. The pressure is enormous and the message is that to be beautiful you need to be thin.

The outcome of this pressure has been the increase in eating disorders such as anorexia nervosa which is a term used to describe a person who although thin, thinks she is fat and that she needs to lose even more weight. There is usually an intense fear of gaining weight and this is controlled not only by restricting food sometimes to the point of starvation but can also be accompanied by an obsession with physical exercise. If any food is consumed which is considered 'too much' then a bout of intense exercise follows to burn off that food.

Women with bulimia nervosa also believe they are overweight but they will have bouts of binge eating where literally they are out of control and stuff whatever food they can into themselves. This is then followed by self-induced vomiting and/or the use of laxatives.

These are serious conditions and the woman involved needs professional help because taken to the extreme, anorexia can be fatal. Psychological help is usually given because it is often viewed as an emotional problem, a lack of self-esteem and maybe the only factor in their life over which they feel they have any control. For further advice contact the Eating Disorders Association (see Useful Addresses).

In recent years, however, scientists have started to look at the physiological aspect of eating disorders instead of just concentrating on the psychological and some interesting research has come out from this. It had been known for a number of years that if animals were placed on a zinc deficient diet they would develop anorexia so the question was asked if people are placed on a zinc deficient diet do they become anorexic and does it follow that people with eating disorders are zinc deficient. The answer to both those question is yes. Studies have shown that people with either anorexia or bulimia are deficient in zinc.[8]

Research then followed where people with anorexia were given zinc supplementation and the eating abnormalities were curbed and significant weight gain followed.[9]

People with eating disorders have been found to have similar chemical imbalances to those with clinical depression. An interesting connection is that symptoms of a zinc deficiency can include depression as well as a loss of taste or smell.

A dietary approach to bulimia has also proved successful where 20 women with bulimia were split into two groups. For the first three weeks 10 of the women were given a 1,400 calories nutrient-rich diet. While they were on this regime they stopped bingeing but the other 10 women not on this diet kept on bingeing. After the three weeks all 20 women were kept on this diet. A follow up 2.5 years later showed that the women were still not bingeing. The diet did not include any sugar, caffeine, white flour and flavour enhancers.[10] Exactly, the same way of eating as in Section 1!

It has been suggested that the zinc supplementation should be given in liquid form rather than tablets or capsules so that it is directly absorbed into the blood. Tablets and capsules have to be broken down by the stomach and then absorbed by the small intestines so in women with eating disorders who may not be digesting nutrients properly it is better to by-pass the digestive system.

CHAPTER 14

Hysterectomy: Making a Decision

It is estimated that over 1,000 hysterectomies are performed each week in the UK and that number totals more than 11,000 in the US. Hysterectomy is the most commonly performed operation, and it has, over the past decades, been used to 'solve' all manner of female problems. Hysterectomies are rarely performed to save lives, many are unnecessary and the most common reason for a hysterectomy is heavy periods. Frankly, the removal of a fundamental part of a woman's body for this reason is nothing short of scandalous.

I firmly believe that hysterectomy should only be offered to women whose lives are at stake if their womb is not removed. If you are suffering from a womb or other cancer, for instance, a hysterectomy can mean the difference between life and death. It may be that you do need a hysterectomy for legitimate medical reasons other than cancer, but before you make that decision you need to know what choices are available to you and whether there are alternative ways of approaching the problem. The majority of hysterectomy operations are not necessary, but many women are unaware that there are viable alternatives. If, in fact, your hysterectomy is necessary, there are still choices to be made. Should you keep your ovaries? Can your cervix be left in place? There are many, many options available to most women, but to make an informed decision, you need to know the facts. All of these points will be covered in detail below.

Some time ago I was speaking at a seminar on pre-menstrual syndrome (PMS). One gynaecologist stood up to outline his solution to the problem, which involved a total hysterectomy, removing the ovaries as well. The logic behind this was that if a woman did not have a cycle, she would not suffer from pre-menstrual symptoms! This 'treatment' was offered even to young women, in the midst of their childbearing years. Certainly the PMS symptoms would be wiped out, but what these women probably would not know is that a radical hysterectomy involving the removal of the womb and the ovaries would plunge them straight into menopause, with all its symptoms. So, for example, the irritability of PMS would be traded for hot flushes. The solution to early menopause and its symptoms? HRT (hormone replacement therapy). It doesn't take a rocket scientist to work out that dealing with the PMS symptoms would be a much more viable, and healthy, solution.

It is this sort of radical 'treatment' option that you need to question. Always remember that it is your body, and you will almost always have choices. Educate yourself on the options, and make your decision after seeking a number of different opinions.

What Your Doctor Might Tell You

It may be suggested that you should have a hysterectomy for any of the conditions below:

- heavy periods
- fibroids
- endometriosis
- prolapse
- pelvic inflammatory disease (PID)
- cancer.

All of the conditions mentioned above, apart from cancer, are covered in separate chapters in this book. In each section, I outline the ways to deal with that condition from both a conventional and a natural point of view. In other words, there are a variety of viable treatment options that do not involve hysterectomy.

In every case, hysterectomy should be a last resort, except in the case of cancer where your life may be at stake. The information detailed below relates to any other condition apart from cancer, where you will not have the same choices available to you.

Female architecture

Your womb and supporting ligaments form an architectural structure. All of the structures in the pelvic cavity support each other, so it's not surprising that removing one or more of these structures can cause mayhem. As things move, the risk of prolapse (see Chapter 6) increases, and this can involve the bladder, rectum and/or the vagina. This isn't unusual. One woman who came to see me had suffered a prolapsed vagina a number of years after a hysterectomy. It was so severe that the vaginal opening had to be sewn up to prevent her vagina from falling out of her body. This is one of the reasons why choosing a sub-total hysterectomy (see below) can make a difference: when the cervix is left intact, the lower genital diaphragm is supported.

QUESTIONS TO ASK YOURSELF BEFORE CONSIDERING A HYSTERECTOMY

1. Can I live with the symptoms?

2. Do the symptoms affect my quality of life to the extent that it prevents me from doing things I would like to do?

3. Have I tried all the alternative medical treatments?

4. Have I tried the natural approach?

5. Do I want to have children or to have more children?

If you decide that a hysterectomy is inevitable then you need to ask yourself two questions:

1. What kind of hysterectomy should I have?

2. Should my ovaries be removed at the same time?

Types of Hysterectomy

Hysterectomy is an operation to the remove the womb (uterus), and sometimes other parts, or the rest of, your reproductive system. There are six main types, and the extent of surgery usually depends on the reason why a hysterectomy has been suggested. Remember that a hysterectomy involves a general anaesthetic with all its associated risks, including blood clots and infections.

Total abdominal hysterectomy

In this procedure, the womb and cervix are removed through an incision made in the abdomen. This is a major operation, and you will need at least three months to recover. Some women experience pain and do not feel completely recovered and back to their normal selves for up to a year after surgery. Because the cervix is removed, there is no risk of cervical cancer, and you will not need any more smears. However, some women find it harder to reach orgasm without a cervix.

Total abdominal hysterectomy with bilateral salpingo-oophorectomy (ovaries removed)

This is the most drastic option and unfortunately the most common. In this procedure, the womb and cervix are removed as above, as well as both ovaries and the Fallopian tubes. Because the ovaries are removed as well, you will literally go into a surgical menopause overnight and probably be given HRT while you are in the hospital.

Sub-total abdominal hysterectomy

In this procedure, only the womb is removed. The ovaries and the cervix are left intact. This is a simpler operation to perform and carries less risk of bladder damage and infection. Because the cervix remains in place, you will need to continue to monitor for cervical cancer; however, most women prefer this choice because it may help to maintain sexual relations with normal sensations. It may also lessen the risk of a future vaginal prolapse because the cervix is left intact.

Vaginal hysterectomy

In this procedure, the womb and cervix are removed through the vagina rather than abdominally. Because it is performed vaginally certain layers of muscle don't have to heal, which means that there is less post-operative pain and recovery is quicker. Furthermore, the operation is less invasive, requiring less anaesthetic.

Less than 5 per cent of hysterectomies are performed this way, largely because British and US or European doctors are routinely trained in abdominal surgery, and vaginal surgery is technically more difficult.

This method can't be used if the womb is very large, if it is stuck down inside the pelvis because of scar tissue, or if the ovaries need to be removed.

Laparascopically assisted vaginal hysterectomy

This involves using keyhole techniques to separate the womb from the abdomen through tiny incisions in the abdomen. After this, the womb and cervix are removed vaginally. The recovery time is faster, but the operation is complex and takes longer to perform than an ordinary abdominal hysterectomy or vaginal hysterectomy.

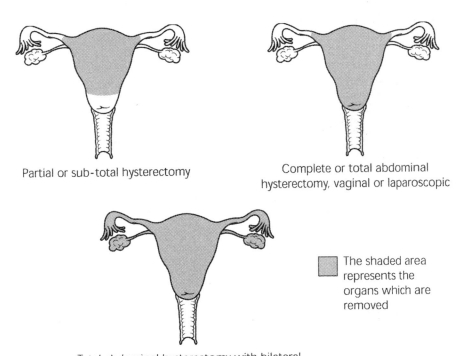

Partial or sub-total hysterectomy

Complete or total abdominal hysterectomy, vaginal or laparoscopic

The shaded area represents the organs which are removed

Total abdominal hysterectomy with bilateral salpingo-oophorectomy (ovaries removed), vaginal or laparoscopic

Different kinds of hysterectomy

Radical hysterectomy

This type of hysterectomy is usually indicated for cancerous conditions, and it involves the removal of the womb, cervix, ovaries, Fallopian tubes, the upper portions of the vagina and pelvic lymph nodes.

WHICH TYPE OF HYSTERECTOMY?

The choice will depend on the reason why you need the hysterectomy. You'll need to find a conservative doctor who will remove only what is necessary and preserve healthy tissue and organs.

- If the reason that you need the hysterectomy is because of very large fibroids, you will probably need an **abdominal hysterectomy**, because the fibroids might be too large to remove through the vagina.

- An **abdominal hysterectomy** will be necessary if cancer is the reason for the operation. The surgeon must remove as much of the cancerous tissue as possible, wherever it is situated.

- A **vaginal hysterectomy** will allow you to leave the hospital more quickly, and you will be back on your feet sooner. However, the cervix is usually removed because it is difficult to preserve when the operation is performed vaginally. If there is no medical reason why your cervix needs to be removed, your decision will depend upon your personal needs. Is it important for you to be back on your feet as soon as possible after the operation or would you rather keep your cervix but experience a longer recovery time? Financially you may need to get back to work as soon as possible. Or, you may be a single mother who needs to be up and about as soon as you can. If you have a history of abnormal smears, then it may be better for you if your cervix is removed. Everybody's circumstances are different and yours need to be taken into account when making any choices. Bearing these in mind, your doctor can guide you to the type of hysterectomy that is right for you. Don't hesitate to get a second opinion. Remember that the choice you make will be irrevocable. There is no turning back.

I recommend the following: if a hysterectomy is necessary, opt for the choice that involves keeping as many healthy parts of your reproductive system as possible. This would include the cervix. Although it might mean a longer stay in hospital, and a longer recovery time, the effects of the operation will be with you for the rest of your life.

Keeping Your Ovaries

Your ovaries produce the hormones oestrogen, progesterone and testosterone. If your ovaries are removed, your body will suddenly enter a state of surgical menopause, which can be enormously traumatic both physically and emotionally. When the female hormone supply from the ovaries is cut off, your body literally goes into menopause overnight. On the other hand, a natural menopause (even if you don't have a womb) can take anywhere from 15 to 20 years, as hormone levels gradually decline.

Premature menopause is normally classed as taking place before the age of 40. If you are younger than 40, and require a hysterectomy with your ovaries removed, you will be pushed into a premature menopause. That means beginning HRT because you cannot risk being without important female hormones for a long period of time. It has serious implications for your bones (see Chapter 12), among other things.

A hysterectomy with the ovaries removed, over the age of 50 (the average age of menopause), won't have quite the same implications because you will have a naturally lower level of oestrogen in your body, and will be unlikely to experience such a shock as the supply is cut off. It may be enough to use the natural alternatives to HRT, and to ensure that your bones are regularly monitored for signs of osteoporosis (see Chapter 12).

Protocol in some hospitals dictates that whenever the ovaries are removed during a hysterectomy, oestrogen implants are inserted straight after surgery. These implants have now been outlawed in the US because of serious concerns over their safety. The pellets that are inserted contain a type of oestrogen that does not dissolve evenly, and it appears that controlled doses are not always maintained, causing risk of overdosing.

When a woman has had a hysterectomy she is given HRT in the form of oestrogen only and not as combined oestrogen and progestogen. If you take HRT after a hysterectomy, you will only be given oestrogen. Normally HRT is a combination of oestrogen and progestogen, because if oestrogen is given on its own there is a risk of womb cancer (because oestrogen will build up the lining of the womb). When the womb is removed progestogen is not needed so only oestrogen is prescribed.

This also raises the issue of whether or not you want to go down the HRT route. If you do decide to try hormone replacement therapy, there are a number of different ways that it can be administered (see page 404).

ENDOMETRIOSIS AND HRT

If you have undergone a hysterectomy because of endometriosis, it is important to remember that HRT is *not* appropriate for at least six to nine months after surgery. Endometriosis is oestrogen-dependent – in other words, the endometrial patches require oestrogen to grow. Some of these patches will undoubtedly remain in the body, even after surgery, and if you take HRT, they can begin to grow again. If you do decide to take HRT following the operation, it is essential that you allow time for any endometrial patches to clear.

Does keeping your ovaries prevent an early menopause?

Unfortunately, even if you keep your ovaries there is a 50 per cent chance of starting the menopause within five years of a hysterectomy.[1] It is believed that this happens because of the change in blood supply to the ovaries after the surgery. For the same reason, an early menopause can result from sterilisation, where the Fallopian tubes are cut as a contraceptive measure.[2]

But it's important to remember that when the ovaries are removed, *all* women suffer from an immediate menopause. If given the choice, it's much better to leave the ovaries in place and work towards keeping the menopause at bay through natural remedies. There is every chance that you'll be in that 50 per cent who don't suffer an early menopause.

PREVENTIVE MEDICINE?

Many women are told to have their ovaries removed 'just in case'. In other words, it is suggested that their removal is a form of preventive medicine. Given that your womb is being removed, which would prevent future conception, the whole 'works' might as well be removed at the same time. There would, obviously, be no risk of ovarian cancer if there are no ovaries present.

This may sound like a sensible approach, but the wisdom behind it is undoubtedly flawed. The American College of Obstetricians and Gynecologists have estimated that 700 'just in case' ovaries would have to be removed in order to prevent a single case of ovarian cancer.[3] Yes, ovarian cancer is one of those 'silent killers' and it's not easy to detect. However, if there is no strong family history of the disease, there is very little – if any – value in removing the ovaries during a hysterectomy. Imagine suggesting that you should have your breasts removed to prevent the development of breast cancer, or your liver, or indeed any other organ. That proposal is ludicrous.

Furthermore, if you have healthy ovaries removed, forcing you to take HRT because of the abrupt and strong menopausal symptoms, you will be increasing the risk of breast cancer (see page 405). In my opinion, this is an unacceptable risk.

Surgical menopause presents a dramatic and traumatic change for your body, and its effects are much more profound than those experienced through natural menopause. If your ovaries are healthy, keep them.

Informed consent?

If you are due for a hysterectomy and have decided to keep your ovaries, it is essential that you read the consent form before signing it prior to your operation. Consent forms are designed to allow surgeons to make decisions on your behalf during the operation. For example, if they open you up and find a cancerous ovary, they need to be able to remove it. That's fair enough, but the problem is that this trust is being abused. You may also want somebody else there to help you read the consent form as you are going to be fairly anxious waiting for the operation.

An organisation called Campaign for Informed Consent (see Useful Addressess) is campaigning to ensure that women are provided with the information they need in order to give truly informed consent – in other words, to let women know exactly what they are consenting to. In recent years, there have been a number of cases where women have not consented to have their ovaries removed during a hysterectomy, only to find out, following surgery, that they had been removed on 'clinical grounds'. These same women have later discovered that their ovaries had been perfectly healthy, and that their removal had been unnecessary.

Make sure that your doctor knows your views and, if necessary, express those views in writing before the operation.

Coping With Surgery

One of the best things you can do following surgery, and even leading up to the operation itself, is to see a good homeopath for remedies suitable to your specific needs. These can make a big difference to how you feel after surgery, and improve your rate of recovery dramatically. Examples of useful homeopathic remedies are arnica, which helps traumatised tissue to heal, relieves pain and prevents infections, and phosphorus, which helps with the nausea after anaesthetic.

Here are more suggestions to help you cope well:

- You want to be as healthy as possible before, during and after the surgery to allow your body to recover quickly and to fight off any infections. Follow the dietary recommendations in Chapter 1 (see page 16). Unless you have an emergency hysterectomy (which is not common, unless cancer has been diagnosed), you will have time to begin eating well long before you go into hospital. This can make a great deal of difference to the healing process.

- In particular, it is important that you give up alcohol in the lead-up to the operation. You will be given drugs, anaesthetics, painkillers and many other toxins over the course of the operation and follow-up treatment, and you will need your liver to work efficiently to eliminate these from your system.

- Start weaning yourself off tea and coffee and anything else containing caffeine (such as colas, chocolate and others) as soon as possible. It is now known certain post-operative symptoms are not caused by the effects of the anaesthetic, as previously thought, but by caffeine withdrawal. Before a general anaesthetic, patients are asked not to eat or drink for a number of hours and by the time they come round from the operation the withdrawal symptoms have already started.

- Eat foods that help to boost your immune system. These include plenty of fresh fruits and vegetables. Include fresh garlic in your diet for its immune-boosting properties.

- While you are in hospital, do the best you can with the hospital food and choose the healthiest options.

Supplements

It's a good idea to take a programme of supplements leading up to the operation and start them again after the surgery (see page 482). The aim is to keep you in good health in order for your body to cope as comfortably as possible with the trauma of the operation.

Certain nutrients, such as vitamin C, zinc and garlic, are included to boost your immune system. I have also included acidophilus (a probiotic; see page 268), which you should take before and after the operation. You will probably be given antibiotics after the surgery, to prevent infection, but these can, unfortunately, upset the balance of bacteria in your gut and give you an attack of thrush. There can also be distressing digestive side-effects, such as nausea and diarrhoea. Acidophilus helps to build up the 'healthy' bacteria in the gut, which can minimise later problems.

Vitamin E can be extremely useful to speed up wound healing and to reduce scarring. Get some pure vitamin E oil or buy capsules of vitamin E, which can be broken open and rubbed into the scar. Check with your doctor before doing this.

Vitamin E can be taken by mouth as well after the surgery and this can help post-operative complications caused by blood clots. Once again, however, check with your doctor before taking this vitamin, especially if you have already been given medication to thin your blood, such as aspirin.

Herbs

Herbs can be taken before you enter hospital, in order to encourage healing and to increase your chances of avoiding post-operative infections.

Echinacea

Echinacea is useful for boosting immune system function as it can increase white blood cell count and activity. This increase can help the body engulf abnormal cells.[4] Echinacea appears to be more effective when taken on and off. Take for ten days, stop taking it for three, and then take it for another ten days.

Counselling

Having a hysterectomy is a big decision. There will be psychological and emotional issues that you may need to address. For some women having a hysterectomy is the best decision they have ever made. Other women have regretted the decision. Others know it was the right decision to make, but still feel a sense of bereavement that they have lost part of themselves.

Many women have found that counselling can be very beneficial both before and/or after the surgery.

Your Supplement Plan

- A good multivitamin and mineral supplement, e.g. The Healthy Woman by the Natural Health Practice
- Vitamin C (1,000mg per day)
- Zinc citrate (30mg per day)
- Garlic capsules
- Acidophilus (with approximately 4 million bacteria)

References

Chapter 1 Nutrition and Lifestyle

1. Schroeder, H. A., 'Losses of vitamins and trace minerals, resulting from processing and preservation of foods', *American Journal of Clinical Nutrition*, vol. 24 (1971), pp. 562–73.
2. *Journal of Nutrition*, vol. 125 (1995), pp. 437–45.
3. Cassidy, A. et al, 'Biological effects of a diet of soy protein rich in isoflavones on the menstrual cycle of premenopausal women', *American Journal of Clinical Nutrition*, vol. 60 (1994), pp. 333–40.
4. Coleman, M. P. et al, *Trends in Cancer Incidence and Mortality*, IARC Publication no. 121, Lyon, France, (1993).
5. Phillimore, J., 'Soya bean crisis', *The Observer Magazine* (27 August 2000).
6. Aldercreutz et al, 'Dietary phytoestrogens and cancer: in vitro and in vivo studies', *Journal of Steroid Chemistry and Molecular Biology*, vol. 41 (1992), pp. 331–7.
7. Ingram, D. J., *Journal of the National Cancer Institute*, vol. 79 (1987), p. 1225.
8. *The Lancet* (21 May 1994).
9. *American Journal of Clinical Nutrition*, vol. 71 (2000), pp. 103–8.
10. Hikon, H. et al, 'Antihepatotoxic actions of flavonolignans from *Silybum marianum* fruits', Planta *Medica*, vol. 50 (1984), pp. 248–50.
    Wagner, H. in Bean, J. L. and Reinhard, E. (eds), *Natural Products as Medicinal Agents*, Hippokrates-Verlag, Stuttgart (1981).
11. Boyce, N., 'Growing up too soon', *New Scientist* (2 August 1997), p. 5.
12. Bernstein, L., *Journal of the National Cancer Institute*, vol. 86 (1994), p. 18.
13. Campbell, J. M. and Harrison, 'Smoking and infertility', *Medical Journal of Australia*, vol. 1 (1979), pp. 342–3.

14. Jick, H. et al, 'Relation between smoking and age of natural menopause', *The Lancet*, vol. 1 (1979), pp. 1345–5.
15. Barnea, E. R. and Tal, J., 'Stress-related reproductive failure', *Journal of In Vitro Fertilisation and Embryo Transfer*, vol. 8 (1991), pp. 15–23.

Chapter 4 Testing Your Health

1. Suzuki, T. and Yamamoto, P., 'Organic mercury levels in human hair with and without storage for eleven years', *Bull Environ Contam Toxicol*, vol. 28 (1982), pp. 186–8.
2. James, V., 'Using hair to screen for breast cancer', *Nature*, vol. 398 (1999), pp. 33–4.
3. Dickman, M. D. and Leung, K. M., 'Mercury and organochlorine exposure from fish consumption in Hong Kong', *Chemosphere*, vol. 35 (5) (1998), pp. 991–1015.

Chapter 5 The Menstrual Cycle

1. Walker, A., 'Theory and methodology in pre-menstrual syndrome research', *Social Sciences and Medicine*, vol. 41(6) (1995), pp. 793–800.
2. Trott, A. et al, 'Pre-menstrual syndrome: diagnosis and treatment', *Delaware Medical Journal*, vol. 68(7) (1996), pp. 357–63.
3. Thomas, S. and Ellertson, C., 'Nuisance or natural and healthy: should monthly menstruation be optional for women?', *The Lancet*, vol. 355 (2000), pp. 9222–4.
4. Watson, N. R. et al, 'Treatment of severe pre-menstrual syndrome with oestradiol patches and cyclicaloral noresthisterone', *The Lancet*, vol. 2 (1989), pp. 730–2.
5. Magos et al, 'Treatment of the pre-menstrual syndrome by subcutaneous oestradiol implants and cycle oral noresthisterone: placebo controlled study', *British Medical Journal*, vol. 292 (1986), pp. 1629–33.
6. Schagen van Leeuwen, J. H. et al, 'Is pre-menstrual syndrome an endocrine disorder?', *Journal of Psychosomatic Obstetrics and Gynaecology*, vol. 14(2) (1993), pp. 91–109.
7. Rossignol, A. M. and Bonnlander, H., 'Prevalence and severity of the pre-menstrual syndrome. Effects of foods and beverages that are sweet or high in sugar content', *Journal of Reproductive Medicine*, vol. 36(2) (1991), pp. 131–6.
8. Wurtman, J. J. et al, 'Effect of nutrient intake on pre-menstrual depression', *American Journal of Obstetrics and Gynecology*, vol. 161(5) (1989), pp. 1228–34.

9. Minton, J. P. et al, 'Clinical and biochemical studies of methylxanthine-related fibrocystic breast disease', *Surgery*, vol. 90 (1981), pp. 299–304.

10. Adams, P. et al 'The effect of pyridoxine hydrochloride (vitamin B6) upon depression associated with oral contraception', *The Lancet*, vol. 1 (1973), pp. 897–904.

11. Wyatt, K. M., 'Efficacy of vitamin B6 in the treatment of pre-menstrual syndrome: systematic review', *British Medical Journal*, vol. 318 (1999), pp. 1375–81.

12. London, R. S. et al, 'Efficacy of alpha-tocopherol in the treatment of pre-menstrual syndrome', *Journal of Reproductive Medicine*, vol. 32 (1987), pp. 400–4.

13. Choung, C. J., 'Vitamin E levels in pre-menstrual syndrome', *American Journal of Obstetrics and Gynecology*, vol. 164 (1990), pp. 1591–5.

14. Abraham, G. E. and Lubran, M. M., 'Serum and red cell magnesium levels in patients with pre-menstrual tension', *American Journal of Clinical Nutrition*, vol. 34 (1981), pp. 2364–66.

15. De Souza, M. C., 'A synergistic effect of magnesium and vitamin B6 supplementation for the relief of symptoms of the pre-menstrual syndrome', *Proceedings of the Nutrition Society*, vol. 56 (1996), p. 193 (75A).

16. Chuong, C. J. and Dawson, E. B., 'Zinc and copper levels in pre-menstrual syndrome', *Fertility and Sterility*, vol. 62 (1994), pp. 313–20.

17. Horrobin, D. F. et al, 'Abnormalities in plasma essential fatty acid levels in women with pre-menstrual syndrome and with non-malignant breast disease', *Journal of Nutritional Medicine*, vol. 2 (1991), pp. 259–64.

18. Puolakka, J. et al, 'Biochemical and clinical effects of treating the pre-menstrual syndrome with prostaglandin synthesis precursors', *Journal of Reproductive Medicine*, vol. 30 (1985), pp. 149–53.

19. Graham, J., *Evening Primrose Oil*, Thorsons (1984), pp. 37–8.

20. McFayden, I. J. et al, 'Cyclical breast pain – some observations and the difficulties in treatment', *British Journal of Clinical Practice*, vol. 46 (1992), pp. 161–4.

21. Lauritzen, C. et al, 'Treatment of pre-menstrual tension syndrome with Vitex agnus castus. Controlled double-blind study versus pyridoxine', *Phytomedicine*, vol. 4 (1997), pp. 183–9.

22. Qi-bing, M. et al, 'Advance in the pharmacological studies of radix Angelica sinensis (olic) diels (Chinese danggui)', *Chinese Medical Journal*, vol. 104 (1991), pp. 776–81.

23. Cooper, K. et al, 'Comparison of microwave endometrial ablation and transcervical resection of the endometrium for treatment of heavy menstrual loss: a randomised trial', *The Lancet*, vol. 354 (1999), p. 1859.

24. Lithgow, D. and Politzer, W. , 'Vitamin A in the treatment of menorrhagia', *South African Medical Journal*, vol. 51 (1977), pp. 191–3.

25. Cohen, J. and Rubin, H., 'Functional menorrhagia, treatment with bioflavonoids and vitamin C', *Current Therapeutic Research*, vol. 2(11) (1960), pp. 539–42.

26. Kelly, R. W. et al, 'The relationship between menstrual blood loss and prostaglandin production in the human: evidence for increased availability of arachidonic acid in women suffering from menorrhagia', *Prost Leuk Med*, vol. 16 (1984), pp. 69–77.

27. Ozaki, Y., 'Anti-inflammatory effect of tetramethylpryazine and ferulic acid', *Chem Pharm Bull*, vol. 40(4) (1992), pp. 954–6.

28. Petcu, P. et al, 'Treatment of juvenile menorrhagia with *Alchemilla vulgaris* L. fluid extract', *Clujul Med*, vol. 52(3) (1979), pp. 266–70.

29. Mowrey, D. B., *The Scientific Validation of Herbal Medicine*, Keats Publishing, New Canaan, Connecticut (1986).

30. Vander Walt, L. A. et al, 'Unusual sex hormone pattern among desert-dwelling hunter-gatherers', *J Clin Endocrinol Metab*, vol. 46 (1978), p. 658.

31. Barnea and Tal, 'Stress-related reproductive failure', pp. 15–23.

32. Phipps, W. R. et al, 'Effect of flaxseed ingestion on the menstrual cycle', *Journal Clin Endocrinol Metab*, vol. 77(5) (1993), pp. 1215–19.

33. Aldercreutz, 'Dietary phytoestrogens and cancer', pp. 331–7.

34. Clark, A. M. et al, 'Weight loss results in significant improvement in pregnancy and ovulation rates in anovulatory obese women', *Human Reproduction*, vol. 10(10) (1995), pp. 2705–12.

35. Drozdz, M. et al, 'Concentration of selenium and vitamin E in the serum of women with malignant neoplasms and their family members', *Ginekol Pol*, vol. 60(6) (1989), pp. 301–5.

36. Cahill, D. J. et al, 'Multiple follicular development associate with herbal medicine', *Human Reproduction (UK)*, vol. 9(8) (1994), pp. 1469–70.

37. Probst, V. and Roth, O., 'On a plant extract with a hormone-like effect', *Dtsch Me Wschr*, vol. 79(35) (1954), pp. 1271–4.

38. Rivlin, M. E., 'Endometrial hyperplasic', in Rivlin, M. E. and Martin, R. W. (eds), *Manual of Clinical Problems in Obstetrics and Gynaecology*, Little, Brown and Company, Boston (19xx), pp. 433–7.

39. Clark, 'Weight loss results in significant improvement in pregnancy and ovulation rates in anovulatory obese women', pp. 2705–12.

40. Berga, S. L., 'Stress and amenorrhoea', *The Endocrinologist*, vol. 5(6) (1995), pp. 416–21.

41. Webb, J., 'Nutritional effects of oral contraceptive use: a review', *Journal of Reproductive Medicine,* vol. 25(4) (1980), pp. 150–6.

42. Vallee, B., 'Zinc' in Comar, C. L. and Bonner, C. S. (eds), *Mineral Metabolism*, vol. IIB, Academic Press (1965).

43. Schwabe, J. W. R and Rhodes, D., 'Beyond zinc fingers: steroid hormone receptor have a novel motif for DNA recognition', *Trends in Biochemical Science*, vol. 15 (1991), pp. 291–6.

44. Losh, E. and Kayser, E., 'Diagnosis and treatment of dyshormonal menstrual periods in the general practice', *Gynakol Praxis*, vol. 14(3) (1990), pp. 489–95.

45. Milewica, A. et al, '*Vitex agnus castus* extract in the treatment of luteal phase defects due to hyperprolactinemia. Results of a randomised placebo-controlled double-blind study', *Arzneim-Forsch Drug Res*, vol. 43 (1993), pp. 752–6.

46. Powell, A. M. et al, 'Menstrual-PGF2 alpha, PGE2 and TXA2 in normal and dysmenorrheic women and their temporal relationship to dysmenorrhoea', *Prostaglandins*, vol. 29 (2), 1985), pp. 273–90.

47. Horrobin, 'Abnormalities in plasma essential fatty acid levels in women with pre-menstrual syndrome and with non-malignant breast disease', pp. 259–64.

48. Abraham, G. E., 'Primary dysmenorrhoea', *Clinical Obstetrical Gynaecology*, vol. 21(1) (1978), pp. 139–45.

49. Gokhale, L. B., 'Curative treatment of primary (spasmodic) dysmenorrhoea', *Indian Journal of Medical Research*, vol. 103 (1996), pp. 227–31.

50. *Nutrition Research*, vol. 20 (2000), pp. 621–32.

51. Butler, E. B. and McKnight, E., 'Vitamin E in the treatment of primary dysmenorrhoea', *The Lancet*, vol. 1 (1955), pp. 844–7.

52. Columbo, D. and Vescorini, R., 'Controlled trial of anthodyanosides from *Vaccinium myrtillus* in primary dysmenorrhoea', *G Ital Obstet Ginecol*, vol. 7 (1985), p. 1033.

53. Fontana-Klatber, H. and Hogg, B., 'Therapeutic effects of magnesium in dysmenorrhoea', *Schweiz Runhdsch Med Prax*, vol. 79(16) (1990), pp. 491–4.

54. Seifert, B. et al, 'Magnesium – a new therapeutic alternative in primary dysmenorrhoea', *Zentralbl Gynakol*, vol. 111(11) (1989), pp. 755–60.

55. Deutch, B., 'Menstrual pain in Danish women correlated with low n-3 polyunsaturated fatty acid intake', *European Journal of Clinical Nutrition*, vol. 49 (1995), pp. 508–16.

56. Taussig, S. J. and Batkin, S., 'Bromelain, the enzyme complex of pineapple (*Ananas comosus*) and its clinical application', *Ethnopharmacol*, vol. 22 (1988), pp. 191–203.

57. Hardy, M. L., 'Women's health series: herbs of special interest to women', *Journal of the American Pharmaceutical Association*, vol. 40(2) (2000), pp. 234–42.

58. Ozaki, 'Anti-inflammatory effect of tetramethylpryazine and ferulic acid', pp. 954–6.

59. Hardy, 'Women's health series: herbs of special interest to women', pp.234–42.

60. Nicholson, J. A. et al, 'Viopudial, a hypotensive and smooth muscle antispasmodic from *Viburnum opulus*' *Proc Soc Exp Biol Med*, vol. 40 (1972), pp. 457–61.

61. Mowrey, *The Scientific Validation of Herbal Medicine*.

62. Bolomb, L. M. et al, 'Primary dysmenorrhoea and physical activity', *Med Sci Sports Exerc*, vol. 30 (1998), pp. 906–9.

63. Ben-Manachem, M., 'Treatment of dysmenorrhoea: a relaxation therapy program', *International Journal of Gynecology and Obstetrics*, vol. 17 (1980), pp. 340–2.

Chapter 6 The Womb

1. Dmowski, W. P. et al, 'The role of cell-mediated immunity in pathogenesis of endometriosis', *Acta Obstetricia et Gynecologica Scandinavica Supplement*, vol. 159 (1994), pp. 7–14.

2. Oliker, A. J. and Harries, A. E., 'Endometriosis of the bladder in a male patient', *Journal of Urology*, vol. 106 (1971), pp. 858. O'Connor, D. T., *Endometriosis: Current review in Obstetrics and Gynaecology 12*, Churchill Livingstone (1987), p. 20.

3. Dmowski, W. P., 'Women with endometriosis: dismissed, devalued, ignored', Second International Symposium on Endometriosis, Fin, Program P-045:54.

4. Knapp, V. J., *Fertility and Sterility*, vol. 72 (July 1999), pp. 10–14.

5. Igarashi, M. et al, 'Novel vaginal danazol ring therapy for pelvic endometriosis, in particular deeply infiltrating endometriosis', *Human Reproduction*, vol. 13(7) (1998), pp. 1952–6.

6. Grodstein, F. et al, 'Relation of female infertility to consumption of caffeinated beverages', *American Journal of Epidemiology*, vol. 137 (1993), pp. 1353–60.

7. Abraham, 'Primary dysmenorrhoea', pp. 139–45.

8. Butler and McKnight, 'Vitamin E in the treatment of primary dysmenorrhoea', pp. 844–7.

9. Columbo and Vescorini, 'Controlled trial of anthocyanosides from *Vaccinium myrtillus* in primary dysmenorrhoea', p. 1033.

10. Fontana-Klatber and Hogg, 'Therapeutic effects of magnesium in dysmenorrhoea', pp. 491–4.

11. Mathias, J. R. et al, 'Relation of endometriosis and neuromuscular disease of the gastrointestinal tract: new insights', *Fertility and Sterility*, vol. 70 (1998), pp. 81–7.

12. Wagner, in *Natural Products as Medicinal Agents*.

13. Gibbons, A., 'Dioxin tied to endometriosis', *Science*, vol. 262 (1993), p. 1373.

14. Goodwin, S. C. and Walker, W. J., 'Uterine artery embolisation for the treatment of uterine fibroids', *Curr Opin Obstet Gynecol*, vol. 10(4) (1998), pp. 315–20.

15. Vashisht, A. et al, 'Fatal septicaemia after fibroid embolisation' (letter), *The Lancet*, vol. 354 (1999), pp. 307–8.

16. Law, P et al, 'Magnetic-resonance-guided percutaneous laser ablation of uterine fibroids' (letter), *The Lancet*, vol. 354 (1999), pp. 2049–50.

17. Stalder, R. et al, 'A carcinogenicity study of instant coffee in Swiss mice', *Food Chem Toxicol*, vol. 28(12) (1990), pp. 829–37.

18. Aldercreutz, 'Dietary phytoestrogens and cancer', pp. 331–7.

19. Saxena, S. P. et al, 'DDT and its metabolites in leiomyomatous and normal human uterine tissue', *Arch Toxicol*, vol. 59(6) (1987), pp. 453–5.

20. Kelly, 'The relationship between menstrual blood loss and prostaglandin production in the human', pp. 69–77.

21. Sakamoto et al, 'Pharmacotherapeutic effects of Kue-chih-fu-ling-wan (Keishi-bukuryo-gan) on human uterine myomas', *American Journal of Chinese Medicine*, vol. 20(3–4) (1992), pp. 313–17.

22. Mowrey, *The Scientific Validation of Herbal Medicine*.

23. Dellas, A. and Drewe, J., 'Conservative therapy of female genuine stress incontinence with vaginal cones', *European Journal of Obstetrics and Gynaecology and Reproductive Biology*, vol. 62 (1995), pp. 213–15.

24. 'Vitamin C, cancer and ageing', *Age*, vol. 16 (1993), pp. 55–8.

Chapter 7 The Ovaries

1. Wyshak, G. et al, 'Smoking and cysts of the ovary', *International Journal of Fertility*, vol. 33(6) (1988), pp. 398–404.

2. Hatcher, R. et al, *Contraceptive Technology*, 16th edn, Irvinton Publishers, Inc, Contraceptive Technology Communications, Inc, New York (1994).

3. Aldercreutz, 'Dietary phytoestrogens and cancer', pp. 331–7.

4. Stimpel, M. et al, *Infection Immunity*, vol. 46 (1984), pp. 845–9.

5. Insler, V. and Lunenfeld, B., 'Pathophysiology of polycystic ovarian disease: new insights', *Hum Reprod*, vol. 6(8) (1991), pp. 1025–9.

6. Kiddy, D. S. et al, 'Differences in clinical and endocrine features between obese and non-obese subjects with polycystic ovary syndrome: an analysis of 263 consecutive cases', *Clinical Endocrinology*, vol. 32 (1990), pp. 213–20.

7. Regan, L., *Miscarriage*, Bloomsbury (1997).

8. Kiddy, D. S. et al, 'Diet-induced changes in sex hormone binding globulin and free testosterone in women with normal or polycystic ovaries', pp. 757–63
Pasquali, R. et al, 'Clinical and hormonal characteristics of obese amenorrheic hyperandrogenic women before and after weight loss', *Journal of Clinical Endocrinology and Metabolism*, vol. 68(1) (1989), pp. 173–9.

9. Kiddy, D. S. et al, 'Improvement in endocrine and ovarian function

during dietary treatment of obese women with polycystic ovary syndrome', *Clinical Endocrinology*, vol. 36 (1992), pp. 105–11.

10. Clark, 'Weight loss results in significant improvement in pregnancy and ovulation rates in anovulatory obese women', pp. 2705–12.

11. Kiddy, 'Differences in clinical and endocrine features between obese and non-obese subjects with polycystic ovary syndrome', pp. 213–20.

12. Clark, 'Weight loss in obese infertile women results in improvement in reproductive outcome for all forms of fertility treatment', pp. 1502–5.

13. Foreyt, J.P. and Poston, W. S., 'Obesity: a never-ending cycle?', *International Journal of Fertility and Women's Medicine*, vol. 43(2) (1998), pp. 111–16.

14. Aldercreutz, 'Dietary phytoestrogens and cancer', pp. 331–7.

15. Evans, G. W. and Pouchnik, D. J., 'Composition and biological activity of chromium-pyridine carbosylate complexes', *Journal of Inorganic Biochemistry*, vol. 49 (1993), pp. 177–87.

16. American Diabetes Association, 'Magnesium supplementation in the treatment of diabetes', *Diabetes Care*, vol. 15 (1992), pp. 1065–7.

17. Van Gall, L. et al, 'Biomedical and clinical aspects of coenzyme Q10', vol. 4 (1984), p. 369.

18. Shigeta, Y. et al, 'Effect of coenzyme Q10 treatment on blood sugar and ketone bodies of diabetics', *Journal of Vitaminology*, vol. 12 (1966), pp. 293–8.

19. DiSilverio, F. et al, 'Evidence that Serenoa repens extract displays aniestrogenic activity in prostatic tissue of benign prostatic hypertrophy', *Euro Urol*, vol. 21 (1992), pp. 309–14.

Chapter 8 Infections and Other Problems

1. Gomez, C. et al, 'Attachment of Neisseria gonorrhoea to human sperm', *Br J Ven Dis*, vol. 55 (1979), pp. 245–55.

2. Neri, A. et al, 'Bacterial vaginosis: drugs versus alternative treatment', *Obstetrical and Gynecological Survey (US)*, vol. 49(12) (1994), pp. 809–13.

3. Alexander, M. et al, 'Oral beta-carotene can increase the number of OKT4+ cells in human blood', *Immunol Letters*, vol. 9 (1985), pp. 221–4.

4. Stephens, L. et al, 'Improved recovery of vitamin E treated lambs that have been experimentally infected with intertracheal Chlamydia', *Br Vet J*, vol. 135 (1979), pp. 291–3.

5. Sharma, V. D. et al, 'Antibacterial property of *Allium sativum Linn.*: in vivo and in vitro studies', *Indian Journal of Experimental Biology*, vol. 15 (1977), pp. 466–8.

6. Klebanoff, S. et al, 'Control of the microbial flora of the vagina by H202-generating lactobacilli', *J Infec Dis*, vol. 164 (1991), pp. 94–100.

7. Hilton et al, 'Lactobacillus GG vaginal suppositories and vaginitis', *J Clin Microbiol*, vol. 33(5) (1995), p. 1433.

8. Amin, A. et al, 'Berberine sulfate: antimicrobial activity, bioassay and mode of action', *Canadian Journal of Microbiology*, vol. 15 (1969), pp. 1067–76.

9. Pena, E., '*Melaleuca alternifolia* oil: its use for trichomonal vaginitis and other vaginal infections', *Obstetrics and Gynaecology*, vol. 19(6) (1962), pp. 793–5.

10. Shafter, M. et al, 'Acute salpingitis in the adolescent female', *J Ped*, vol. 100 (1982), pp. 339–50.

11. Hilton, E. et al, 'Ingestion of yoghurt containing *Lactobacillus acidophilus* as prophylaxis for candidal vaginitis', *Annals of Internal Medicine*, vol. 116(5) (1992), pp. 353–7.

12. Mikhail, M. S. et al, 'Decreased beta-carotene levels in exfoliated vaginal epithelia cells in women with vaginal candidiasis', *American Journal of Reproductive Immunology*, vol. 32 (1994), pp. 221–5.

13. Edman, J. et al, 'Zinc status in women with recurrent vulvovaginal candidiasis', *American Journal of Obstetrics and Gynecology*, vol. 155(5) (1986), pp. 1082–5.

14. Das, U. N., 'Antibiotic-like action of essential fatty acids', *Canadian Medical Association Journal*, vol. 132(12) (1985), p. 1350.

15. Adetumbi, M. et al, '*Allium sativum* (garlic) inhibits lipid synthesis by *Candida albicans*', *Antimicrob Agents and Chemother*, vol. 30(3) (1986), pp. 499–501.

16. Amin, 'Berberine sulfate', pp. 1067–76.

17. Pena, '*Melaleuca alternifolia* oil', pp. 793–5.

18. Coeuginet, E. and Kuhnast, R., 'Recurrent candidiasis: adjuvant immunotherapy with different formulations of Echinacin (R)', *Therapiewoche*, vol. 36 (1986), pp. 3352–8.

19. Heldrich, F et al, 'Clothing factors and vaginitis', *Journal of the Family Practitioner*, vol. 19 (1984), pp. 491–4.

20. Palacios, A. S. et al, 'Eosinophilic food-induced cystitis', *Allergol Et Immunopathol*, vol. 12 (1984), pp. 463–9.

21. Lidefelt, K. J. et al, 'Changes in periurethral microflora after antimicrobial drugs', *Archives of Disease in Children*, vol. 66 (1991), pp. 683–5.

22. Avorn, J. et al, 'Reduction of bacteriuria and pyuria after ingestion of cranberry juice', *Journal of the American Medical Association*, vol. 271(10) (1994), pp. 751–4.

23. Howell, A. B. et al, 'Inhibition of the adherence of P-fimbriated *Escherichia coli* to uroepithelia-cell surfaces by proanthocyanidin extracts from cranberries', *New England Journal of Medicine*, vol. 339(15) (1998), pp. 1085–6.

24. Ringsdorf, W. et al, 'Sucrose, neutrophil phagocytosis and resistance to disease', *Dent Surv*, vol. 52 (1976), pp. 46–8.

25. Sharma, 'Antibacterial property of *Allium sativum Linn.*', pp. 466–8.

26. De La Fuente, M. et al, 'Immune function in aged women is improved by ingestion of vitamins C and E', *Canadian J J Physiol Pharmaco*, vol. 76(4) (1998), pp. 373–80.
    Hughes, D. A., 'Effects of dietary antioxidants on the immune function of middle-aged adults', *Proc Nut Soc (England)*, vol. 58(1) (1999), pp. 79–84.

27. Sirsi, M., 'Antimicrobial action of vitamin C on M. tuberculosis and some other pathogenic organisms', *Indian J Med Sci*, vol. 6 (1952), pp. 252–5.

28. Mori et al, 'The clinical effect of proteolytic enzyme containing bromelain and trypsin on urinary tract infection evaluated by double blind methods', *Acta Obstet Gynaecol Jpn*, vol. 19 (1972), pp. 147–53.

29. Walsh, C. T. et al, *Environmental Perspectives*, vol. 102 (suppl. 2) (1994), pp. 4–46.

30. Reid, G. et al, 'Influence of three-day antimicrobial therapy and lactobacillus vaginal suppositories on recurrence of urinary tract infections', *Clinical Therapies*, vol. 14 (1992), pp. 11–16.

31. Amin, 'Berberine sulfate', pp. 1067–76.

32. Stimpel, *Infection Immunity*, pp. 845–9.

33. Aziz-Fam, A., 'Use of titrated extract of *Centella asiatica* (TECA), in bilharzial bladder lesions', *Int Surg*, vol. 58 (1973), pp. 451–2.

34. Smith, S. D. et al, 'Improvement in interstitial cystitis syndrome scores during treatment with oral L-arginine', *Journal of Urology*, vol. 158 (1997), p. 3.

35. Walboomers, J. M. M. et al, 'Human papillomavirus is a necessary cause of invasive cervical cancer worldwide', *Journal of Pathology*, vol. 189 (1999), pp. 12–19.

36. Schiffman, Mark H., 'Latest HPV findings: some clinical implications', *Contemporary OB/GYN*, vol. 38 (1993), pp. 27–40.

37. *The What Doctors Don't Tell You Guide to Screening Tests*, publisher, (date).

38. *The Lancet* (10 July 1993).

39. Clavel, C. et al, 'Hybrid capture II-based human papillomavirus detection, a sensitive test to detect in routine high-grade cervical lesions: a preliminary study on 1,518 women', *British Journal of Cancer*, vol. 80(9) (1999), pp. 1306–11.

40. Lyon, J. et al, 'Smoking and carcinoma in situ of the uterine cervix', *American Journal of Public Health*, vol. 73 (1983), pp. 558–62.

41. Orr, J. et al, 'Nutritional status of patients with untreated cervical cancer, II, vitamin assessment', *American Journal of Obstetrics and Gynecology*, vol. 151 (1985), pp. 632–5.

42. Dawson, E. et al, 'Serum vitamin and selenium changes in cervical dysplasia', *Feb Proc*, vol. 46 (1984), p. 612.

43. Palan, P. et al, 'Decreased plasma beta-carotene levels in women with uterine cervical dysplasias and cancer', *Journal of the National Cancer Institute*, vol. 80(6) (1988), pp. 454–5.

44. Van Enwick, J. et al, 'Dietary and serum carotenoids and cervical intraepithelial neoplasia', *International Journal of Cancer*, vol. 48 (1991), pp. 34–8.

45. Levy, J. et al, 'Carotene and antioxidant vitamins in the prevention of oral cancer', *New York Academy of Sciences*, (1992), pp. 260–9.

46. Kwasniewska et al, 'Content of alpha-tocopherol in blood serum of human papillomavirus-infected women with cervical dysplasias', *Nutrition and Cancer*, vol. 28(3) (1997), pp. 248–51.

47. Romney, S. et al, 'Plasma vitamin C and uterine cervical dysplasia', *American Journal of Obstetrics and Gynecology*, vol. 151 (1985), pp. 978–80.

48. Wassertheil-Smoller, S. et al, 'Dietary vitamin C and uterine cervical dysplasia', *American Journal of Epidemiology*, vol. 114 (1981), pp. 714–24.

49. Basu, J. et al, 'Smoking and the antioxidant ascorbic acid: plasma, leukocyte and cervicovaginal cell concentrations in normal healthy women', *American Journal of Obstetrics and Gynecology*, vol. 163(6 part 1) (1990), pp. 1948–52.

50. Ramaswamy, P. and Natarajan, R., 'Vitamin B6 status in patients with cancer of the uterine cervix', *Nutrition and Cancer*, vol. 6 (1984), pp. 176–80.

51. Van Niekerk, V., 'Cervical cytological abnormalities caused by folic acid deficiency', *Acta Cytol*, vol. 10 (1966), pp. 67–73.

52. Butterworth, C. D. et al, 'Folate deficiency and cervical dysplasia', *Journal of the American Medical Association*, vol. 367(4) (1992), pp. 528–34.

53. Lindenbaum, J. et al, 'Oral contraceptive hormones, folate, metabolism and the cervical epithelium', *American Journal of Clinical Nutrition*, vol. 28(4) (1975), pp. 346–53.

54. Whitehead, N. et al, 'Megaloblastic changes in the cervical epithelium: association with oral contraceptive therapy and reversal with folic acid', *Journal of the American Medical Association*, vol. 226 (1973), pp. 1421–4.

55. Dawson, 'Serum vitamin and selenium changes in cervical dysplasia', p. 612.

56. Stimpel, *Infection Immunity*, pp. 845–9.

57. *Journal of Ethnopharmacology*, vol. 38(1) (1993), pp. 63–77.

58. Chu, D. et al, *Clinical Immunology and Immunopathology*, vol. 45 (1987), pp. 48–57.

59. Gerhausser, C. et al, 'What is the active antiviral principle of Thuja occidentalis', *Pharm Pharmacol Lett*, vol. 2 (1992), pp. 127–30.

Chapter 9 Breasts

1. Janiger, O. et al, 'Cross cultural study of premenstrual symptoms', *Psychosomatics*, vol. 13 (1972), pp. 226–35.
2. Grimes, D., *Fertility and Sterility*, vol. 57(3) (1992), pp. 492–3.
3. Minton, 'Clinical and biochemical studies of methylxanthines-related fibrocystic breast disease', pp. 299–304.
4. Boyd, E. M. F. et al, 'The effect of a low-fat, high complex carbohydrate diet on symptoms of cyclical mastopathy', *The Lancet*, vol. 2 (1988), pp. 128–32.
5. Petrakis, N. L. and King, E. E., 'Cytological abnormalities in nipple aspirates of breast fluid from women with severe constipation', *The Lancet*, vol. ii(1) (1981), pp. 203–5.
6. London, R. et al, 'Mammary dysplasia: endocrine parameters and tocopherol therapy', *Nutrition Research*, vol. 7 (1982), p. 243.
7. Pye, J. K. et al, 'Clinical experience of drug treatments for mastalgia', *The Lancet*, vol. 2 (1985), pp. 373–7.
8. Kaiser, L. et al, 'Fish consumption and breast cancer risk', *Nutrition and Cancer*, vol. 12 (1989),pp. 61–8.
   Cave, W. T., 'Dietary Omega-3 polyunsaturated fats and breast cancer', *Nutrition*, vol. 12(1) (1996), pp. S39–S42.
9. Bohnert, K. J. and Hahn, G., 'Phytotherapy in gynaecology and obstetrics –Vitex agnus castus', *Erfahrungsheilkunde*, vol. 39 (1990), pp. 494–502.
   Dittmar, F. W. et al, 'Pre-menstrual syndrome: treatment with a phytopharmaceutical', *Therapiwoche Gynakol*, vol. 5, pp. 60–8.
10. Tamborini, A. and Taurelle, R., 'Value of standardised ginkgo biloba extract (EGB 761) in the management of congestive symptoms of premenstrual syndrome', *Rev Fr Gynaecol Obstet*, vol. 88(7–9) (1993), pp. 447–57.
11. Singer, R. and Grismaijer, S., *Dressed to Kill – the link between breast cancer and bras*, Avery (19xx).
12. Chen, C. et al, 'Antioxidant status and cancer mortality in China', *Int J Epidemiology*, vol. 21 (4) (1992), pp. 625–35.
13. Lockwood, K. et al, 'Apparent partial remission of breast cancer in "high risk" patients supplemented with nutritional antioxidants, essential fatty acids and co-enzyme Q10', *Molec Aspects Med*, vol. 15 (supplement) (1994), pp. S231–s240.
14. Coleman, *Trends in Cancer Incidence and Mortality*.
15. Aldercreutz, 'Dietary phytoestrogens and cancer', pp. 331–7.
16. Schairer, C., 'Menopausal oestrogen and oestrogen-progestogen replacement therapy and breast cancer risk', *Journal of the American Medical Association*, vol. 283(4) (2000), pp. 485–91.
17. *American Journal of Epidemiology*, (December 1991).

18. Herbert, J. and Rosen, A., 'Nutritional, socioeconomic and reproductive factors in relation to female breast cancer mortality: findings from a cross-national study', *Cancer Detect Preven.*, vol. 20(3) (1996), pp. 234–44.

19. Boyd, N. F. and McGuire, V., 'The possible role of lipid peroxidation in breast cancer risk', *Free Radic Biol Med.*, vol. 10(3–4) (1991), pp. 185–90.

20. Willett, W. C., 'Fat, energy and breast cancer', *Journal of Nutrition*, vol. 127(5) (1997), pp. 921S–923S.

21. Chen, C. et al, 'Adverse life events and breast cancer: case-controlled study', *British Medical Journal*, vol. 311 (1995), pp. 1527–30.

22. Aronson, K. J., 'Breast adipose tissue concentrations of polychlorinated biphenyls and other organochlorines and breast cancer risk', *Cancer Epidemiol Biomarkers Prev*, vol. 9(1) (2000), pp. 55–63.

23. Verma, S. P., 'Curcumin and genistein, plant natural products, show synergistic inhibitory effects on the growth of human breast cancer MCF-7 cells', *Biophysical Research Communications*, vol. 233(3) (1997), pp. 692–6.

24. Stomper, P. and Gelman, R., *Hematol Oncol Clin N Am*, vol. 3 (1989), pp. 611–40.
Canadian Journal of Public Health, vol. 84 (1993), pp. 14–16.

25. Gotzche, P. C. and Olsen, O., 'Is screening for breast cancer with mammography justifiable', *the Lancet*, vol. 355 (2000), pp. 129–34.

26. James, 'Using hair to screen for breast cancer', pp. 33–4.

27. Cuzick, J. et al, 'Electropotential measurements a s new diagnostic modality for breast cancer', *the Lancet*, vol. 352 (1998), p. 359.

Chapter 10 Infertility

1. Rossing, M. A. et al, 'Ovarian tumours in a cohort of infertile women', *New England Journal of Medicine*, vol. 331 (1994), pp. 771–6.

2. Kurinczuk, J. J. and Bower, C., 'Birth defects in infants conceived by ICSI: an alternative interpretation', *British Medical Journal*, vol. 315 (1997), pp. 1260–6.

3. Shusham, A. et al, 'Human menopausal gonadotrophin and the risk of epithelial ovarian cancer', *Fertility and Sterility*, vol. 65 (1996), pp. 13–18.

4. Potashnik, G., 'Fertility drugs and the risk of breast and ovarian cancers: result of a long-term follow-up study', *Fertility and Sterility*, vol. 71(5) (1999), pp. 853–9.

5. Ward, N., 'Preconceptual care and pregnancy outcome', *Journal of Nutritional and Environmental Medicine*, vol. 5 (1995), pp. 205–8.

6. Hakim, R. et al, 'Alcohol and caffeine consumption and decreased fertility', *Fertility and Sterility*, vol. 70(4) (1998), pp. 632–7.

7. Jensen, T. et al, 'Does moderate alcohol consumption affect fertility?

Follow-up study among couples planning first pregnancy', *British Medical Journal*, vol. 317 (998), pp. 505–10.

8. Bennet, H. S. et al, 'Breast and prostate in men who die of cirrhosis of the liver', *American Journal of Clinical Pathology*, vol. 20 (1950), pp. 814–28.

9. Wilcox, A. et al, 'Caffeinated beverages and decreased fertility', *the Lancet*, vol. 2 (1988), pp. 1453–5.

10. Parazzini, F. et al, 'Risk factors for unexplained dyspermia in infertile men: a case-control study', *Archives of Andrology*, vol. 31(2) (1993), pp. 105–13.

11. Campbell and Harrison, 'Smoking and infertility', pp. 342–3.

12. Jick, 'Relation between smoking and age of natural menopause', pp. 1354–5.

13. Ford, W. C. I. et al, 'Smoking by men and women linked to delayed conception" *Fertility and Sterility*, vol. 74 (2000), pp. 724–32.

14. Abraham, G. E. and Hargrove, J. T., report in *Medical World News* (19 March 1979).

15. Sandler, B. and Faragher, B., 'Treatment of oliogspermia with vitamin B12', *Infertility*, vol. 7 (1984), pp. 133–8.

16. Schwabe and Rhodes, 'Beyond zinc fingers: steroid hormone receptors have a novel structure motif for DNA recognition', pp. 291–6.

17. Abbasi, A. A. et al, 'Experimental zinc deficiency in man: effect on testicular function', *Journal of Laboratory and Clinical Medicine*, vol. 96(3) (1980), pp. 544–50.

18. Krznjavi, H. et al, 'Selenium and fertility in men', *Trace Elements in Medicine*, vol. 9(2) (1992), pp. 107–8.

19. Srivastava, K. C. et al, 'Prostaglandin E and 19-hydroxy-prostaglandin E content in the semen of men with normal sperm characteristics, men with abnormal sperm characteristics, vasectomised men and poly-zoospermic men', *Danish Medical Bulletin*, vol. 28 (1981), pp. 201–3.

20. Bayer, R. 'Treatment of infertility with vitamin E', *International Journal of Infertility*, vol. 5 (1960), pp. 70–8.

21. Geva, E. et al, 'The effect of antioxidant treatment on human sperma-tozoa and fertilisation rate in an invitro fertilisation program', *Fertility and Sterility*, vol. 66(3) (1996), pp. 430–4.

22. Fraga, C. G. et al, 'Ascorbic acid protects against endogenous oxidative DNA damage in human sperm', *Proceedings of the National Academy of Science*, vol. 88 (1991), pp. 11003–6.

23. Igarashi, I., 'Augmentative effects of ascorbic acid upon induction of human ovulation in clomiphene ineffective anovulatory women', *International Journal of Fertility*, vol. 22 (3) (1977), pp. 68–73.

24. De Aloysio, D. et al, 'The clinical use of arginine aspartate in male infertility', *Alta Europaea Fertilitatis*, vol. 13 (1982), pp. 133–67.

25. Gaby, A. R., *Townsend Letters for Doctors and Patients*, (April 1996), p. 20.

26. Jennings, I., *Vitamins in Endocrine Metabolism*, Heinemann (1972).

27.   Rothman et al, *New England Journal of Medicine*, vol. 333 (21) (1995), pp. 157–9.

28.   Propping, D. and Katzorke, T., 'Treatment of corpus luteum insufficiency', *Zeitschr Allgemein medizin*, vol. 63 (19987), pp. 932–3.

Chapter 11 Pregnancy

1.   Rice, R., 'Fish and healthy pregnancy: more than just a red herring', *Professional Care of Mother and Baby*, vol. 6(6) (1996), pp. 171–3.

2.   Reece, M. S. et al, 'Maternal and perinatal long-chain fatty acids: possible roles in preterm birth', *American Journal of Obstetric and Gynecology*, vol. 176(4) (1997), pp. 907–14.

3.   Sahakian, V. et al, 'Vitamin B6 is effective therapy for nausea and vomiting of pregnancy: a randomised, double-blind placebo-controlled study', *Obstetrics and Gynaecology*, vol. 78(1) (1991), pp. 33–6.

4.   Fischer-Rasmussen, W. et al, 'Ginger treatment of hyperemesis gravidarum', *Eur J Obstet Gyn Reprod Biol*, vol. 38(1) (1991), pp. 19–24.

5.   Poston et al, 'Effect of antioxidants on the occurrence of pre-eclampsia in women at increased risk: a randomised trial', *The Lancet*, vol. 354 (1999), pp. 810–19.

6.   Jendrycsko, A. and Drozdz, M., 'Plasma retinol, beta-carotene and vitamin E levels in relation to the future risk of pre-eclampsia,' *Zent bl Gynakol*, vol. 111 (1989), pp. 1121–3.

7.   Williams, M. A. et al, 'Omega-3 fatty acids in maternal erythrocytes and risk of pre-eclampsia', *Epidemiology*, vol. 6(3) (1995), pp. 232–7.

8.   Ehrenberg, A., 'Non-medical prevention of pre-eclampsia', *Acta Obstetricia et Gynecologica Scandinavica – Supplement*, vol. 164 (1997), pp. 108–10.

9.   Bassiuoni, B. A. et al, 'Maternal and foetal plasma zinc in pre-eclampsia', *Eur J Obstet Gynaecol Reprod Biol,* vol. 9 (1979), pp. 75–80.

10.   Dura-Trave, T. et al, 'Relation between maternal plasmatic zinc levels and uterine contractibility', *Gynaecol Obstet Ivest*, vol. 17 (1984), pp. 247–51.

11.   Barker, D. J. and Martyn, C. N. 'The maternal and foetal origins of cardiovascular disease', *J Epdemiol Community Health*, vol. 46 (1992), pp.8–11.

12.   Barker, D. J. P. et al, 'Foetal and placental size and risk of hypertension in adult life', *Brit Med J*, vol. 301 (1990), pp. 259–62.

13.   Barker, D. J. P. et al, 'Weight in infancy and death from coronary heart disease', *The Lancet*, vol. 11 (1989), pp. 577–80.

14.   Hales, C. N. et al, 'Foetal and infant growth and impaired glucose tolerance at age 64', *Brit Med J*, vol. 303 (1991), pp. 1019–22.

15.   Conf Review, *Nutrition and Health*, vol. 8 (1992), pp. 45–55.

16. Schaefer, C. et al, 'Illnesses in infants born to women with *Chlamydia trachomatis* infection', *AJDC*, vol. 139 (1985), pp. 127–33.
    Sollecito, D., 'Prenatal *Chlamydia trachomatis* infection with postnatal respiratory disease in a preterm infant', *Acta Paediatri Scand*, vol. 76 (1987), p. 532.

17. Library, The Royal College of Physicians (1725).

18. Smith, D. W., 'Alcohol effects in foetus', in *Foetal Drug Syndrome: Effects of ethanol, and hydantoins, Paediatrics in Review 1*, American Academy of Paediatrics (1979).

19. Tuormaa, T. , 'The adverse effects of alcohol on reproduction', *Journal of Nutritional and Environmental Medicine*, vol. 6 (1996), pp. 379–91.

20. Streissguth, A. P., 'Foetal alcohol syndrome: an epidemiological perspective', *Am J Epidemiol*, vol. 107 (1978), pp. 467–78.

21. Streissguth, A. P. et al, 'Neurobehavioral effects of prenatal alcohol: Part I, research strategy (review of the literature)', *Neurotoxicol Teratol*, vol. 11 (1989) pp. 461–76.

22. Streissguth, A. P. et al, 'Moderate prenatal alcohol exposure: effects on child IQ and learning problems at age 7.5 years', *Alcohol Clin Exp Res*, vol. 14 (1990), pp. 662–9.

23. Sullivan, J. F. and Lankford, H. G., 'Urinary excretion of zinc in chronic alcoholism', *Am J Clin Pathol*, vol. 45 (1962), pp. 156–9.

24. Flynn, A. et al, 'Zinc status of pregnancy alcohol women: a determination of foetal outcome', *The Lancet*, (14 March 1981), pp. 572–5.

25. Laurence, K. M. et al, 'Double-blind randomised controlled trial of folate treatment before conception to prevent recurrence of neural-tube defects', *Brit Med J*, vol. 282 (1981), pp. 1509–51.

26. Tuormaa, 'The adverse effects of tobacco smoking on reproduction and health', pp. 105–20.

27. Carmichael, N. G. et al, 'Teratogenicity, toxicity and perinatal effects of cadmium', *Human Toxicol*, vol. 1 (1982), pp. 159–86.

28. *Journal of the American Medical Association*, vol. 281 (1999), pp. 1106–9.

29. Gerhard, I. et al, 'Toxic pollutants and fertility disorders: solvents and pesticides', *Geburtshilfe – Frauenheilkd*, vol. 53(3) (1993), pp. 147–60.

30. Stenchever, M. A. et al, 'Chromosome breakages in users of marijuana', *Am J Obstet Gynaecol*, vol. 118 (1974), pp. 106–13.

31. Bongol, N. et al, 'Teratogenicity of cocaine in humans' *J Pediatr*, vol. 1 (1987), pp. 93–6.

32. Ostrea, E. M. and Chavez, C. J., 'Perinatal problems (excluding neonatal withdrawal in maternal drug addiction: a study of 830 cases', *J Pediatr*, vol. 94 (1979), pp. 292–5.

33. Watanabe, G. 'Environmental determinants of birth defects prevalence', *Contributions to Epidemiology and Biostatistics*, vol. 1 (1979), pp. 91–100.

34. Kocisova, J. et al, 'Mutagenicity studies on paracetamol in human

volunteers: I Cytogenetic analysis of peripheral lymphocytes and lipid peroxidation in plasmas', *Mutat Res*, vol. 209 (1988) pp. 161–5.

35. *Psychosomatics*, vol. 30 (1989), pp. 25–31.

36. Yanai (ed), *Neurobehavioural Teratology*, Elsevier Science Publishers BV (1984).
    The Initial Investigation and Management of the Infertile Couple, Evidence-based Clinical Guidelines No. 2, Royal College of Obstetricians and Gynaecologists (February 1998).

37. Tamura, T. et al, 'Maternal serum folate and zinc concentrations and their relationships to pregnancy outcome', *American Journal of Clinical Nutrition*, vol. 56 (1992), pp. 365–70.

38. *British Journal of Obstetrics and Gynaecology*, vol. 107 (2000), pp. 1149–54.

39. Rothman, *New England Journal of Medicine*, pp. 1369–73.

40. Jennings, *Vitamins in Endocrine Metabolism*, (1972).

41. Jendrycsko and Drozdz, 'Plasma retinol, beta-carotene and vitamin E levels in relation to the future risk of pre-eclampsia', pp. 1121–3.

42. Goel, M. et al, 'Serum magnesium level in pregnancy', *Indian Veterinarian Medical Journal*, vol. 15 (1991), pp. 83–7.

43. Zrcone, R. et al, 'Role of magnesium in pregnancy', *Panminerva Medica*, vol. 36(4) (1994), pp. 168–70.

44. Ritchie, L. et al, 'A longitudinal study of calcium homeostasis during human pregnancy and lactation and after the resumption of menses', *American Journal of Clinical Nutrition*, vol. 67 (1998), pp. 693–701.

45. Bergman, K. et al, 'Abnormalities of hair zinc concentration in mothers of newborn infants with spina bifida', *American Journal of Clinical Nutrition*, vol. 3 (1980), p. 2145.
    Buamah, P. et al, 'Maternal zinc status: a determinant of central nervous system malformation', *British Journal of Obstetrics and Gynaecology*, vol. 91 (1984), pp. 788–90.

46. Hay, P. E. et al, 'Abnormal bacterial colonisation of the genital tract and subsequent pre-term delivery and late miscarriage', *British Medical Journal*, vol. 308 (1994), pp. 295–8.

47. Ralph, S. G. et al, 'Influence of bacterial vaginosis on conception and miscarriage in the first trimester: cohort study', *British Medical Journal*, vol. 319 (1991), pp. 220–3.

48. Regan, *Miscarriage* (1997).

49. Clark, 'Weight loss in obese infertile women results in improvement in reproductive outcome for all forms of fertility treatment', pp. 1502–5.

50. Furuhjelm et al, 'The quality of human semen in spontaneous abortion', *International Journal of Fertility*, vol. 7 (1962), pp. 17–21.

51. Sorahan, T. et al, 'Childhood cancer and parental use of tobacco: deaths from 1971 to 1976', *British Journal of Cancer*, vol. 76(11) (1997), pp. 1525–31.

52. Himmelberger, D. U. et al, 'Cigarette smoking during pregnancy and the occurrence of spontaneous abortion and congenital abnormality', *American Journal of Epidemiology*, vol. 108 (1998), pp. 470–9.

53. Bennet, 'Breast and prostate in men who die of cirrhosis of the liver', pp. 814–28.
Kulikauskas, V. et al, 'Cigarette smoking and its possible effect on sperm', *Fertility and Sterility*, vol. 44 (1985), pp. 526–8.

54. Kaufman, M., 'Alcohol threat to babies', *The Sunday Times* (31 January 1988).

55. Kline, J. et al, 'Drinking during pregnancy and spontaneous abortion', *The Lancet*, vol. 2 (1980), pp. 176–80.
Windham, G. C. et al, 'Moderate maternal alcohol consumption and risk of spontaneous abortion', *Epidemiology*, vol. 5 (1997), pp. 509–14.

56. Zhang, H. and Bracken, M. B., 'Tree-based, two-stage risk factor analysis for spontaneous abortion', *American Journal of Epidemiology*, vol. 144(10) (1996), pp. 989–96.

57. Infante Rivard, C., *Journal of the American Medical Association* (22 December 1993).

58. Furuhashi, N. et al, 'Effects of caffeine ingestion during pregnancy', *Gynecologial and Obstetric Investigation*, vol. 19 (1985), pp. 187–91.
Wichit, S. and Bracken, M. B., 'Caffeine consumption during pregnancy and association with late abortion', *American Journal of Obstetrics and Gynecology*, vol. 154 (1985), pp. 14–20.

59. Fenster, L. et al, 'A prospective study of caffeine consumption and spontaneous abortion', *American Journal of Epidemiology*, vol. 143(11), 525, abstract no. 99 (1996).

60. Parazzini, 'Risk factors for unexplained dyspermia in infertile men', pp. 105–13.

61. Webb, T., reported in Stuttaford, T., 'The screen of fear', *The Times* (15 November 1984).

62. De Matteo, *The Terminal Shock*, NC Press, Toronto (1985).

63. Ward, 'Preconceptual care and pregnancy outcome', pp. 205–8.

64. Stephens, N. G. et al, 'Randomised controlled trial of vitamin E in patients with coronary disease: Cambridge Heart Antioxidant Study (CHAOS)', *The Lancet*, vol. 347 (1996), pp. 781–6.

65. Barrington, J. W. et al, 'Selenium deficiency and miscarriage: a possible link?', *British Journal of Obstetrics and Gynaecology*, vol. 103 (1996), pp. 130–2.

66. Propping, P. et al, 'Diagnosis and therapy of corpus luteum deficiency in general practice', *Therapiewoche*, vol. 38 (1988), pp. 2992–3001.

Chapter 12 Menopause

1. Hoover, R. et al, *New England Journal of Medicine*, vol. 295 (1976), pp. 401–5.
2. Smith et al, *New England Journal of Medicine*, vol. 293 (1975), pp. 1164–72.
3. Grady, D. et al, 'Hormone replacement therapy and endometrial cancer risk: a meta-analysis', *Obs Gynec*, vol. 85(2) (1995), pp. 304–13.
4. Hoover, *New England Journal of Medicine*, pp. 401–5.
5. Beral, V., 'Breast cancer and HRT: collaborative reanalysis of date from 51 epidemiological studies of 52,705 women with breast cancer and 108, 411 without breast cancer', *the Lancet*, vol. 350 (1997), pp. 1047–59.
6. Schairer, 'Menopausal oestrogen and oestrogen-progestogen replacement therapy and breast cancer risk', pp. 485–91.
7. Daly, E. et al, *The Lancet*, vol. 348 (1996), pp. 977–80.
    Jick, H. et al, *The Lancet*, vol. 348 (1996), pp. 981–3.
    Guttham et al, *Br Med J*, vol. 314 (1997), pp. 796–800.
8. Stampfer, M. J. et al, *New England Journal of Medicine*, vol. 313 (1985), pp. 1044–9.
9. Hulley, S. et al, 'Randomised trial of oestrogen plus progestogen for secondary prevention of coronary heart disease in postmenopausal women', *Journal American Medical Association*, vol. 280 (1998), pp. 6–5–13.
10. Rossouw, J., National Heart, Lung and Blood Institute Press Statement (April 2000).
11. Barbour, M., 'Hormone replacement therapy should not be used as secondary prevention of coronary heart disease', *Pharmacotherapy*, vol. 20(9) (2000), pp. 1021–7.
12. Coleman, *Trends in Cancer Incidence and Mortality*.
13. Wilcox, F. et al, 'Oestrogenic effects of plant foods in postmenopausal women', *British Medical Journal*, vol. 301 (1990), pp. 905–6.
14. Albertazzi, P. et al, 'The effect of dietary soy-supplementation on hot flushes', *Obstetrics and Gynaecology*, vol. 91 (1998), p. 1.
15. *Journal of Nutrition*, vol. 125 (1995), pp. 437–45.
16. Anderson, J. et al, 'Meta-analysis of the effects of soy protein intake on serum lipids', vol. 333(5) (1995), pp. 276–82.
17. Smith, C., 'Non-hormonal control of vaso-motor flushing in menopausal patients, '*Chicago Medicine*, vol. 67 (1964), pp. 193–5.
18. Christy, C., 'Vitamin E in menopause: preliminary report of experimental and clinical study', *American Journal of Obstetrics and Gynaecology*, vol. 50 (1945), pp. 84–7.
    Finkler, R., 'The effect of vitamin E in the menopause', *Journal of Clin Endocrin Metab*, vol. 9 (1949), pp. 89–94.
    McLaren, H., 'Vitamin E in the menopause', *British Medical Journal* (1949), pp. 1378–82.

19. Stephens, 'Randomised controlled trial of vitamin E in patients with coronary disease', pp. 781–6.

20. Houghton, P., 'Agnus castus', *The Pharmaceutical Journal*, vol. 19 (1994), pp. 720–1.

21. Stolze, H., 'An alternative to treat menopausal symptoms', *Gynaecology*, vol. 3 (1982), pp. 14–16.

22. Hofferberth, B. 'Simultanerfassung elektrophysiologischer, psychometrischer und rheologischer Parameter bei Patienten mit hirnorganischem Psychosyndrom und erhöhtem Gerfässrisko? Eine Placebo-kontrollierte Doppleblindstudie mit Ginkgo biloba-Extrakt EGB 761', in Stodtmesiter, R, Pillunat, L (eds), *Mikrozirkulation in Gehirn und Sinnesorgananen*, Ferdinand Enke, Stuttgart (1991), pp. 64–74.

23. Yeater, R. and Martin R., *Postgraduate Medicine*, vol. 75 (1984), pp. 147–9.

24. Jick, 'Relation between smoking and age of natural menopause', pp. 1345–5.

25. Rose, L., *Osteoporosis*, Allen & Unwin (1994).

26. Kin, K. et al, *Calcification Tissue International* vol. 49 (1991), pp. 101–6.

27. Wynn, A. and Wynn, M., *Journal of Nutritional and Environmental Medicine,* vol. 5 (1995), pp. 41–53.

28. Kreiger, N. et al, *American Journal of Epidemiology*, vol. 116 (1982), pp. 141–8.

29. Sanchez, V. et al, 'Bone mineral mass in elderly vegetarian females', *American Journal of Roentgenol*, vol. 131 (1978), p. 542.

30. Ellis, F, et al, 'Incidence of osteoporosis in vegetarians and omnivores', *American Journal of Clinical Nutrition*, vol. 25 (1972), pp. 55–8.

31. Holbook, T. L. and Barrett-Conner, E., *British Medical Journal* (1993), pp. 1056–8.

32. Felson, D. et al, 'Alcohol consumption and hip fractures: The Framingham study', *American Journal of Epidemiology*, vol. 128 (1988), pp. 1102–10.

33. Felson, D. T. et al, *New England Journal of Medicine*, vol. 329 (1993), pp. 1141–6.

34. Grimes, *Fertility and Sterility*, pp. 492–3.

35. Horwitz, K. B. et al, 'Surprises with antiprogestins: novel mechanisms of progesterone receptor action', *Ciba Foundation Symposium*, vol. 191 (1995), pp. 235–49; (discussion), pp. 250–3.

36. Brattstrom, L. et al, 'Folic acid responsive postmenopausal homcysteinemia', *Metab*, (1985), pp. 1073–7.

37. Benke, P. J. et al, 'Osteoporotic bone disease in the pyridoxine-deficient rat', *Biochem Med*, vol. 6 (1972), pp. 526–35.

38. Harvey, J. A. et al, *Journal of Bone Mineral Research*, vol. 3(3) (1988) pp. 253–8.

39. *Current Research in Osteoporosis and Bone Mineral Measurement II*, British Institute of Radiology (1992).
40. Abraham, G. E., *Journal of Nutritional Medicine*, vol. 2 (1991), pp. 165–78.
41. Marier, J., 'Magnesium content of the food supply in the modern-day world', *Magnesium*, vol. 5 (1986), pp. 1–8.
42. Abraham, *Journal of Nutritional Medicine*, (1991), pp. 165–78.
43. Calhoun, N. R. et al, 'The effects of zinc on ectopic bone formation', *Oral Surg*, vol. 39 (1975), pp. 698–706.
44. Atik, O. S., 'Zinc and senile osteoporosis', *J Am Geriatr Soc*, vol. 31 (1983), pp. 790–1.
45. Gennari, C. et al, 'Effect of chronic treatment with ipriflavone in postmenopausal women with low bone mass', *Calcif Tissue Int*, vol. 61 (1997), pp. 519–22.

Chapter 13 Weight

1. Yamamoto, I. et al, 'Anti-tumour effect of seaweed', *Japanese Journal of Experimental Medicine*, vol. 44 (1974), pp. 543–6.
2. Iritani, N. and Nagi, S., 'Effects of spinach and wakame on cholesterol turnover in the rat', *Atherosclerosis*, vol. 15 (1972), pp. 87–92.
3. Olivieri, O. et al, 'Low selenium status in the elderly influences thyroid hormones', *Clinical Science*, vol. 89 (1995), pp. 637–42.
4. Blundell, J. E. and Hill, A. J., 'Paradoxical effects of an intense sweetner (aspartame) on appetite', *The Lancet*, vol. 1 (1986), pp. 1092–3).
5. Wurtman, R. J., 'Neurochemical changes following high dose aspartame with dietary carbohydrates', *New England Journal of Medicine*, (1983), pp. 429–30.
6. Evans and Pouchnik, 'Composition and biological activity of chromium-pyridine carbosylate complexes', pp. 177–87.
7. Van Gaal, L. et al, Biomedical and clinical aspects of coenzyme Q10, vol. 4 (1984), p. 369.
8. Humphries, L. et al, 'Zinc deficiency and eating disorders', Journal of Clinical Psychiatry, vol. 50(12) (1989), pp. 456–9.
9. Safai-Kutti, S., 'Oral zinc supplementation in anorexia nervosa', ACTA Psychiatri Scand, vol. 361(82 suppl.) (1990), pp. 14–17.
10. Davit-McPhillips, S., 'A dietary approach to bulimia treatment', Physiol Behav, vol. 33(5) (1984), pp. 769–75.

Chapter 14 Hysterectomy

1. Siddle, N. et al, 'The effect of hysterectomy on the age of ovarian failure: identification of a subgroup of women with premature loss of ovarian function and literature review', *Fertility and Sterility*, vol. 47 (1987), pp. 94–100.
2. Turney, L., 'Risk and contraception: what women are not told about tubal ligation', *Women's Studies International Forum*, vol. 16 (1993), pp. 471–86.
3. Goldfarb, H. A., *The No-Hysterectomy Option*, John Wiley & Sons (1997).
4. Stimpel, *Infection Immunity*

Useful Addresses

National Endometriosis Society
50 Westminster Palace Gardens
Artillery Row
London SW1P 1RL
Tel: 020 7222 2776

The Daisy Network
(for premature menopause)
PO Box 392
High Wycombe
Bucks HP15 7SH

Menorrhagia (heavy periods) Information Service
Tel: 0906 470 0187

For information on microwave ablation for heavy periods
Microsulis helpline
Tel: 0800 328 3025

Campaign against Hysterectomy and Unnecessary Operations on Women
PO Box 30
Woking
Surrey GU22 0YE
Tel: 01483 715435

Fax: 01483 722446
Works towards eliminating all unnecessary surgery on women, particularly hysterectomies, removal of ovaries, breast surgery and Caesarean sections.

Campaign for Informed Consent
19 St Edward Gardens
Eggbuckland
Plymouth PL6 5PB
Campaigns on major women's issues, e.g. surgery without consent and medication without consent – and presses for the provision of the information women need in order to give truly informed consent.

Women's Healthcare
St John's Wood
27A Queens Terrace
London NW8 5EA
Tel: 020 7483 0099

Nutri Centre
7 Park Crescent
London W1N 3HF
Tel: 020 7436 5122

Human Fertilisation and Embryology Authority (HFEA)
Paxton House
30 Artillery Lane
London E1 7LS
Tel: 020 7377 5077

Verity – The Polycystic Self-Help Group
Trindlemanor
52–54 Featherstone Street
London EC1Y 8RT

What Doctors Don't Tell You (monthly newsletter, sold by subscription)
Satellite House
2 Salisbury Road
London SW19 4EZ
For subscriptions tel: 01858 438894

Active Birth Centre
25 Bickerton Road
London N19 5JT
Tel: 020 7561 9006

BACUP
Cancer charity
Tel: 020 7613 2121/0808 8001234
www.cancerbacup.org.uk

Eating Disorders Association
Sackville Place
44–46 Magdalen Street
Norwich
Norfolk NR3 1JE
Under 18s Tel: 01603 765050
Adults Tel: 01603 621414

Natural Medicine Organisations

Nutrition
British Association of Nutritional Therapists
27 Old Gloucester Street
London WC1N 3XX
Tel/fax: 0870 6061284

Acupuncture
The British Acupuncture Council
63 Jeddo Road
London W12 9HQ
Tel: 020 8735 0400
Fax: 020 8735 0404

Homeopathy
Society of Homeopaths
4a Artizan Road
Northampton NN1 4HU
Tel: 01604 621400

Medical Herbalism
National Institute of Medical Herbalism
56 Longbrook Street
Exeter EX4 6AH
Tel: 01392 426022

Osteopathy
General Osteopathic Council
Osteopathy House
176 Tower Bridge Road
London SE1 3LU
Tel: 020 7357 6655

Staying in Touch

If you have any health problems and are interested in finding a more natural approach to treating them or would like to find out what supplements and tests are available to you, please feel free to contact me and I will send you more information on how you can help yourself.

Workshops, Cassettes and Videos

I give workshops and talks around the world, and have produced cassettes and videos from some of these. Please call if you would like to find out more about future workshops and/or recordings and you will be sent an information pack.

Consultations

If you want to see or talk to someone personally, I am available for private consultations at the following clinics and postal consultations can be arranged:

The Hale Clinic, Regents Park, London
and
Women's Healthcare, St John's Wood, London

For Appointments and Enquiries:

Dr Marilyn Glenville
Nevill Estate, Danegate, Eridge Green, Tunbridge Wells,
Kent, TN3 9JA

Tel: 01892 750511 Fax: 01892 750533
website: www.marilynglenville.com
email: health@marilynglenville.com

If you would like to hear more advice from Dr Glenville on any of the following subjects:

- **Natural Alternatives to Dieting** *How to lose weight naturally*

- **Natural Alternatives to HRT** *How to stay healthy through the menopause and prevent osteoporosis*

- **Natural Solutions to Infertility** *How to increase your chances of conceiving and preventing miscarriages*

Then call
0906 7010030
and select your choice for the information you would
like to hear about.

Calls are charged at 50p per minute at all times. Helpline No: 01892 750511

Other books by Marilyn Glenville
Natural Solutions to Infertility (Piatkus, 2000)
Natural Alternatives to HRT (Kyle Cathie, 1997)
Natural Alternatives to HRT Cookbook (Kyle Cathie, 2000)
Natural Alternatives to Dieting (Kyle Cathie, 1999)
Natural Choices for Menopause (St Martin's Press, 1999)

Index

* Reference to diagrams or illustrations are in italics.